# CHILDREN WHO FAIL TO THRIVE

# CHILDREN WHO FAIL TO THRIVE

## A Practice Guide

Dorota Iwaniec

*Institute of Child Care Research, Queen's University of Belfast,
Northern Ireland*

With best
wishes

Dorota Iwaniec

John Wiley & Sons, Ltd

*Other Wiley Editorial Offices*

John Wiley & Sons Inc., 111 River Street, Hoboken, NJ 07030, USA

Jossey-Bass, 989 Market Street, San Francisco, CA 94103-1741, USA

Wiley-VCH Verlag GmbH, Boschstr. 12, D-69469 Weinheim, Germany

John Wiley & Sons Australia Ltd, 33 Park Road, Milton, Queensland 4064, Australia

John Wiley & Sons (Asia) Pte Ltd, 2 Clementi Loop #02-01, Jin Xing Distripark, Singapore 129809

John Wiley & Sons Canada Ltd, 22 Worcester Road, Etobicoke, Ontario, Canada M9W 1L1

Wiley also publishes its books in a variety of electronic formats. Some content that appears in print may not be available is electronic books.

*Library of Congress Cataloging-in-Publication Data*

Iwaniec, Dorota.
Children who fail to thrive : a practice guide / Dorota Iwaniec.
    p. cm.
Includes bibliographical references.
ISBN 0-471-49720-7 (Paper : alk. paper)
    1. Failure to thrive syndrome.    2. Parent and child.    I. Title.
RJ135.I95    2004
618.92–dc22                                              2003016091

*British Library Cataloguing in Publication Data*

A catalogue record for this book is available from the British Library

ISBN 0-470-87077-X (hbk)

ISBN 0-471-49720-7 (pbk)

Typeset in 10/12pt Palatino by TechBooks, New Delhi, India
Printed and bound in Great Britain by Biddles Ltd, King's Lynn
This book is printed on acid-free paper responsibly manufactured from sustainable forestry in which at least two trees are planted for each one used for paper production.

For my grandchildren
**Ben** and **Elena**

# CONTENTS

**SECTION III:   INTERVENTION AND TREATMENT OF FAILURE-
                 TO-THRIVE CHILDREN AND THEIR FAMILIES**

# LIST OF ILLUSTRATIONS

## FIGURES

## TABLES

# ABOUT THE AUTHOR

**Dorota Iwaniec** MA, DipEd, DipSW, CQSW, PhD, AcSS

*Institute of Child Care Research, Queen's University of Belfast,*
*5a Lennoxvale, Belfast BT9 5BY, Northern Ireland*

**Dorota Iwaniec** is a Professor of Social Work and Director of the Institute of Child Care Research at Queen's University of Belfast. She has extensive clinical and research experience of working with children and their families and, in particular, in failure to thrive, neglect, emotional abuse, and behavioural and emotional problems of children and adolescents. She has been researching failure-to-thrive children for the last 25 years and has recently completed a 20-year follow-up study. Prior to coming to Queen's University she worked as a social worker, researcher, and trainer in Leicester for nearly 30 years, both at the Social Services Department and at the Department of Child Health at Leicester Royal Infirmary.

# LIST OF EPIGRAPHS

# ACKNOWLEDGEMENTS

I acknowledge, most warmly and with gratitude, the unfailing support given by my husband, Professor James Stevens Curl, during the writing of this book. Without his help, this book would never have been completed. I am also very grateful and indebted to Mrs Maura Dunn for the production of the text and illustrations and her continuous loyal assistance during the 'long journey' involved in writing and rewriting the text. A big 'thank you' goes to Dr Helga Sneddon, who, as my research assistant, helped with the data analysis of the 20-year follow-up study and literature review on the subject. She has worked closely with me for a considerable time. Dr Emma Larkin has contributed to the literature review on intervention, and Dr Sarah Allen has also helped: they have my thanks. I am also grateful to my colleagues at Queen's University of Belfast for their encouragement and interest in my research and writing. Last, but not least, I am greatly indebted to former failure-to-thrive clients and their families for generously making the 20-year follow-up study possible.

The publisher would like to thank the Child Growth Foundation for permission to reproduce some of their growth reference charts. The Foundation is not the source of the growth curves superimposed. The charts in the book are not intended for practice use. If required, you may obtain the latest release of the charts from Harlow Printing (Maxwell Street, South Shields, NE33 49U, UK, Tel: 0191 427 4379, Contact: Ms Diane Hall)

**Dorota Iwaniec**
Holywood, Co Down
2002–3

# Section I

## THE PROBLEM

# 1

# INTRODUCTION

*Nourish thy children, O thou good nurse; 'stablish their feet.*
Apocrypha, II *Esdras* Ch. 2, v. 25

## PREAMBLE

This book is based on more than a quarter of a century of research, clinical work, and independent assessment work concerning children who fail to thrive. It also draws upon a 20-year follow-up study of 31 subjects, and so contributes to an understanding of the problems of such children, as well as shedding light on parental perceptions and management of difficulties associated with failure to thrive.

Many years of direct contact with these children and their families provided invaluable experience and the accumulation of knowledge about characteristics of children and parents, family dynamics, and problems associated with growth and development. Most importantly, it became clear that there were many aspects of failure to thrive, ranging from mild problems of weight-faltering (due to some feeding problems, parental anxiety, and lack of experience in rearing children) to far more persistent and difficult failure to thrive (associated with inadequate parenting, distorted perceptions and relationships, and neglect and abuse).

Since the mid-1970s, when the present writer began to study children who fail to thrive, knowledge has expanded enormously, and many well-designed studies have been carried out, examining different facets of the subject, in several parts of the world. We now know far more about the prevalence of failure to thrive (FTT), as a result of community-based studies, than we knew years ago when most samples were drawn from hospitalised children with severe failure to thrive. We have also learned that children identified during the early onset of weight-faltering can be helped relatively quickly without any long-term negative effects. But, equally, we have established that some children with more severe FTT may have had the condition induced because of poor or inadequate parenting, and may require more extensive intervention: such children tend to show a very poor prognosis for improvement or recovery. Longitudinal studies have confirmed these findings.

For these reasons, all those who have responsibilities for overseeing children's growth and development should take the first signs of growth-faltering very seriously indeed. 'Prevention is better than cure' may be a cliché, but the sooner the problem is recognised, the better it is for both baby and care-giver. Some children may grow out of early difficulties, but some do not; for them, their problems grow as they do.

During the author's involvement in this field, it became apparent that the failure-to-thrive syndrome can have many shades, and is not a simple matter of faltering growth during the first few months of a child's life. If that were the case, most problems would be resolved by recourse to services and resources available to everybody. However, despite the fact that mandatory help is given by health visitors, many children fail to thrive, so there must be other psychosocial factors at work which create the problems and prove resistant to nutritional treatment alone. Such factors are many and varied, and so no two cases will be exactly the same, although there may be similarities between them. All children displaying symptoms of FTT are undernourished, and all fail to grow according to expected norms, but that is where the similarities end.

There are substantial variations in reasons why certain children fail to thrive, not least those connected with poor nutrition. Some children may have sucking/eating problems, or mild oral-motor dysfunction, while others may not be acquiring sufficient nutrition because of parental lack of understanding of what and how to feed, or because of neglect. In addition, some parents may react to presenting problems and to caring tasks in many different ways. Some worry and become anxious about their children's poor intake of food and poor growth; others become angry and frustrated; some may perceive their children's refusal of food as personal affronts, involving rejection by the children themselves; others may assume that their children are simply not hungry.

Parental attitudes to food will play roles as well. How food is presented to children, and what is fed to them will often establish that fears concerning potential obesity of children will be important factors in those parental attitudes. Some will deliberately withhold food, and some will fabricate illnesses: in both instances the children will fail to thrive.

On the other hand, children will also react to parental behaviour: some will be anxious, apprehensive, and fearful; while others will withdraw, becoming lethargic and detached. Thus, the behaviours of parents and of children may influence each other and create tension, a sense of lack of achievement (and therefore of disappointment), and trigger feelings of depression. Such problems are not conducive to healthy growth, and vicious circles may be created which produce major difficulties requiring complex remedies.

To illustrate different routes to under-nutrition resulting in FTT, a few examples are given below:

### Examples

- Previn, who was referred when he was 3 months old, was not given a sufficient amount of food and the right formula as his mother did not like fat babies or fat people in general;
- Indira was referred when she was 2 years and 3 months old. She had presented with feeding difficulties from birth. Her mother would spend hours trying to feed her. Indira would spit out food, heave, store food in her mouth, and refuse to chew and swallow;
- At the age of 1 year 11 months, Kevin looked extremely thin, and sick, and developmentally was delayed. His mother abandoned him after birth, but was forced to take him back by her parents. He was an unwanted child;
- Penny's birth-weight was 4.1 kg (9 lb. 1 oz.). At $2\frac{1}{2}$ months her weight dropped to 3.75 kg (8 lb. 3 oz.). Her mother was informed two days after Penny was born that her 32-year-old sister had died of cancer;
- Rose was 13 months old, the third child in the family. She looked thin, small, lethargic, and withdrawn. Rose's weight dropped to under the 2nd percentile from the 25th percentile, and at 6 weeks she still was under the 2nd percentile. Her mother suffered from post-natal depression;
- Rebecca's birth-weight was on the 25th percentile. She stopped gaining weight at 5 months, and fell below the 2nd percentile at 7 months. Parental worries that there might be an organic reason for poor intake of food and poor growth were dismissed. At 16 months it was discovered that she suffered from severe neuromuscular incoordination of the oesophagus;
- Nancy, aged 6 months, gained only just under 1 kg (2 lb. 2 oz.) following her birth. Her mother was 16 years old and had spent all her life in care. She was an immature person and there was nobody to help her.

All these children failed to thrive, and they had one thing in common: they did not get a sufficient amount of nutrition into their systems and all of them were undernourished. The reasons why they were underfed, however, differ from case to case.

Previn was underfed because of maternal and paternal attitudes towards food and preoccupation with weight. Penny did not gain weight in spite of unsuccessful attempts by her mother to feed her: this was associated with her mother's depression connected with sudden bereavement and trauma. Rebecca did not thrive because of physical illness which was not detected and dealt with early on. Kevin's physical and psychosocial growth was poor because of severe neglect and rejection. Indira was extremely difficult to feed from birth and demonstrated oral-motor dysfunction. Nancy was starved unintentionally, as her mother proved unable to read her signals of hunger and did not know much about the nutritional needs of children and generally about parenting.

Many of these children presented feeding problems of one kind or another: some were not fed regularly, sufficiently, and in a manner which would facilitate interest and enjoyment of food; some, because of illness, found swallowing and digestion painful; some had mothers who, because of their depressed state, could not tune into their babies' emotional and nutritional needs; some mothers did not know what their children's nutritional needs were; and a few mothers were simply neglectful or rejectful. Many children are difficult to feed and to care for, so parent–child interaction might be influenced by unexpected problems.

Nowadays, support from the extended family generally has diminished: children tend to live far away from their parents (whence traditional child care support came), and there is often no one to turn to for regular help and advice. Many young parents (particularly mothers) may find child-rearing difficult as they have little experience and even less knowledge about the challenges of child care. They may be unaccustomed to infants because they were brought up in small families and were not given responsibilities for caring for their younger siblings, as older children of yesteryear were obliged to do. They may themselves have been brought up in neglectful and uncaring homes, and had no opportunities to acquire parenting skills or any understanding of children's developmental needs. They may live in adverse social and economic circumstances that may affect the quality of everyday child care. Growing numbers of single, young, and immature mothers (often living in poverty), who are socially isolated and unsupported, are unprepared for the demands of child-rearing, and therefore unable to provide basic physical and emotional nurturance and to meet adequately the nutritional needs of small infants. Most parents, however, successfully carry out the complex tasks involved in child-rearing, using a variety of methods in very diverse family, cultural, and social circumstances.

It must be said that the majority of parents of FTT children do their best and provide adequate care and attention for their offspring, but for one reason or another are not successful in feeding them. Failing to feed a child is a devastating experience for most mothers, as they feel inadequate as carers and worry about the child's health and even survival. They also fear that they may be judged by others as neglectful and uncaring, so they become anxious and overwhelmed with the tasks associated with child care, but more specifically with the baby's feeding behaviour and poor weight gain.

All these children and their families need help. Furthermore, help is needed early on to prevent escalation of problems associated with attachment, interaction, relationships, and inadequate growth and development. Unresolved early difficulties can have a long-term negative effect on children and parents. These children are not always identified as potentially at risk at the onset of presenting nutritional and interactional problems. A 'wait-and-see' approach is often favoured, leaving vulnerable children and equally vulnerable parents at a chance juncture. Some of them do survive but some do not. 'Survival' here

is used to mean a healthy and relatively problem-free childho
who enjoy parenthood, and the sense of a job well done.

## WHAT IS FAILURE TO THRIVE?

From the day a baby is born, parents will focus their attention on the child's growth and development: their major preoccupation will be connected with feeding, health, and the baby's contentment, and they will be eager to see how much weight the baby gains, how it responds to their nurturing, and what developmental progress it makes.

In order for a baby to grow adequately and according to expected norms, it will need to get sufficient nutrition on a regular basis: this should be provided in a manner which will be anxiety-free, enjoyable, and satisfying. So, to give and accept nutrition is at the core of the emerging relationship and interactional synchrony between mother and child. The mutual satisfaction and success of feeding and caring will determine not only the speed of physical growth but also psychomotor development and general responsiveness and alertness. In a secure, caring home, and fuelled by adequate nutrition, children will thrive, giving parents pleasure and confidence in their parenting. In homes riddled with conflict, stress, and chaos, or where parents are ill informed, the children's progress might be slowed down or even impaired if nutritional intake and the quality of nurturing are inadequate for their chronological ages.

Early childhood is a very busy and demanding time where growth and development are concerned, for children grow rapidly, both physically and psychologically. Growth in the first year of life will be quicker than at any other stage during childhood, decreasing rapidly until the end of the third year, then continuing at about one-third of its post-natal rate until puberty (Bee, 1985).

Not all children grow at the same rate. There are considerable variations in rates of growth, and some children have very poor rates of growth. These children have been labelled as FTT and, compared with children of the same age, are significantly smaller and thinner, and can be expected to have poor outcomes. They can be found in all social classes and levels of society. Without early detection and help, the likelihood is that their physical growth, cognitive progress, and emotional development will suffer, and that these negative effects will be long-lasting (Iwaniec & Sneddon, 2002). Additionally, failure to identify these children at an early stage, and failure to take appropriate action to provide suitable help, may lead to distortion of the parent–child relationship, attachment disorders, disturbed behaviour, and developmental (especially cognitive) impairment (Iwaniec, 1995).

Failure to thrive can emerge at different times in an infant's life, as the result of illness or trauma, but under-nutrition during early infancy can have the most detrimental effects as the nutritional requirements at that time are at their most critical. Given the period of rapid growth, particularly brain growth, which occurs during the first few years, particular attention should be given to sufficient and appropriate provision of food (Wynne, 1996; Wright (C.M.), 2000).

So what is failure to thrive? In children it is seen as failure to grow because of under-nutrition in terms of weight gain, height, and head circumference according to expected standards and speed for the child's age. Aetiological factors of inadequate intake of food are complex and varied, but the fact remains that all children who fail to thrive (for whatever reason) do not get sufficient calories into their systems.

The phrase 'failure to thrive' was used as early as 1887 and was introduced by Holt in the first edition of *Diseases of Infancy and Childhood* to describe babies who fail to grow after weaning from the breast. The following quotation from his book described chronic disorder of those children:

> The history in severe cases is strikingly uniform. The following is the story most frequently told. 'At birth the infant was plump and well-nourished and continued to thrive for a month or six weeks while the mother was nursing him; at the end of that period *circumstances* made weaning necessary. From that time on the child *ceased to thrive*. He began to lose weight and strength, at first slowly then rapidly, in spite of the fact that every known infant food was tried.' As a last resort the child, wasted to a skeleton, is brought to hospital.

The term has changed its meaning substantially and has been interpreted in many different ways over the last century. Until the first part of the twentieth century the condition of a wasted body was called *marasmus*, and was always associated with some known or unknown physical disease: it was only a few decades ago (when growth began to be studied scientifically) that failure to thrive was recognised as not necessarily a disease, but as an amalgamation of symptoms which might have many causes. Aetiological factors are varied, but the *primary* reason is inadequate nutrition. Contributory factors include: malabsorption, chronic infection, major structural congenital abnormalities, and metabolic and endocrine defects. However, there are some infants and young children who fail to thrive in whom none of the above factors is obvious (apart from inadequate nutrition), who do not grow, and whose well-being gives cause for concern. This is referred to as *non-organic failure to thrive*. It has been recognised in recent years, however, that making a distinction between organic and non-organic failure to thrive is not useful, because it is better to view failure to thrive as a syndrome of malnutrition associated with all possible roots (Taylor & Daniel, 1999). Ill children who are failing to thrive might be neglected or inadequately cared for as well, so both organic and non-organic factors should be investigated.

The term 'failure to thrive' is not generally used (although often applicable) when speaking of a large population of children world-wide who suffer from serious malnutrition as a result of the shortage of food for themselves or their breast-feeding mothers. Where there is total food deficiency resulting in the stunting of growth, we still refer to it as *marasmus*. It has been estimated by the World Health Organisation (1999) that more than 150 million small children throughout the world are severely or moderately malnourished. Most of these children are living in the under-developed countries where famine, war, widespread poverty, and, in some cases, corruption, make food scarce. Yet we know that malnutrition is not exclusively located in the Third World. In Britain and other well-developed countries many children suffer from malnutrition, which is often undetected because of inadequate screening or lack of child-friendly social policies.

Failure to thrive as a diagnosis becomes significant in a society which can presume food will be available to all its children and where knowledge of childhood illnesses and normal growth and development have become sufficiently precise to define the reasons for growth failure. Failure to thrive over the last six decades has acquired various labels, such as:

- *maternal deprivation* (Bowlby, 1953);
- *environmental retardation* (Coleman & Provence, 1957);
- *mask deprivation* (Prugh & Harlow, 1962);
- *environmental failure to thrive* (Barbero & Shaheen, 1967);
- *deprivation-dwarfism* (Silver & Finkelstein, 1967);
- *psychosocial dwarfism* (Wolff & Money, 1973); and
- *psychosocial short stature and stunting of growth* (MacCarthy & Booth, 1970).

Following the introduction of maternal-deprivation theory and studies of the effects on children living in institutions, new theories and new interpretations and practice policies were evolved. Maternal-deprivation theory had long been disregarded in relation to failure to thrive. Before it was rejected, however, the child-abuse syndrome emerged, which firmly pointed a finger at the mother as a main contributory factor in child growth failure. Various small-scale, uncontrolled studies (mostly based on clinical observation in the 1960s and 1970s) were closely linked theoretically to child-abuse and neglect cases. Although there is an undoubted association between abuse, neglect, and failure to thrive, it applies only in some cases. From the 1980s onwards, control studies began to emerge, as well as the results of the first long-term follow-up studies, shedding new light on the problem and greatly expanding current knowledge.

## AIMS OF THE BOOK

In the present book the author aims to review existing research and practice literature and to share with readers personal experiences acquired over many years. This book is written for busy practitioners to assist them in finding some facts, assessment tools, and various intervention and treatment strategies and methods to help these children and their parents. It is hoped that multi-disciplinary teams will find a few things of interest and that inter-agency work associated with failure to thrive will be informed by tips and ideas provided in the book.

As failure to thrive is multi-factorial, and, therefore, multi-disciplinary in assessment and treatment, the book might be of interest and help to health visitors, paediatricians, GPs, paediatric nurses, social workers, dieticians, psychologists, day-nursery staff, teachers, and others who work or have some responsibility to this client group.

It is also anticipated that the book will provide useful material for teaching in professional courses, as well as in multi-disciplinary child care and child-protection courses.

## ORGANISATION OF THE BOOK

The book is organised in three sections.

**Section I** **The Problem** deals with various causal factors and manifestations of failure-to-thrive syndrome.

**Section II** **The Framework of Assessment** examines issues and presenting problems associated with children, their families, and the environment in which they live. Ecological theory-based assessment is described.

**Section III** **Intervention and Treatment** discusses various methods, techniques, and approaches to helping these children and their families. It also puts forward some recommendations for future practice and research.

## SECTION I: THE PROBLEM

**Chapter 1** is an introduction to the book, briefly discussing the complexity of failure to thrive and different aetiological factors leading to inadequate nutrition and subsequent faltering of growth.

**Chapter 2** looks at the history of child care over many centuries, and discusses the development of knowledge of the failure-to-thrive concept through research and practice.

**Chapter 3** discusses difficulties of defining failure to thrive and problems associated with measuring growth and development. It provides a profile and characteristics of these children and their carers, as well as different types of failure to thrive. Case studies are also presented.

Chapter 4   describes characteristic features of children suffering from psychosocial short-stature syndrome, and draws attention to the emotional abuse of such children, the plight of whom is illustrated by case studies.

Chapter 5   outlines various feeding/eating problems in infancy and early childhood. Parental attitudes to food, oral-motor dysfunctions, faddiness, force-feeding, weaning and transition, and parental feeding styles are reviewed.

Chapter 6   examines parent–child interaction generally, and during feeding time specifically. Children's and parental temperamental attributes and how they affect each other are discussed. A pilot study examining FTT parent–child interaction compared with thriving siblings is included.

Chapter 7   describes different attachment styles in children and adults, and discusses why many failure-to-thrive children are insecurely attached to their mothers. Case studies to illustrate insecure attachment styles are provided. A comparison between childhood attachment style with attachment style in adulthood is presented, based on the author's longitudinal study of FTT children.

Chapter 8   describes fabricated or induced illnesses which can lead to failure to thrive. It includes deliberate withholding of food due to fabricated symptoms (such as non-existing allergies or other illnesses).

## SECTION II: THE FRAMEWORK OF ASSESSMENT

Chapter 9   This extensive chapter deals with the assessment of FTT in a holistic and comprehensive way. It includes factors associated with the children's developmental needs, parental capacity, and family and environmental issues. The child-centred assessment is based on the ecological theory recommended by the Department of Health in 2000.

## SECTION III: INTERVENTION AND TREATMENT

Chapter 10   describes four levels of intervention: universal level—available to all; targeted level—available to those in need of family support; selected level of intervention—for those who are causing concern and may be at risk; and Civil Court intervention—for those who are suffering or may suffer significant harm.

**Chapter 11**   appraises examples of interventions based on ecological, behavioural, cognitive, and attachment theories. It also briefly explains why children fail to thrive from each theoretical point of view.

**Chapter 12**   provides a multidimensional model of intervention developed by the author using behavioural, cognitive, and psychosocial methods of treatment, as well as a number of services to promote positive change in children and parents.

**Chapter 13**   reviews approaches to failure-to-thrive interventions, such as multi-disciplinary and inter-agency approaches as well as the suitability and effectiveness of the involvement of health visitors and social workers. Additionally, a brief discussion of the necessity to view failure to thrive as a psychosocial problem (and not just as a health problem) is provided.

**Chapter 14**   puts forward considerations arising from FTT intervention research such as: parental beliefs, parental history of nurturance, psychosocial issues, parental competence and compliance, self-efficacy, individual differences, and methodological issues. The chapter ends with recommendations regarding practice and research.

**Epilogue**   sums up current practice.

# 2

# HISTORICAL PERSPECTIVE OF FAILURE TO THRIVE

*Truth lies wrapped up and hidden in the depths.*

Lucius Annæus Seneca

## INTRODUCTION

Looking into the history of various civilisations, we can see that infanticide has been accepted by many cultures and has been practised in cases where children were deformed, handicapped, or who failed to thrive. Both Aristotle and Plato approved of it as an appropriate solution to various problems. It was sometimes employed for economic reasons (as in Polynesia, where the relative smallness of the islands ensured the practice was imposed on all families without distinction). It was also common in advanced ancient civilisations, such as those of Egypt, Greece, and Rome to ensure destruction of weak, deformed, or unsightly children.

Among early recorded investigations of infant deprivation and failure to thrive were those carried out by Frederick II of Hohenstaufen (1194–1250),[1] Holy Roman Emperor, King of Sicily and Jerusalem, and *Stupor Mundi et Immutator Mirabilis* ('wonder of the world and transformer to be marvelled at'), as he was called by Matthew Paris (*c.*1200–59), the historian and monk.[2] His Sicilian court (1215–50) was a centre of intellectual activity and attracted the translator, mathematician and astrologer, Michael Scott (*c.*1175–*c.*1234), known as the Scottish Merlin,[3] as well as Leonardo of Pisa (Leonardus Pisanus or Fibonacci—author of *Liber abaci* and *Practica Geometria*, whose work secured the introduction of Arabic notation into Europe and provided the basis for works on algebra and arithmetic in the following centuries). Scott tended

---

[1] For Kaiser Frederick *see Encyclopædia Britannica* (London: Encyclopædia Britannica Ltd, 1959), **ix**, 711–13.

[2] *D.N.B.* (1917), **xv**, 207–13.

[3] *D.N.B.* (1917), **xvii**, 997–1001.

to guide Frederick away from occult, magic, and secret paths, and directed him to more dispassionate scientific experimentation. At that time Frederick developed a rigorous approach to design, measurements, and evaluation. Under Frederick's aegis, studies were made of the effects of deprivation in children, albeit in the realms of language acquisition: in order to establish what was the original language of mankind, new-born infants were reared by foster-mothers who suckled and bathed the children, but were not permitted to speak to them so that they would not learn a language from the foster-mothers. No spontaneous acquisition of Hebrew, Greek, Latin, Arabic, or the languages of the parents to whom the children were born occurred, for in those silent domains the subjects of the experiment all died, although it is not recorded if infection, lack of hygiene, disease, or silence caused their passing.

The conclusion was that Frederick II had the will and intellectual wisdom to seek the truth by means of experimentation at a time when passive acceptance was the established order of the day. Frederick is seen as the first scholar to observe and document the serious effects of deprivation in children, but, like many other curious and inquisitive observers who followed, he failed to find appropriate answers to the questions he asked. There were sundry studies on the fringes of Renaissance enquiry, but in the seventeenth century Sir John Harington (1561–1612)[4] published his famous book *The Englishman's Doctor Or, The Schools of Salerne* (1607), in which he proposed that digestion was encouraged by pleasurable emotions but inhibited by stressful ones. He recommended 'three Doctors' (figuratively speaking of course) to increase an awareness and to suggest what to eat, how much to consume, when to eat, and under what conditions to fully benefit from the taken nutrition. He stated that the quality and amount of food we eat (proper diet) will be beneficial if we consume it in an atmosphere which is relaxed, calm and happy. As he put it:

> Use three Physicians still, First Doctor Quiet, next Doctor Merryman, and Doctor Diet.

Those who work with children who fail to thrive and their families will find this quotation very apposite, as it clearly emphasises the importance of adequate nutrition and the atmospheres that should surround it. The quotation indicates that those 'three wise men' are often absent from the nutritional lives of what are often sad, undernourished children, and of parents who may be anxious, frustrated, demoralised, unsuccessfully trying to feed the child, or neglectful and ill informed about the child's nutritional and nurturing needs.

Documentation of child deprivation and its outcome is very scarce and we know that during the Middle Ages children were portrayed as adults in small bodies (Ariès, 1973). The artist William Hogarth (1697–1764) pictured many

---

[4]*D.N.B.* (1917), **viii**, 1269–72.

aspects of child abuse and deprivation in his widely disseminated engravings, such as 'Gin Lane' (1751): his work portrayed cruelty, neglect, and abuse of all kinds. This included nutritional starvation as deprivation-dwarfism syndrome by showing a child eating garbage, Münchausen Syndrome by Proxy, overt abuse, and acute neglect of children's nutritional, emotional, and physical needs. Hogarth tried to draw public attention to the plight of children by depicting different accidents which he observed and which had an enormous effect on him. In 1738 he produced an engraving entitled 'The Four Times of Day'. The etching entitled 'Noon' portrays a boy carrying a dish of food, but he has dropped it, spilling the contents. In his distress the boy, who knows he is going to be severely punished for it, does not even notice the ragged girl helping herself to the food on the ground.

Institutions for the care of 'foundlings' (children, usually illegitimate, who were abandoned) have a long history. There were 'foundling hospitals' in numerous European cities, and these have been documented. As early as the seventh and eighth centuries there were such establishments in Trier on the Mosel (Augusta Treverorum, the oldest town in Germany), Milan, and Mont-pellier (to name but three such), and in the fourteenth century a famous foundling hospital was created in Venice. Paris and Lyons acquired important foundling hospitals in the seventeenth century, and from 1704 to 1740 Antonio Vivaldi (c.1675–1741) was director of the Conservatorio dell' Ospedale della Pietà, one of four celebrated Venetian music-schools for orphaned or ille-gitimate girls (or girls whose parents were unable to support them). These State-supported schools provided very high standards of education, and the Ospedale della Pietà's musical performances were much appreciated and justly renowned (Blom, 1966).

Indeed, interest in disadvantaged children accelerated during the eigh-teenth century, a time when rational enquiry of all kinds proceeded apace. One of the best-known foundling hospitals was that established by Captain Thomas Coram (c.1668–1751), shipwright, seafarer, trader, colonist (he was involved in both Georgia and Nova Scotia), and philanthropist.[5] Shocked by the common sight of infants exposed and dying in the streets of London, he agitated for the creation of a foundling hospital, and laboured for 17 years to that end. A Charter was obtained, considerable sums subscribed, and the first meeting of the guardians was held in 1739. Some houses were acquired at Hatton Garden, and the first children were admitted in 1741. Eventually, a larger parcel of land was purchased north of Lamb's Conduit Street, and build-ings were erected (1742–52, demolished 1928) under the direction of James Horne (d.1756) to designs by Theodore Jacobsen (d.1772). The first children were removed from Hatton Garden and settled there in 1745.

Huge interest was excited by the undertaking, and support was given by numerous individuals, including Hogarth, who presented his fine portrait of

---

[5]*D.N.B.* (1917), **iv**, 1119–20.

Coram to that hospital in 1740. Georg Friederich Händel (1685–1759) gave concerts there between 1749 and 1750, and composed the Foundling Hospital Anthem, *Blessed are they that consider the poor* (*Händel-Gesellschaft*, vol. 36, 1749), especially for the benefit of the charity (Arnold, 2001; Blom, 1966).

At first, the London Foundling Hospital[6] admitted any child under 2 months of age who was free from certain specified diseases, without question or any attempt to identify its parentage. A basket was suspended outside the entrance-gate in which unwanted infants were deposited, and a bell rung to inform staff of new arrivals. So great was demand that a system of balloting for admission had to be introduced, as fights had occurred outside the gates among those mothers wishing to get rid of their unwanted babies. Grants were made by Parliament from 1756, on condition that all children orphaned were admitted, and in 1757 branch-hospitals had to be opened at Ackworth, Shrewsbury, Westerham, Aylesbury, and Barnet to cope with the 3,727 children for whom admission was sought. This general admission was soon found to be a mistake, for of the 14,934 children received during the three years it was in force, no fewer than 10,389 died. Parents even brought dying children in order to have them buried at the expense of the hospital, and persons were paid by parents to bring infants from all over the country to the London Hospital, but few of those children, through brutality or criminal negligence, ever even reached 'Coram's Fields' alive. So abused was the system that State grants ceased entirely in 1771, and from then onwards the foundation had to depend on private philanthropy for its funds, and admission was changed to a process of selection. Eventually, a child could only be admitted upon the personal application of the mother, and the children of married women or widows were not received. No application was entertained before the birth, nor after a child reached 12 months.

The Coram Foundation was among the first to recognise that there were advantages in keeping mother and child together for at least the first year, for infant mortality rates could thereby be greatly reduced. The herding together of children in larger institutions was also gradually perceived as risky, not only because of the danger of infection, but because an institutionalised environment, except for very short periods, became recognised as being bad for any child. Thus a system of boarding out or fostering was developed. The London Foundling Hospital was a pioneer in boarding out, and by the middle of the twentieth century *all* children admitted to what had become the Thomas Coram Foundation for Children were boarded out.

Drawing on the well-documented archives of Coram's Foundling Hospital, Harry Chapin, in 1915, pointed out the susceptibility of infants to inadequate caring environments, and their undoubted need for *individual* care. Thus it began to be recognised at the beginning of the twentieth century that the outcomes of children deprived of individual care were shocking, in that they

---

[6]*Encyclopædia Britannica* (1959), **ix**, 559–60.

were poor. In some places, such as Romania, the quality of care was found to be equally poor, even at the end of the second millennium. Nutritional and emotional deprivation of children in Romanian orphanages and the levels of suffering to which they were exposed have been well documented, and shocked all who saw the horrific pictures of those children and the environments in which they lived. Malnourishment, lack of stimulation, and all-round gross negligence affected their physical, cognitive, emotional, and social development (in many cases beyond the probability of repair and help).

In Britain the problem of child abuse was beginning to be recognised when the *Offences Against the Person Act* (24 & 25 Vict., *c*.100) became law in 1861: it forbade the abandonment and exposure of infants under 2 years of age, but this enactment was difficult to enforce. The *Poor Law Amendment Act* (31 & 32 Vict., *c*.122, of 1868) stated that parents would be punished if they wilfully neglected their children in terms of failing to provide adequate food, clothing, medical aid, or lodgings for those under 14 years of age, whereby the health of the child was likely to be seriously impaired. In spite of this legislation, very little in reality happened to protect the children, and very few parents or carers were prosecuted for cruelty and negligence of their charges. Children were considered as private property, so interference in child-rearing tended to be avoided. However, in 1889 a statute (52 & 53 Vict., *c*.44) was passed clearly specifying prevention of cruelty to children; this was superseded by a number of similar enactments leading up to the more modern and comprehensive *Children Act* (8 Edw. 7, *c*.67) of 1908.

Abandoned, rejected, neglected, cruelly treated and orphaned children were cared for in the large orphanages or hospitals. The poor outcomes of institutional care were widely acknowledged, and many professionals and researchers expressed their concerns. However, Holt and Fales (1923) stated that, given the appropriate conditions,

> strikingly good health and excellent nutrition can be maintained in children obliged to live in institutions.

After outlining the hazards and dangers for children being cared for in the infant ward, Joseph Bremeau (1932) made eight recommendations for prevention, one of which was 'one nurse for two babies, minimum'.

Apart from stressing the nutritional needs of children, doctors increasingly began to emphasise the nurturing aspect of daily care and the need for interaction with adults. It began to be recognised that in order to grow healthily and vigorously and to recover more quickly from illnesses, babies need appropriate physical and emotional contact with care-givers, as the absence of such continuing nurturance and physical intimacy can bring about anxiety and fretting in children, disrupting biological functions.

Development of awareness for the necessity of emotional care was well described by Montagu (1978). In his chapter on 'Tender Loving Care' he described high mortality rates in institutions, and related an interesting anecdote. In a German hospital before the 1939–45 war, a visiting American doctor, while being shown over the wards in one of the hospitals, noticed an ancient hag-like woman who was carrying a very undernourished infant. The doctor enquired of the director the identity of the old woman and was told that she was 'Old Anna': when the staff at the hospital had done everything medically they could do for a baby, and it still failed to thrive, they handed it over to 'Old Anna', who succeeded in remedying matters every time. She fed the child, encouraged it to eat, was patient, held it gently, talked to it, rocked, giving tender attention plus the close physical contact which every baby needs: it is small wonder that babies passed to her, who had been near death's door, began to thrive due to the increased intake of food and the manner in which she fed and looked after them.

## SOCIO- AND PSYCHO-GENESIS

The hypothesis of a psychological aetiology for failure to thrive has its roots in the extensive literature on the effects of institutionalisation, hospitalisation, and maternal deprivation on infants. During the 1940s studies began to emerge postulating that emotional deprivation *per se* could affect physical growth, and many claimed that deprivation in infancy would lead to irreversible impairment of psychosocial functioning in later life. Some of the best accounts of growth failure at the time were those of Spitz (1945), Talbot *et al.* (1947), Bakwin (1949), and Widdowson (1951). The 'disorder of hospitalism' (as Spitz termed it) occurred in institutionalised children in the first five years of life, and the major manifestation involved emotional disturbance, failure to gain weight, and developmental retardation resulting in poor performance during tests. Spitz compared a group of infants cared for by their mothers with a group raised in virtual isolation from other infants and adults. Spitz stated that physical illnesses, including infections, are contracted more frequently by infants deprived of environmental stimulation and maternal care than those not so deprived. The failure-to-thrive syndrome, according to Spitz, is a direct result of inadequate nurturance: indeed he actually documented long-term intellectual deficit in the survivors of the non-nurtured group. Of the deprived group, 37% had died by 2 years of age, compared with none in the adequately mothered group. Spitz stated that a condition of anaclitic depression manifested itself in severe developmental retardation, extreme friendliness to any persons, anxious avoidance of inanimate objects, anxiety expressed by blood-curdling screams, bizarre stereotyped motor patterns resembling catatonia, failure to thrive, insomnia, and sadness. It should be noted that Spitz's work has been severely criticised for methodological and other weaknesses, and it would be inappropriate to link failure to thrive (as we observe and know it now) to the cases of children studied by Spitz. A comparison of the effects of institutionalised rearing, as described by Spitz, with conditions in Romanian orphanages (where children were incarcerated in badly run, impoverished, and ill-informed institutions rather than by parents in their natural homes) would be more appropriate. Nevertheless, these studies proved (with the addition of Bowlby's work) to be significant in a heuristic sense, and have been important catalysts in generating research and informing policy and practice.

## CAUSAL MECHANISMS

The association between maternal deprivation and failure to thrive has led some investigators to hypothesise the existence of a physiological pathway whereby emotional deprivation affects the neuro-endocrine system regulating growth.

Several studies were done to test growth-hormone efficiency. The mechanism in dwarfism was studied extensively in attempts to answer the question 'what factors play a role in growth-hormone arrest and what happens and under what circumstances are they switched on again?'. These studies concentrated on various forms of growth failure, but particularly on dwarfism without organic cause. Dwarf children were defined by Patton and Gardner (1962) as being below the 3rd percentile in height, with weight below that expected for the height (though exceptionally that weight may be appropriate for the height), and the child might appear well nourished. However, such appearances may be deceptive because neither weight nor height is normal for the chronological age. Patton and Gardner postulated that emotional disturbances might have direct effects on intermediary metabolism so as to interfere with the anabolic processes. The production and release of several anterior pituitary hormones are influenced by hypothalamic centres, which are, in turn, recipients of pathways from higher neural centres, particularly the limbic cortex (also thought to be the focus of emotional feelings and behaviour). These authors, on the basis of six very thoroughly studied children, favoured a theory of emotional influence on growth with secondary hormonal insufficiencies as the main cause of the dwarfism.

Apley et al. (1971) made penetrating enquiries based on paediatric, psychiatric, and social-work team-work information to discover the truth about the food-intake of individuals with dwarfism syndrome in Bristol. Their exhaustive clinical, biochemical, and endocrine tests on all the children ruled out the operation of pathological causes in the stunting of growth, and, by inference, they pointed to under-feeding as the cause.

In 1947 Nathan Talbot and his co-workers reported on the concept of dwarfism in healthy children and its possible relationship to emotional, nutritional, and endocrine disturbances. Their work foreshadowed much of what is now known about these children. They found that children studied were physically healthy, were small with a height-age less than 80% of actual age, were underweight for height, had low caloric intake, were anorexic secondary to emotional disturbance, had no significant history of short stature, and had scanty subcutaneous tissue. They were the first to point to 'chronic grief' as one of the causes of dwarfism. They studied over one hundred individuals with dwarfism syndrome between $2\frac{1}{2}$ and 15 years of age, but were not able to find any organic cause for the stunting in growth. The nutritional history of these children clearly indicated that there were feeding problems for a major part of their lives (and in some cases since birth): the authors postulated that once a child became undersized, it continued with basically reduced protein and calorific requirements, and, the pituitary function having become adaptively reduced, it failed to function normally when the diet improved. Some children, therefore, remained small though apparently well nourished. Talbot and his colleagues treated them with pituitary hormones and discovered that some of these children, both the well-nourished and thin ones, were capable of good growth over many months thereafter.

However, they discovered through psychiatric and social studies that the backgrounds of these children were grossly problematic, and listed the following features in 24 of them:

- 34% rejection;
- 14% poverty;
- 14% mental deficiency;
- 19% chronic grief;
- 14% maternal delinquency; and
- breakdown in family and marital relationship in 14% of cases.

No abnormality was found in only 5% of cases. In seven well-nourished children no abnormality was found in three cases, maternal delinquency or breakdown in three, and rejection in one. Four of these children with disturbed maternal relationships were stunted in growth, but on the surface appeared well nourished. The outcomes suggested that the intake of food was not the whole answer to the cause of the dwarfism, and led other researchers to pursue the hormone studies.

In 1949 Bakwin concluded that failure to thrive in institutions is the result of emotional deprivation, and that emotional reactions arise principally in response to sensory stimuli. He believed that children who are hospitalised should receive attention and affection, and should often be held in the arms of adults. He proposed that the mother should be at the baby's bedside most of the time and that preoccupation with infection was ill founded. He described the appearance and psychological expression in the following ways:

| Appearance | Psychological expression |
|---|---|
| Listlessness | No interest in food, accepted passively |
| Quietness | Emaciation |
| Poor appetite | Immobility |
| Unhappiness | Withdrawal |
| Absence of sucking habits | Unresponsiveness |
| No interest in surroundings | Insomnia |
| Poor tone | Miserableness |
| Seldom crying | Lying motionless in bed |
| Slow movement | Sunken cheeks |

Bakwin associated poor growth development and psychological presentation with emotional deprivation and absence of maternal care while in hospital. He questioned the aetiology as being directly linked to nutrition, infection, and the psychological make-up of a child.

Widdowson (1951) reported in *The Lancet* the effects of psychosocial deprivation on children's physical growth. She replicated Spitz's findings that adequate calorific provision in an unfavourable psychological environment (due to harsh and unsympathetic handling) may seriously curtail growth-rates. Just after the Second World War, Widdowson studied children in two German orphanages where she was stationed as a British Army medical officer. Each orphanage accommodated around 50 boys and girls of a wide age range between 4 and 14 years. A dietary supplement, which was expected to produce faster weight gain, was introduced as an experiment in one orphanage, using the other as a control. Contrary to expectation, it was the control group which gained weight and grew a little faster during the experimental period of six months. Afterwards it was discovered that the matrons of the two orphanages had swapped over at about the time of the start of the dietary supplement. The matron in charge of the experimental group (who had transferred to the control group) had been a kindly, caring, and warm person, but the matron originally in charge of the control group (who had transferred to the experimental group) was harsh, a hard disciplinarian who tended to harass the children at meal-times. Such harsh behaviour could well have caused some achlorhydria and also anorexia (though it is unlikely that the children would have been allowed to leave anything on their plates).

One may speculate that the dietary supplement was wasted. This study suggests that nutritional intake (to be beneficial) has to take place in relative calmness and in an anxiety-free state, and that non-nutritional emotional factors play an important role in digestion and absorption. Indeed, one of the indices of basic trust and security in an infant (in Erikson's sense) is stable feeding behaviour, and eating (to be beneficial nutritionally and enjoyable) requires conditions conducive to a relatively benign and calm state of psychosomatic harmony. But without adequate consumption of food a child will not put on weight, so feeding it quantities needed for its age is the first requirement. The second requirement is calm and friendly interaction during feeding/eating times, and the third is sensitivity and awareness of a child's personal characteristics, i.e. temperament, and of some feeding difficulties (such as oral-motor problems or other illnesses) which make eating uncomfortable or painful.

In her wise paper (ibid.), Widdowson's biblical quotation (Better is a dinner of herbs where love is, than a stalled ox and hatred therewith [Proverbs, xv, 17]) is very pertinent—all of us can identify with it to some extent. We enjoy food more and are more eager to eat when we are happy and in the company of people we like than when we are stressed, anxious, and miserable.

## MATERNAL PATHOLOGY AND GROWTH-FAILURE

In the late 1950s and 1960s, studies of growth failure and developmental delays, similar to those found among institutionalised children, were replicated on infants and young children living at home. Studies of such children and their families have shown that the most commonly identified precursors to these growth problems are emotional disturbance and environmental deprivation—with the wide range of psychosocial disorganisation that these concepts imply. Deprivation often involves rejection, isolation from social contact, and neglect. These associations with poor growth have been delineated in the context of maternal personality problems, stemming from the mother's own early background, family dysfunction, immaturity, social isolation, and mental-health problems. Other psychological difficulties have been found to stem from the manner in which mothers nurture their small infants. The prevailing view was that socio-emotional deprivation could be the cause of some cases of short stature, and that the most likely aetiology was deprivation or inadequate, disturbed mothering in general (Coleman & Provence, 1957; Patton & Gardner, 1962), and that failure to thrive was occasioned either through diminished intestinal absorption, faulty conservation of nutrients, or possible abnormality of endocrine function (Leonard et al., 1966).

## POINTING THE FINGER AT THE MOTHER

In cases considered with the concept of the Battered Child Syndrome introduced by Henry Kempe and his colleagues in 1962, theorists, researchers, and clinicians have explored the causes of child abuse and neglect, including failure to thrive. For a considerable time the medical–psychiatric model of the causation and treatment was favoured, attributing the blame for its occurrence to the pathological personality structure of the mother and her history of having herself been abused and neglected as a child. Let us look at a few studies conducted at the time and their preoccupation with maternal failings.

Coleman and Provence (1957) presented detailed reports of two infants from middle-class families in whom they postulated retardation of both growth and development resulting from insufficient stimulation from the mother and insufficient maternal care. In the first case the child was difficult to feed and presented as generally passive and difficult to enjoy. When the infant was 7 months old the mother was pregnant again. During that time, the mother's father committed suicide. The mother showed grief, depression, and anger over a prolonged period and further neglected the child.

In the second case the mother was isolated and emotionally detached from her infant: she stopped breast-feeding on the fourth day after birth because she said she was afraid she would smother the child, and spanked the infant because its crying drove her wild. She alternated between feelings of depression and helplessness over the baby's poor development. The baby was not planned or wanted and the mother resented breaking her career. The authors did not make any distinction between these two infants and mothers. It is clear, however, that both babies were undernourished and failed to thrive: one presumably because of feeding difficulties and maternal grief; and the second because of rejection and inadequate provision of food.

Fischhoff *et al.* (1971) conducted a study of 12 mothers of 3- to 24-month-old infants. Their findings were based on two interviews with the mothers, brief contacts on the wards, social-work reports, unstructured interviews with the fathers, and reported observations by paediatricians and nurses. They concluded that 10 out of 12 mothers presented enough behavioural signs to warrant diagnoses of character disorder. These women (according to the authors) presented a constellation of psychological failures conducive to inadequate mothering, including:

- limited abilities to perceive accurately the environment, their own needs, or those of their children;
- limitations of adaptability to changes in their lives;
- adverse affective states;
- defective object-relationships; and
- limited capacity for concern.

Since character disorders (in the view of many) are untreatable, they suggest that some of these failure-to-thrive children may be better off in foster-homes. Although mothers in their small sample were found to present character disorders, it would be wrong to say that all mothers or the majority of mothers whose children fail to thrive have personality disorders. The label can also be a facile and meaningless designation, devoid of useful implications.

Similar and different signs of psychopathology have been identified among mothers of failure-to-thrive children. Barbero and Shaheen (1967) found mothers in their sample depressed, angry, helpless, and desperate, and suffering from low self-esteem. However, they drew professional attention to those children who might be at risk of being inappropriately diagnosed, noted that there were some who failed to thrive because of abuse or neglect, and that such children should be referred to appropriate helping agencies. They postulated that those mothers lived with significant environmental and psychological disruption, such as alcoholism, childhood abuse, family violence, and general family dysfunction.

Again, Leonard et al. (1966) described similar characteristics found in 13 mothers of infants who failed to thrive: these included tension, anger, anxiety, and depression, but it proved difficult to disentangle cause and effect because, for example, failure to thrive in an infant might have contributed to such states in the women. Mothers in this comprehensive study were poorly mothered themselves, were sexually traumatised as children, and had experienced family instability. The authors found that those mothers were lacking in self-esteem, unable to assess their babies' needs and their own self-worth realistically, and were lonely, isolated, and depressed. The authors described these mothers as severely malfunctioning and disturbed.

Spinetta and Rigler (1972) have hypothesised on the basis of their studies that the parents of failure-to-thrive children (like parents who have physically abused their children) have themselves been physically abused and neglected in childhood. Bullard et al. (1967) found from their study of 50 FTT children that neglect (identified as lack of interest by parents) is the major cause of that condition. They identified factors contributing to neglect, such as instability of lifestyle, severe marital strife, erratic living habits, alcoholism, a history of entanglements with the law, and inability to maintain employment or to provide financial support for the care of the children. The mothers tended to describe lack of feelings for their children, and admitted to leaving them unattended or with strangers for long periods. The authors questioned the appropriateness of using the blanket term 'maternal deprivation' when applied to failure-to-thrive children, feeling it should be used more specifically and should refer to possible inadequacies in feeding, holding, and other care-taking activities of the mother. The proposition emerged at that time that failure to thrive (as secondary to maternal deprivation) was based on evidence that the child had little physical handling by the mother, or no appropriate social contact. Such mothers were said rarely to hold, cuddle, smile at, play with, or communicate with their children. The researchers observed that those mothers might lack positive feelings for their children, and could be insensitive to and unable to assess their needs, particularly with regard to hunger. These aspects have been highlighted by several researchers (Coleman & Provence, 1957; Leonard *et al.*, 1966; Bullard *et al.*, 1967; Fischhoff *et al.*, 1971). In these studies feeding was singled out as a time of major conflict between mother and child: none of them, however, examined or measured how much food was consumed by the children.

In 1967 Powell and his colleagues (Powell *et al.*, 1967) measured growth-hormone response along with other endocrine studies in 13 children. They described many of the common social circumstances in families of children who failed to thrive (which included divorce, marital difficulties, alcoholism, and extra-marital affairs), and they noted that the fathers spent little time with the children. In addition to their endocrine studies they made interesting observations of the children's behaviour, such as soiling and wetting; stealing food; eating non-food items; eating from garbage cans; gorging and vomiting; wandering around the house at night; playing alone; and having temper-tantrums. Such children tended to be malnourished, thin, and short, with weight-for-height appearing normal or greater. All children in their sample were observed to be short, with weight-ages ranging between 30% and 66% of the chronological age. The oldest boy, when initially seen, was $11\frac{1}{2}$ years old, with a height-age of $5\frac{1}{2}$ years: his weight was normal for his height. The head circumferences were $-1$ to $-11\%$ of the average head circumference for the chronological age and $+1$ to $-9\%$ of the average circumference expected for the actual height. All had protuberant abdomens and some had decreased muscle bulk. Many had retarded bone-ages commensurate with their height-ages. All the children had depressed or infantile nasal bridges, giving a younger naso-orbital configuration than expected for their age. The researchers concluded that aetiology of the growth failure and possible hypopituitarism was unresolved.

In 1969 Whitten and his associates (Whitten *et al.*, 1969) began to question some of the concepts of subtle influence of deprivation or neglect upon metabolic functioning. They postulated that growth-failure occurs because of under-nutrition, and they presented evidence arising from a study of children hospitalised because of their failure to thrive: they found that 11 out of 13 children gained weight at an accelerated rate when adequately fed while living in a hospital environment where personal care was given to them. In addition, seven out of seven depressed infants rapidly gained weight in their own homes when given an adequate diet by their mothers in the presence of an observer. They went further to say that children gained weight when fed the appropriate amount of food regardless of whether or not they received extra stimulation or attention. They concluded that maternally deprived infants are underweight because of under-eating, which is secondary to not being offered adequate food or to not accepting it, and not because of some psychologically induced defect in absorption or metabolism.

The findings of Whitten *et al.'s* study of 1969 was a turning-point for many researchers. The emphasis was put on the energy intake, rather than on concentrating exclusively on emotional deprivation and abuse, although both could be in operation. It was recognised that maternal perceptions and statements on how much a child consumed in terms of calories were not always accurate, and that some children were simply starved. MacCarthy and Booth (1970) studied the influence of deprivation on somatic growth, and concluded that deprivation-dwarfism is caused by malnutrition because of inadequate intake of food. They suggested it is likely that these children are not given enough food by the mother, and that, consequently, because of chronic underfeeding, they become undemanding.

The studies conducted in the 1960s and 1970s showed striking similarities in clinical observations of personalities and behavioural features of the mothers of failure-to-thrive children. These observations, however, are somewhat questionable because of the absence of contrast or control groups. As we know, clinic-attending patients make for a notoriously biased sample. A further weakness of much of the work is the absence of evidence on the reliability or validity of the procedures used for data collection. Most of the studies then (as well as now) are based on retrospective data and therefore have to be interpreted with caution. Early studies have been based on observations of children and parents mainly in hospitals or clinics, so observations of interactions and quality of care at home, including feeding style and nutritional intake, were not taken into consideration. It is well known that people behave differently, present a different picture of themselves, and tell different stories when away from their natural habitats. Nevertheless, much has been learned from those small, hospital-based studies. They were not different in quality and validity to those of child abuse. The mother was seen as all-powerful, as well as wicked, who was wholly responsible for good and bad in the child's outcomes. The next chapter will deal with more recent studies and the changing philosophy about aetiology and controlling mechanisms of failure to thrive.

## SUMMARY

Failure to thrive is as old as human history. There have always been children who fail to thrive, and, although they were not labelled as such, they were described as 'sickly', 'weak', or 'defective', and their fate, as a rule, was death. This chapter provides glimpses only of child-rearing, care and protection over the centuries. It aims to put into context the development of child welfare and the long and painful journey to reach current views of a complicated matter. Failure to thrive (as it was coined by Holt in 1897) has gone through various stages of knowledge-development as well, and these stages have been briefly summarised above.

It was once argued that hospitalised and institutionalised children failed to thrive because they did not receive maternal nurturing and attention as a result of separation from their mothers. However, when children who failed to thrive began to be studied in their own homes, they showed the same outcomes, and it was assumed that their condition had developed because of neglect or abuse. As will be demonstrated below, neither simplistic view embraced the full picture.

# 3

# FAILURE TO THRIVE: DEFINITION, PREVALENCE, MANIFESTATION, AND EFFECT

*Use three Physicians still, First Doctor Quiet, next Doctor Merryman, and Doctor Diet.*

Sir John Harington, 1607

## INTRODUCTION

The term 'failure to thrive' is applied to infants and young children whose weight, height, head circumference, and general psychosocial development are significantly below age-related norms, and whose well-being causes concern. It is conceived as a variable syndrome of severe growth retardation, delayed skeletal maturation, and problematic psychomotor development, which is associated with under-nutrition (Iwaniec, 1995). There are, however, various reasons why children are undernourished: they include acute feeding difficulties including oral-motor dysfunction, disturbed mother–child interaction, insecure disoriented attachment, family dysfunction, neglect, rejection, poverty, and various illnesses (Iwaniec, 1995). The definition adapted by the author (and which will be used throughout this book) is: *failure to thrive in infants and children is failure to develop in terms of weight-gain and growth at the normal speed and amount for their ages as a result of inadequate calorie intake.*

Failure to thrive (or under-nutrition during infancy and early childhood) is a common problem and is usually identified during the first three years of life. When children are undernourished they will fail to gain the required weight. After a while their growth in terms of height also falters. On the growth-chart they remain or drop below the 2nd percentile (or the lowest line) of weight or height. Most children are diagnosed as failing to thrive when their weight- and height-percentiles are low and remain low for two to three months. Others are diagnosed when growth drops down across two or more percentiles, and when there has not been any obvious reason for this, such as illness or the normal slimming associated with extended mobility and activity-levels during the crawling and walking stages of development.

Additionally, genetic growth expectation is considered (e.g. the parents' heights and weights), so for a small child who has small parents to be labelled as failing to thrive, that child would have to be low in weight for height, or demonstrate poor weight-gain velocity, since weight-for-age would normally be low. However, it needs to be remembered that parental height might not represent actual genetic potential, as those parents might have failed to thrive as children, and their growths could possibly have been stunted.

The causes of FTT are often divided into three categories: organic, non-organic, and combined. Organic failure to thrive is thought to result from illnesses or genetic conditions, whilst non-organic failure to thrive may derive from inadequate parenting and from various environmental factors. Combined FTT may have both organic and non-organic origins. Whatever the sources of failure to thrive, it is always associated with under-nutrition, whether that is caused by a disease that blocks or interferes with the absorption of nutrients or by an inadequate food intake in quantity and quality for the child's age and size (Dykman *et al.*, 2000).

Different terms are used to describe failings in weight and height as stated by the World Health Organisation (WHO) Expert Committee (1995). These are:

1. low height-for-age (called *stunting*), considered to be an indicator of long-term malnutrition and poor growth;
2. low weight-for-height (called *wasting*), a result of recent severe weight loss; and
3. low weight-for-age (called *underweight*), found in both stunting or wasting.

As a rule, researchers use the measure of low height-for-age (stunting) as the selection criterion for growth deficit (Walker *et al.*, 1992; Voss, 1995). It is generally recognised that stunting is the most widespread indicator of growth deficiency across the globe, even though weight-for-age is the usual screening parameter for undernourished children (Reifsnider *et al.*, 2000). Stunting can be *discriminated* from failure to thrive (which is a symptom rather than a diagnosis), because, as a rule, FTT shows low weight-for-age or weight-for-height (WHO Expert Committee, 1995).

## PREVALENCE OF FAILURE TO THRIVE

Although failure to thrive usually occurs early in a child's life, its effects and consequences can be observed at the older toddler stage, middle childhood, or even adulthood (Sneddon & Iwaniec, 2002; Iwaniec & Sneddon, 2002).

- Estimates of prevalence have varied from as much as 10% of the poor children (both from rural and urban areas) seen in out-patients' clinics, to 1% of all paediatric hospitalisation cases (Bithoney & Newberger, 1987).
- It has been estimated that between 3 and 5% of all infants under one year of age who are hospitalised are diagnosed as FTT.
- At the primary setting its occurrence was calculated as 9.5%. Berwick (1980) reported that out of 1% of hospitalised children, 80% of infants are younger than 18 months.
- MacMillan (1984) stated that FTT probably affects 1–3% of the child population at some time.
- The breakdown of the population of children with FTT is suggested to range from 32 to 58% (non-organic), and from 17 to 58% (organic) (Spinner & Siegel, 1987).
- In the United Kingdom, Skuse et al. (1992, 1994a, b), from a series of epidemiological studies, estimated a 3.3% incident rate of failure to thrive. The criterion for admission to the study was a weight below the 3rd percentile at the age of one year and being in evidence for at least three months.
- In their community study conducted in Israel, Wilensky et al. (1996) found similar prevalence rates of 3.9% in children who failed to thrive. The calculations were based on a sample taken from all children born in 1991.
- Wright et al. (1994), endeavouring to unravel the prevalence and reasons for FTT, examined various environmental factors which they thought might have contributed to an increased rate of occurrence of the syndrome. They classified all children who failed to thrive into three categories, as affluent, intermediate, or deprived by using the census data for the areas covered by the research investigation. They found that deprived children dominated in prevalence, but that failure to thrive was evident in all three groups. This study confirmed the findings of Iwaniec's (1983) investigations that FTT occurred in all social classes, and that aetiological factors leading to under-nutrition did not vary substantially in the sample group.
- Batchelor and Kerslake (1990) found the recognition rate very poor, for one in three children falling below the 3rd percentile were not identified by the health visitors. However, when Batchelor (1996) broadened her criteria for failure to thrive to include those children who had dropped down across two major percentile lines (but not the 3rd percentile), she found that half of these children were not recognised as poor weight-gainers.

It can be seen that prevalence very much depends on the criteria used for admission into the study and on operational definitions of the problem.

Opinions differ as to whether children who drop across the percentiles at the age of increased activity level should be considered as failing to thrive when their behaviour and/or development do not give cause for concern.

They might lose weight because of increased activities and a greater pre-occupation with play, thus redirecting their attention from eating to other curiosity-attracting events or objects. But it may be that something traumatic has occurred in the child's or parents' life which disturbs eating behaviours and slows down the child's growth and development. It has been found that sexual and physical abuse can play a role and lead to more acute stunting of growth as time goes on (Skuse *et al.*, 1996). Sudden bereavement in the family, marital breakdown, loss of employment, serious illnesses, and other events can influence parenting behaviour by reducing the level and quality of inter-action and reduce substantially the amount of interest, time spent, and energy in daily child care. It would seem advisable to assess each case of this kind individually, yet only when the child's behaviour and development indicate deviation from the norm and when intake of food has decreased substantially. If falling across the percentile criterion is used indiscriminately, and seen as a line drawn on the weight chart, then it can lead to erroneous diagnoses of FTT and put unnecessary burdens and pressures on the parents, when in fact the term 'failure to thrive' should not even be used. A more strict medical and developmental definition is required to prevent over-zealousness regarding weight gain or loss and to give confidence to those who have to deal with these children and families on a daily basis.

In Europe and North America, children below the lowest percentile are considered for intervention, but, according to Cole (1994), few get referred as the false/positive rate is exceptionally high: 5% of normal children in Amer-ica and 2% in the United Kingdom fall below the cut-off point. He argues that it might be better to use the –2SD score instead of the 2nd percentile as this measure would reduce the false/positive rate to 2.3%. A realistic cut-off for referral is much lower than the 2nd or 5th percentile. Current weight measurements will be discussed further in the chapter on assessment.

As we can see, the prevalence rate of all FTT children is not clear. It varies according to the definition used, and, since there is no agreement as to when exactly we can say that a child is failing to thrive, confusion and different estimations will be evident. There is also much debate over how growth failure should be diagnosed, what the consequences are for a child and its family, and how practitioners can successfully intervene in FTT cases.

## REASONS FOR GROWTH FAILURE

As was noted above, there are different and many reasons why children eat less than is necessary, and, quite often there may be more than one rea-son why they fail to thrive. Some children will fail to grow at an expected speed because of an illness or some chronic medical condition. It is known that virtually all serious paediatric illnesses and also minor recurrent or chronic ones can result in impeded growth. For example, Aids, cerebral palsy,

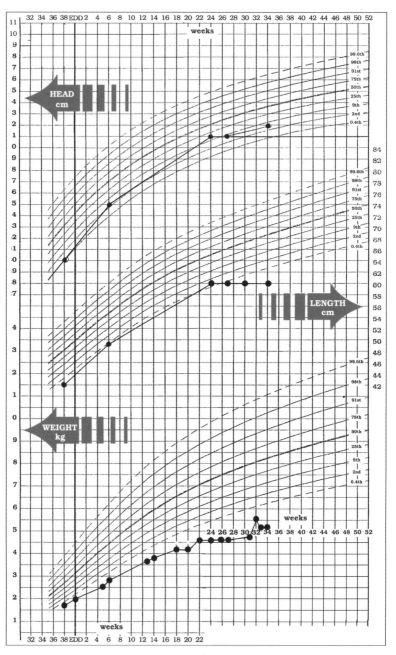

**Figure 3.1** Growth chart illustrating failure to thrive: 0–1 year
Copyright © Child Growth Foundation

malabsorption, congenital heart disease, recurring infection, cystic fibrosis, etc., will all contribute to fluctuations of weight and growth. Neurological problems which interfere with normal growth make up the largest single diagnostic category (Palmer *et al.*, 1993).

Many anatomical malformations of the orofacial structures can also result in growth failure, such as cleft palette and cleft lip. A direct predictable link can normally be observed between the course of the illness and a child's growth patterns, e.g. after a successful course of treatment or an operation the child's growth pattern will gradually stabilise or return to normal. Although the majority of childhood illnesses result, to some degree, in a slowing down of growth, there may also be more subtle organic problems which, if not recognised or taken into account, may lead to unfair and wrong diagnosis that FTT is due to poor parenting, behavioural problems, or sheer neglect. These include factors such as oral-motor dysfunction, prenatal factors, or more serious illnesses, e.g. a tumour. However, it is estimated that fewer than 5% of cases of all failures to thrive are due solely to organic disease (Wynne, 1996; Wright & Talbot, 1996). Diagnoses have to be made carefully to avoid not only a culture of blame, but, more importantly, failure to identify serious illness. Let us look at Isabella's case to see what can happen if behavioural symptoms are not taken as indicators of a serious illness.

---

### Isabella's Case

*Failure to thrive because of serious illness*
Isabella, aged 6 years, was seen in the out-patients' clinic because of loss of weight, diminished appetite, and problematic behaviour (such as irritability, defiance, moodswings, and unpredictable behaviour at school). As preliminary medical investigations did not show anything abnormal, it was assumed that Isabella was simply playing up and needed some behaviour-management intervention, and advice as to how to manage her deteriorating appetite.

The behavioural assessment indicated a number of worrying signs: these included sudden loss of appetite, loss of weight, moodswings, loss of balance, headaches, vomiting, excessive sleep, irritability, and nausea. A request for further medical examination was disregarded as it was believed that the presenting failure to thrive was non-organic, stemming from behavioural mismanagement. Six months later Isabella collapsed, was taken to a different hospital and was diagnosed as having a brain tumour. The tumour was successfully removed, but Isabella lost her sight in one eye. The parents were told that if the problem had been identified earlier, which it could have been, she would not have been thus affected.

---

This tragic case indicates the necessity to respond speedily to worrying signs and to avoid the ideological belief that only very few children fail to thrive because of illness. There were many serious signs indicating the necessity for a more comprehensive medical investigation, but they were not taken on board.

## MALNUTRITION AND FAILURE TO THRIVE

Strictly speaking there is a difference between malnutrition and under-nutrition. When we speak of malnutrition generally we understand that there is a shortage of food resulting in starvation. If, however, it is presumed that food is available (as is the case in the westernised world), malnutrition refers to the absence of one or more essential nutrients in the diet. Under-nutrition refers to insufficient calorific intake: in other words, the child simply does not get enough food to eat. A malnourished child may have an adequate amount of food but the diet is not balanced.

Malnutrition is far more widespread than under-nutrition in the human population and it can happen that an overnourished individual is also mal-nourished. Every human needs a certain combination of essential amino acids, and a diet which lacks one or more of these results in a form of mal-nutrition generally known as protein deficiency. This type of malnutrition is most likely to occur in populations where food supply does not meet population demands. The victims are usually children, who, if they survive infancy, are likely to be retarded in physical and (at times) mental develop-ment (Grantham-McGregor *et al.*, 2000). In Africa this syndrome is known as *kwashiorkor*, meaning 'rejected one', as it is likely to take place when a child is weaned from its mother's milk and given a starchy diet soon after a sibling is born. This almost always results in the onset of impaired physical development. We refer to this type of malnutrition as *marasmus*.

It has been calculated that a malnourished child recovering from growth failure needs approximately 25–30% more nutrition for catch-up growth than a normal child, and the amount of protein needs to be nearly doubled. MacCarthy and Booth (1970) stated that a child weighing 9 kg would need about 14 grams of protein per day, which could be obtained one-third of a pint of milk and three-quarters of an ounce of cheese. A less rich source of protein could be provided from cereal foods.

## NON-ORGANIC FAILURE TO THRIVE

The term 'non-organic failure to thrive' is applied to children whose failure to grow normally is due to psychosocial reasons in their environment rather than as a result of any medical illness. One of the problems in the literature is that traditionally non-organic failure to thrive has been diagnosed on the basis that no medical reason can be found for the child's growth failure. This is often the outcome of negative results from a series of laboratory investiga-tions. However, it is believed that enough is now known about the characteris-tics of non-organic FTT to enable a positive diagnosis to be made, i.e. a diagno-sis made on the basis of observing certain characteristics (such as the quality of the interaction with the primary care-giver and the behaviour of the child), rather than a negative one made on the failure to make a medical diagnosis.

These children show no organic or medical reason for their poor growth patterns, and many different explanations have been offered as to why they fail to grow normally. Initially it was thought that psychological or socio-economic problems of the care-giver (usually taken to be the mother) affected her relationship with the child. The care-giver was thought to be emotionally distant and unresponsive to the child, thus providing an inadequate environment for development and growth (sometimes both physical and psychological). This emotional 'negligence' was not necessarily assumed to be deliberate: sometimes it might be the unfortunate result of a care-giver too distracted by outside concerns (such as financial pressures) to offer the child the attention it deserved. The consequence of these poor-quality interactions was thought to be that the child ate less, was fed less, or was unable to absorb adequate calories (Spinner & Siegel, 1987).

Early explanations of non-organic FTT, as elaborated on in the previous chapter, drew on the extensive literature on the effects of institutionalisation, hospitalisation, and maternal deprivation in children. These ideas were influenced by a society which saw a child's upbringing as being primarily the responsibility of the mother. However, during the last quarter of a century the focus has shifted to recognise the role that other people play in a child's upbringing. Nevertheless, we still know very little about the role that fathers play in the upbringing of their children. Whereas earlier investigations focused almost exclusively on the contribution of the mother to the interaction, researchers also now look at both sides of the dyad and are investigating how subtle characteristics of the infants (such as temperament) may stress relationships with others and result in disturbed interactions. For example, children with non-organic FTT have been described as apathetic, passive and irritable, with poor appetites, histories of feeding problems, and an inability to interact with their physical and emotional environments. These characteristics may make it difficult for people to interact with these children. It has also been documented that some of these children are just not likeable: not only by their parents, but also by teachers and health practitioners (Skuse, 1992; Iwaniec, 1995). The pertinent question is whether these characteristics *precede* or are a *result* of failure to thrive.

Regardless of which comes first, there is little doubt that, over time, stressful interactions can contribute negatively to familial problems. It is still, therefore, useful to summarise some of the characteristics of children and their families where failing growth without organic cause has been observed. It is important to note that there is huge variation in the presentation of these cases, and no two such cases are exactly alike. Some children and families may show most of these characteristics, whereas others may show few of them. Nevertheless, identifying each family's unique problems is the first step in tailoring an intervention to their particular needs. Available evidence suggests that this is a much more successful strategy than adopting a 'one-size-fits-all' approach to helping children and their families (Iwaniec, 1995; Iwaniec & Sneddon, 2001a; Iwaniec & Sneddon, 2002).

## EATING BEHAVIOUR AND UNDER-NUTRITION IN NON-ORGANIC FAILURE TO THRIVE

Of course, not all children who have eating problems are associated with neurological abnormalities or illnesses affecting their appetite and digestive processes, and therefore contributing to reduced growth velocity. Some children live in homes of heightened stress and receive poor quality of care: their parents might know little about children's nutritional and nurturing needs; they might live in an environment which is impoverished economically; and emotionally they might have been born at a difficult time for the parents (e.g. loss of employment, illness, or tragic bereavement—which could have reduced the parental capacity of positive parenting). The list is extensive. These children are commonly termed as suffering from non-organic failure to thrive, and manifest severe components of malnutrition. Hanks and Hobbs (1993) and Hobbs and Hanks (1996) found, through their painstaking observations, recording, and analysis, that intake of food was simply inadequate in such cases, and they concluded that the main issue regarding nutrition was insufficient calories rather than protein or any other specific dietary deficiency. In other words, these children were not being fed adequate food rather than there being a problem with quality of the fare on offer. It has been observed that these children do not show distress because of hunger, do not ask for food, and do not cry because of being hungry. It has been suggested that their apathy and low levels of activity may be a reductive adaptation to their nutritionally inadequate environment (Waterlow, 1984). Malnutrition in itself will result not only in physical stunting, but also in social, cognitive, and behavioural changes. Children who suffer from malnutrition are more likely to be unresponsive, irritable, lethargic, and of lower cognitive abilities than children who are well fed (Oates *et al.*, 1985; Ricciuti, 1991; Reifsnider, 1995), as shown in Figure 3.2 (*see* page 37). The timing of the malnutrition may also mediate its effects: nearly all of a child's brain-growth and synoptic connections occur by age 2, and if protein and calories are not taken to support that growth it cannot occur (Frank & Zeisel, 1988). A further concern is that once stunting takes place and is established, these children may be unable or reluctant to increase their intake even if offered more food at a later stage (Iwaniec, 1991). It would appear that due to prolonged under-nourishment the body adapts to chronic starvation and levels itself for survival. This situation is analogous to being on a drip to sustain life, but it is hardly enough, as far as nutrition is concerned, to provide energy for normal functioning.

## COMBINED FAILURE TO THRIVE

For many years FTT was clearly dichotomised into two categories: organic and non-organic. Diagnosis was seen as either one category or the other: the

## Profile of Children with Non-Organic Failure to Thrive

Child falls below expected norms, usually 3rd percentile for the chronological age in weight, and often in height and head circumference.

### *Physical appearance*
Small, thin, wasted body, thin arms and legs, enlarged stomach, thin, wispy, dull, and falling-out hair, dark circles around the eyes

### *Characteristic features*

- frequent eating problems
- vomiting, heaving
- refusal to chew and swallow
- diarrhoea
- frequent colds and infections
- under-nutrition

### *Insecure, Avoidant, or Disoriented Attachment Style in Many Children*
Tense when in the mother's company; does not show interest and pleasure when with the mother or carer; does not show distress when mother leaves, or is too clingy. Poor relationship with siblings and peers.

### *Developmental retardation*

- motor development
- language development
- social development
- intellectual development
- emotional development
- cognitive development

### *Psychological description and behaviour*

- sadness, withdrawal, and detachment
- expressionless face
- general lethargy
- tearful
- frequent whining
- minimal or no smiling
- diminished vocalisations
- staring blankly at people or objects
- lack of cuddliness
- unresponsiveness
- passivity or over-activity

### *Problematic behaviour*

- whining and crying
- restlessness
- irritability
- anxiety
- resistance to socialisation
- poor sleeping pattern
- feeding and eating problems (in some)

**Figure 3.2** Profile of failure-to-thrive children
*Source:* Iwaniec, D. (1995) *The Emotionally Abused and Neglected Child.* Chichester: John Wiley & Sons Ltd

possibility of an interaction effect between physical factors and psychosocial environmental factors was generally dismissed. However, with the increase of research, and greater attention given by practitioners on a multi-disciplinary basis, it became clear that these divisions were unhelpful. It has been argued that FTT for organic reasons can be exacerbated by social and emotional influences (Iwaniec, 1995). Current opinion suggests that it is not particularly useful to separate them (Humphry, 1995). Infants who fail to thrive may have some organic features that contribute to, but do not explain, their lack of growth. All failure-to-thrive children have at least one organic problem in common, that of malnutrition (Bithoney & Newberger, 1987). This may help to explain why some children with an organic impairment such as cardiac disease or cleft lip may fail to thrive, whereas others, with virtually the same degree of organic impairment, will thrive (Woolston, 1984). The resilience and, conversely, the vulnerability of some children who fail to thrive have long attracted the interest of practitioners and researchers. It has been observed and evidenced that ill children who are well looked after and are nurtured emotionally will thrive in spite of an organic problem (MacMillan, 1984). Equally, those whose psychosocial environment is changed often begin to thrive, although their illness has not been resolved.

Many studies found that between 15% and 35% of infants fell between the organic and non-organic group (Woolston, 1984). Because of the clear overlap it is now accepted that clinically it does not make sense to have such a rigid distinction, but to view FTT as a syndrome of malnutrition associated with both. Malnutrition *per se* causes organically determined irritability, disturbances in biological functioning and temperament, and altered feeding interactions. Malnourished infants are characteristically lethargic and unresponsive. Bithoney and Newberger (1987) argued that behavioural manifestations are the result and not the cause of malnutrition, and often behavioural problems will improve as nutritional requirements are met. It could be argued, however, that the manner in which those nutritional requirements are provided is as important as the nutrition itself. A child who is force-fed more often than not develops, at best, food-avoidance behaviour, and at worst food phobias, which usually necessitates tube-feeding and consequently loss of instrumental eating skills. To illustrate this point let us look at Bob's case.

## Bob's Case

*The Consequences of Aversive Feeding Pattern*

Bob was born at full term weighing 3.3 kg (7 lb. 6 oz.). He was the second child in a well-to-do, skilled, working-class family. At the time of his birth Bob's brother was 4 years old attending nursery and his mother was working at home as an overlocker for the local hosiery factory. Bob proved to be far more difficult to care for than his older brother. He slept badly, waking several times at night, was restless during the day, and took a long time to feed. He required frequent attention as he cried, was sick, or needed changing more often as he had diarrhoea. The mother could not fulfil her obligations regarding the agreed amount of work she was supposed to do because of the constant interruptions, so became frustrated and, as time went on, more angry with Bob. Although she was not desperate for money as her husband had a good income as a plumber, she wanted to have her own income. When Bob cried she would put him upstairs so that she was not disrupted in her work. If Bob did not feed quickly (or was difficult to feed) she would either abandon feeding (assuming that he was not hungry), or hurry him—screaming if he refused to eat—or force-fed him. This type of feeding style persisted for almost six months, and Bob spent most of the time upstairs in his cot or in the pram in the garden.

When Bob was 10 months old he was admitted to hospital via Emergency as he completely stopped taking feeds from his mother, and became so dehydrated and wasted that the GP, fearing for the child's life, called an ambulance. Bob's weight was 'miles' below the lowest percentile: he presented as withdrawn, depressed, and unresponsive, and his well-being was causing concern. While in hospital he never cried, did not indicate hunger, was very passive, unresponsive, never smiled, and was not heard to vocalise. After a week he began to show interest in food, to eat more, and began to respond to nurses and other children. His weight began to increase in the second week. When discharged home, his weight was almost at the 2nd percentile, but dropped down within days to its previous level, while he regressed to his depressed, withdrawn, behavioural state. The mother, out of desperation and awareness that he could consume adequate amounts of food (as shown in hospital), began to push food on him and kept him sitting in the high chair for 2–3 hours until the food was eaten. If he refused, she force-fed him.

At the age of 14 months Bob again was admitted to hospital, but this time he did not take feeds from the nurses. As he was seriously wasted, nostril tube-feeding was introduced which was continued for two months. Although Bob's weight reached the 25th percentile and he became far more responsive, he lost the ability to eat normally by mouth. A specially designed treatment programme to reintroduce him to the intake of food orally had to be implemented to deal with this complicated problem (the treatment programmes in hospital are discussed in Chapter 12).

Needless to say, Bob's attachment to his mother was insecure, and their relationship was poor. The mother worried about his safety: she used to go to his bedroom at night to check whether he was breathing and was alive. She felt extremely guilty about Bob and confused about her feelings and reactions towards him. She blamed Bob for bringing so much stress and unhappiness to the family which, before his birth, was contented. As she said:

'If I had had help and assistance when he was tiny, if someone had told me what I should and should not do, we would have avoided all this, but now it is too late for both of us. The harm is done. I was successful with my first child and I thought I would be successful with this one as well. But he was so different.'

## WHY DOES COMBINED FAILURE TO THRIVE OCCUR?

Goldson (1987) suggested that this group of children with 'mixed' aetiology can be divided into roughly three categories:

## 1 *Children with subtle neuromotor problems*

These children may have difficulty eating because of oral-motor disturbances. For example, neurological abnormalities in oral-motor or gastro-intestinal functioning have been observed by Mathisen *et al.* (1989). Lewis (1982) suggested that oral-motor abnormalities can contribute to non-organic failure to thrive, including difficulties with sucking, chewing and swallowing, tongue-thrusting, involuntary biting of the tongue, spoon, or nipple, excessive drooling, and an intolerance of the textures of developmentally appropriate food. Contextual features (such as inappropriate positioning during feeding) may also compound these problems. Parents and professionals may then mistakenly interpret these eating difficulties as being food refusal on the child's part. This may result in force-feeding which may then lead to serious food refusal and subsequent failure to gain weight. As a result, the child frequently is irritable, resists food, and generally is behaviourally and physiologically disorganised. The parent may feel inadequate or negligent, and further problems in infant–parent interactions occur.

## 2 *Children with aversive eating experiences*

These children may have already had aversive experiences with regard to eating due to allergic reactions or gastro-oesophageal reflux. Other children may have required prolonged parenteral nutrition, and never have had the normal experience of eating. For example, many children who have experienced gavage- or tube-feeding may later experience difficulty in 'normal' feeding. Even though the organic problem which necessitated the tube-feeding has been cured, these difficulties in feeding may persist. One possible mechanism for this is that these children may have limited experience of how to feed normally. For example, Field *et al.* (1982) studied infants in whom gavage- or tube-feeding was used. They compared two groups of infants: one group was given a pacifier during all tube-feedings; and the other group received no pacifiers. Compared with the control group, the treatment-group required fewer tube-feedings, the average weight gain per day was greater, hospitalisation lasted fewer days, and the hospital costs were significantly lower. In addition, the treatment-group infants were easier to feed during later bottle-feedings (as demonstrated by the nurses having to engage in fewer stimulating behaviours such as bottle-jiggling and changes of feeding position). It may be possible that, as a result of their experiences with the pacifier associated with the intake of nutrition, these babies were predisposed to switch to 'normal' feeding practices than those who had no sucking experience. Children who have had organic problems may also react badly to the stress of their illness (and/or environment) and may refuse to eat even after the organic problem has been resolved.

## 3 *Children with significant psychiatric disorders*

These children may suffer from rumination or self-induced gagging resulting in vomiting; they may lose control over themselves and progress to a state of severe protein-energy malnutrition and profound growth failure.

## CHARACTERISTICS OF CHILDREN WHO FAIL TO THRIVE

As indicated in Figure 3.2, failure-to-thrive children present a worrying picture. They look thin, small, and sickly: developmentally, they (not all) are often impaired and can remain delayed for a considerable time, especially in cognitive and emotional areas. Feeding difficulties and mutually stressful interaction during feeding/eating time dominate the problem profile. The psychological expression of these children is marked by withdrawn, lethargic, and depressed behaviour, or by irritability, crying, negative moods, and poor sleeping. Because of the poor intake of food they tend to lack energy, seem to be detached, and do not show curiosity about the environment and people around them. Some appear to be hard work for the parents because of feeding difficulties and negative moods, whilst others do not generate interest in them because of low activity levels and a general lack of responsiveness to parental interaction. Many FTT children were found to be temperamentally either difficult or slow to warm up, which makes child-rearing for many parents challenging or excessively demanding (Pollitt & Eichler, 1976; Iwaniec, 1983). For example, a mother who is passive and quiet may find a child who is irritable, cries a lot, sleeps badly, and presents as difficult to feed, very hard to cope with and to enjoy. Such mothers get very anxious and then depressed, which, in turn, will reduce the time spent with the baby such as verbal interaction and perseverance at doing anything with the child. The length of time spent feeding the child will be substantially cut. Equally, a mother who is energetic, robust, sociable, and outgoing, may find a withdrawn, inactive, and passive baby rather unrewarding, as it will give little feedback. A mismatch between a mother's and baby's temperament in some cases can lead to problematic, incompatible interaction. When these characteristics happen to coincide with an illness or some other dysfunction, such as oral-motor or general eating or sleeping problems, the child is at risk of growth failure, much more so than the one who is more relaxed, has an easy disposition, is adaptable, predictable in biological functioning, and able to signal distress, hunger, and pleasure in a sharper and observable way. Iwaniec *et al.* (1985a) found, on the basis of extensive observations of mother–child interaction in their natural home setting, that ambivalence, confusion, anxiety, distress, disappointments, hopelessness, and sheer frustration were common features presented by the mothers in the index sample. It is of interest to point out that mothers in the first control group (organic failure-to-thrive children) showed far more tolerance and acceptance when faced with feeding problems. They attributed both poor growth and feeding/eating difficulties to the child's health and not to their management of the problems (which often was at fault). Not feeling responsible for the child's FTT enabled them to be more at ease and relaxed, which was in sharp contrast to the index-group mothers, whose reactions were influenced by anxiety, fear of being blamed for the child's poor growth and miserable appearance, feelings of failure as a parent, embarrassment, and anger.

Negatively and anxiety-based interactions can and do influence a baby's feeding behaviour and intake of food. A child who does not take feeds from the mother, but improves substantially when fed by another person in terms of intake of food and reactivity to being fed, indicates at best interactional problems and lack of synchrony in the mother–child dyad and, at worst, neglect and abuse. These interactional problems seem to be triggered by anxiety in response to the inability to feed the child, which either leads to giving up and feeling defeated, or feeling hurt, rejected, and angry. Regardless of parental reaction, the child's response is not to eat, either because of associated stress or some difficulties with the instrumental eating process. Repetition of unpleasant experiences for a considerable time can lead to serious consequences, as demonstrated in Bob's case. Feeding/eating problems will be discussed fully in Chapter 6.

## THE EFFECTS OF FAILURE TO THRIVE ON A CHILD'S GROWTH AND DEVELOPMENT

One can ask if it really matters whether a child is thin or chubby, short or tall, has a good appetite and eats everything that is put in front of him, or is fussy, choosy, picky, and not particularly interested in food. Does it really matter how heavy the baby is and at what speed it puts on weight and grows in centimetres? We know that it matters to parents, as their primary objective is to see the baby grow and develop healthily, vigorously, and happily. It matters, as the baby must be given a chance to have a good start in life. Without an adequate energy intake, generic potentials are not going to be facilitated, to emerge and take off at the right speed and capacity, such as intellectual development or physical growth. Being underfed means being lethargic, withdrawn, or irritable and showing disorganised behaviour and unpredictable rhythmicity in biological functioning. It also means confused, tense, and often reduced parental interaction and stimulation, which is so important for the child's developmental attainments. It matters to professionals who are charged with the duty and responsibility to promote child-health and welfare and to assist parents who are in difficulties.

Let us look at why it is so important to identify failure to thrive in children early in the baby's life and why it needs to be dealt with adequately and speedily.

### Developmental Impairments

Prolonged FTT in early childhood resulting in stunting of growth is strongly associated with an exceptionally poor outcome for intellectual abilities.

Studies on both sides of the Atlantic have shown that severe growth retardation in the first year of life affects later mental development and, the longer the duration of the growth retardation, the greater is the effect (Illingworth, 1983; Colombo *et al.*, 1992).

It has long been known that the crucial developments of the brain and cognitive processes take place during the first few years of a child's life (Wynne, 1996). Infants and small children experience a rapid increase in neuronal connections crucial to language, executive functioning, and other cognitive tasks (Dawson, 1992). Because of quick cerebral growth during this time of the child's life any significant under-nutrition that brings about failure to thrive carries a high risk of negative effects for intellectual development later in life (Iwaniec, 2000).

The serious consequences of failure to thrive or under-nutrition on developmental outcome have been well documented over the years (Oates *et al.*, 1985; Hutcheson *et al.*, 1997; Grantham-McGregor *et al.*, 2000). Children who fail to thrive are thought to be at risk of poor cognitive development indicated by IQ reduction of 10–20 points (Dowdney *et al.*, 1987; Kristiansson & Fällström, 1987; Skuse *et al.*, 1994b). The IQ can improve if the child is nourished properly and if the quality of care and stimulation improves as well (Grantham-McGregor *et al.*, 2000). Reif *et al.* (1995) found in their five-year follow-up study that children who failed to thrive in comparison with a matched control group showed significantly more learning difficulties and developmental delay. Interesting data were presented by Skuse *et al.* (1994a): they found that the timing, duration, and onset of growth failure seem to determine cognitive and psychomotor development in the second year of life. They stated that those babies who showed growth-faltering after six months of age showed better developmental attainments at the age of two years than those whose growth failure was evident soon after birth, in spite of having mothers who were exposed to greater social and psychological adversity. It could be that the level of interaction was more engaging, generating better stimulation regardless of its quality. Equally, good intake of calories while on liquids gave them a good start. As the interaction changes when solids are introduced (and more time, patience and better organisation are required when weaning starts), it is possible that those mothers found it harder to do that than simply making a bottle.

Spinner and Siegel (1987) found (using *Bayley's Mental Developmental Index and Psychomotor Index*) that both organic and non-organic failure-to-thrive groups (compared with hospitalised and non-hospitalised controls) were significantly lower in their development. Both FTT groups scored significantly less on the subscales of vocalisation and social responsiveness, language comprehension, and imitation.

Mackner and Starr (1997) compared three groups of children: those who were neglected; those who failed to thrive; and those with a combination of failure to thrive and neglect. They found that cognitive performance of the group of children who failed to thrive because of neglect was significantly lower than was the case among those from the FTT or neglect-only groups. This study indicates that FTT due to neglect is particularly harmful to intellectual development because of the serious lack of stimulation and attention in addition to under-nutrition. This is well illustrated by Kevin's study described below.

Children hospitalised for FTT with weight-for-ages below the 2nd percentile (as measured in the United Kingdom) or 5th percentile (as measured in the United States of America) perform poorly on measures of cognitive functioning as well. Their scores were below more than one standard deviation on the standardisation sample means on cognitive measures (Field, 1984). Studies of the long-term effects of poor growth and nutrition show similar results. Galler & Ramsey (1987) followed 129 malnourished Barbadian children from infancy into grade school and compared them with a carefully matched control group. They found mean IQ and achievement scores significantly lower in the previously malnourished children, and 60% of that group demonstrated attention deficit disorder (ADD). In a similar follow-up study of 48 pre-school children diagnosed earlier as failing to thrive, Drotar and Sturm (1992) found a deficit in behavioural organisation, ego control, ego resiliency, and problem-solving.

Failure to thrive in childhood has been shown to have long-lasting effects on cognitive and emotional development later in life. Oates and her associates (1985) found that teenagers who were hospitalised for FTT 16–18 years earlier scored significantly lower on a cognitive measure and higher on behavioural problems than a matched comparison group. Iwaniec's (2000) 20-year follow-up study on subjects who failed to thrive as children showed that 40% had poor school attainments, 18% were semi-illiterate in spite of finishing secondary school, 30% were statemented for special education, and 45% had difficulties in maintaining employment because of lack of competency and literacy.

## CASE STUDIES

To illustrate the complexity of failure-to-thrive aetiology a few cases are described. They will also be referred to in the treatment section to show what intervention and treatment methods and techniques have been used to resolve or alleviate problems.

### Penny's Case

Penny was admitted to hospital at 8 weeks of age because of failure to gain weight and parental worries about her well-being. At birth Penny's weight was 4.1 kg (9 lb. 1 oz.). She was a healthy, lively baby. Both parents were in their mid-thirties, both had PhDs in psychology, and had successful careers. They were delighted to have their first child. The baby was breast-fed and mother and baby were discharged home after five days. On discharge Penny's weight dropped slightly to just under 4 kg (8 lb. 3 oz.). At home she did not gain weight as expected. She still weighed 4 kg eight weeks after she was born despite the fact that she was fed for many hours, especially in the evenings. She slept badly during the night and required feeding every hour. Still she was not gaining weight so she was admitted to hospital with the diagnosis of non-organic FTT. Both parents were devastated as the diagnosis implied that they had failed to provide adequate and caring parenting.

While in hospital she was breast- and bottle-fed and gained 0.5 kg within three days. Mother and child were discharged home with various instructions on how to feed and manage Penny. However, the situation did not improve until a friend, whose baby was five weeks older, suggested that she would help the mother to re-establish breast feeding. She breast-fed Penny while Penny's mother breast-fed her friend's baby. After a week of swap-feeding Penny began to suck longer on the mother's breast and the mother became more relaxed and at ease while nursing Penny. She began to put on weight steadily and persistently.

The assessment revealed that the mother's sister (who was only 32 years of age) had died of cancer three days after Penny was born. The mother was devastated and even more disturbed by the fact that she could not attend the funeral, and that she could not see her sister before she died. As a result, she became very depressed.

## Causal Factors

1. Loss of the sister, shock, bereavement, feeling of guilt that she could not be there when she died. Depression.
2. Feeling depressed and unable to tune in to the child emotionally.
3. It is possible that the supply of milk was reduced by shock and depression.

### Rebecca's Case

Rebecca was born at 38 weeks' gestation with a normal delivery. She was a planned and very much-wanted child. Both parents were well educated with established professional careers and a high standard of living. Rebecca's birth-weight was on the 25th percentile. She was breast-fed. At three weeks she developed some colic and posseting, was sucking poorly, and had persistent vomiting. She stopped gaining weight at five months and fell below the 2nd percentile at seven months. In spite of medical advice on how to feed and interact with Rebecca, the vomiting and feeding difficulties continued. She had two admissions to hospital to deal with feeding difficulties. Her poor eating performance was seen by the medical staff as a result of a high maternal anxiety level and mismanagement of feeding. Resistance to eating was perceived by nursing staff as manipulative behaviour which needed firm handling. She began to be force-fed, which resulted in Rebecca's complete food-avoidance behaviour. She was panic-stricken when food appeared: she would scream, push food away, heave, vomit, and have diarrhoea. The feeding interaction was highly aversive, resulting in complete food refusal.

This resistance to eating confirmed the parents' fears that there was something physically wrong with the child, and they decided to seek private medical help.

Further absorptive studies were carried out and severe neuromuscular incoordination of the oesophagus was demonstrated. Surgery was carried out successfully, and it was then hoped that Rebecca would improve psychologically as the memory of the early discomfort when eating and being force-fed faded, but unfortunately this was not the case.

After being told that there was no longer anything wrong with Rebecca, the parents began to be more firm with her, expecting a quick improvement in eating behaviour, with subsequent weight gain. She refused to take food and her physical appearance deteriorated, although her psychosocial development was within norms. Feeding-time became a major battle, and feeding interaction fluctuated between an angry, anxious, and, at times, forceful feeding style, to begging the child to eat, encouraging, bribing, giving up, running after her with the spoon, or allowing Rebecca to do anything she wanted in order to get some food into her.

As a result of faulty interaction and desperation to feed Rebecca she became extremely manipulative and oppositional as she learnt how to get what she wanted. Since there was no improvement in weight-gain and the intake of food was insufficient for the child's age (in spite of determined efforts to feed her), the mother became totally demoralised and depressed. She began to believe very strongly that she was inadequate as a carer, and that she could not do anything right: her self-esteem was at rock bottom. The situation became so serious that the father asked for urgent help for his wife and daughter after the wife left the house one night and was found wandering along the streets confused and very depressed.

To ease the situation at home, Rebecca attended nursery, where the feeding programme was introduced and then extended at home. Rebecca reached the 25th percentile within seven months and her general behaviour became less manipulative and more compliant as a result of treatment (*see* Chapter 12 for discussion on treatment).

## Causal and Maintaining Factors

1. Inadequate intake of food.
2. Feeding difficulties due to severe neuromuscular incoordination of the oesophagus.
3. Deterioration due to the force-feeding in the hospital.
4. Maternal anxiety, depression, and reinforcement of manipulative behaviour.

### Kevin's Case

Kevin, a third child of a single mother, was born at full term without any complications, weighing 3 kg (6 lb. 6 oz.). The mother abandoned the child three days after birth, leaving a note saying that she wanted him to be adopted. Kevin was a result of her one-night stand with someone she did not like, and it happened under the influence of alcohol. She was also worried that her parents would not approve of her having yet another child. She already had two boys, aged 3 and 4 years respectively, and received substantial help from her parents with them.

She managed to hide her pregnancy successfully. However, the grandparents were notified of what happened and they insisted that Kevin's mother keep him and care for him with their assistance.

Kevin's weight gain was causing concern from very early on, as was his very withdrawn behaviour and lack of developmental progress. His weight was well below the 2nd percentile and getting lower each time he was seen by the health visitor or in the health centre. Kevin was admitted to hospital on several occasions because of poor growth, and typically put on weight and became more responsive while there, but rapidly lost weight on returning home.

The quality of care at home, both physical and emotional, was extremely poor. He was fed when the mother happened to remember to feed him, as he almost never indicated hunger. When he was given a bottle it was usually propped up in the pram, and he was seldom picked up to be fed or nursed. On many occasions his older brothers were asked to feed him. Kevin was not attended to when he was distressed, and received no attention whatsoever. After a while he was not heard crying. He spent most of the time lying in the pram and, when older, strapped in the buggy. He was often tormented by his siblings and there was nobody to protect him. By the age of two Kevin could hardly walk, had no recognisable words, and his social behaviour was extremely poor. He looked very small, thin, and unhealthy. Kevin's general growth and development were globally impaired, and his psychological expression was that of a severely rejected and neglected child who required urgent attention and a firm decision regarding his future.

Kevin was received into care on a *Place of Safety Order* and placed in a foster-home with a view to adoption. Although his weight reached the 50th percentile within a few months and he grew well in height, approaching the 50th percentile as well, his psychomotor development was seriously impaired. He also showed (at the point of being placed in the foster-home) very worrying emotional disturbances such as hiding his face and screaming if anybody walked into his room when he was in bed, being panic-stricken when put in the bath, and staring into space or sitting quietly with his head down. He seemed totally detached from his surroundings. He never smiled or showed interest or curiosity about anything. It took well over a year before he became more alert, responsive, and showed pleasure and interest in toys and in people's company. His physical failure to thrive was resolved relatively quickly after being rescued from an abusive home, but his psychosocial failure to thrive was very much in evidence and was likely to continue for years to come. Given that he was an easy child to look after, had a placid temperament, and was physically attractive, he was lucky to be adopted by people who would help him further to overcome his earlier deprivation. He needed help with cognitive and emotional development, which were badly affected by under-nutrition and lack of emotional care and attention. His mother failed to show any insight or understanding about her parenting failures, and perceived Kevin as 'a bit slow but otherwise fine'.

## Causal and Maintaining Factors

1. Under-nutrition.
2. Rejection and neglect.
3. Emotional abuse.
4. Persistent starvation.

## Rose's Case

Rose was a 16-month-old baby who had just started to walk. She looked very skinny and thin. She appeared to be oblivious to the things going on around her, her face was expressionless, and her eyes were fixed on the big teddy-bear twice her size which stayed in the corner of the room. There were two older children in the family, one already at school, and the middle girl was 4 years of age.

Rose's mother developed post-natal depression after she was born and found caring and interacting with her children very difficult. She lacked energy and emotional drive to do anything. The mother seemed to resemble Rose: she was thin, sad, and detached. Due to the mother's depression, Rose was very seldom spoken to, played with, or picked up. As a rule she was fed lying in the pram or in the cot, and if she refused to feed or struggled while being fed, the bottle was propped up for Rose to feed herself when she wanted.

Rose failed to thrive almost from birth, although this was not spotted until she was almost 5 months old because her mother did not take her to the baby clinic at the required times. As the quality of parenting with her other children (when they were babies) was very good, there was no concern about Rose's growth and development. The health visitor thought that things would get better once the mother's health improved. However, they did not improve, and the mother had to be hospitalised for depression. Rose went to stay with her grandparents for eight months, and within that time she recovered physically and emotionally. Her weight reached the required level for her age, she accelerated developmentally, and became a lively and responsive child. She ate well after initial reluctance to try different things.

It was apparent that Rose failed to thrive because her mother was unable to provide the care, attention, and stimulation that she needed. There was a severe lack of interaction of any kind, apart from absolute essentials. Her poor physical growth resulted from inadequate calorific provision, which lasted a long time. Lack of interaction and stimulation brought about delayed psychomotor development and striking withdrawal and sadness.

## Causal and Maintaining Factors

1. Inadequate nutrition.
2. Lack of stimulation.
3. Emotional and physical neglect.
4. Maternal depression.

## Previn's Case

Previn, a first child in the family, was born at full term weighing 9 lb. 4 oz. (4.25 kg) after a long labour and difficult delivery. Both parents decided to bottle-feed Previn as they felt it would be easier to monitor his intake of milk and that the mother would get into shape more quickly and easily, so breast-feeding was not even considered.

Previn began to lose weight soon after being discharged from the hospital. At 6 weeks his weight was 1 lb. 2 oz. lower than at birth. The health visitor became quite concerned when Previn's weight dropped to the 2nd percentile at 2½ months and he progressively became more lethargic and irritable. The health visitor discovered that Previn was not given enough milk for his size and age and that the formula was watered down to reduce the fatness of the milk so he would not become an obese baby. Both parents stated that they did not like fat children and fat people generally, and that Previn would be healthier if he was leaner and they wanted to build up a culture of body trimness from the start of their son's life. The mother said that she was told while attending neo-natal clinic that parents should not overfeed their babies and that food given should be healthy and not excessive. She interpreted the neo-natal clinic advice according to her attitudes towards food.

It was observed that the intake of food was very much controlled by both parents and that they were preoccupied to the point of obsession with their own weight-intake of food, the type of food they ate, and their appearance. The mother spent about three hours a day in the fitness centre, while Previn was looked after by an elderly man living in the neighbourhood. The parents became very concerned when they were told about the negative consequences of under-nutrition, but were reluctant to accept help in terms of nutritional consultation for themselves. Previn's weight gradually climbed up to the 25th percentile within 2½ months, with the health visitors closely monitoring his progress and parental behaviour.

## Causal Factors

1. Inadequate provision of food, both in quantity and quality.
2. Previn was starved as the parents did not like big/fat babies and felt it was good for his health.
3. Parental attitudes to food and body image were extreme.

## SUMMARY

This chapter discussed problems in defining FTT and lack of a unified world-wide definition, which makes prevalence calculation difficult and probably inaccurate. The issues of classifying FTT in three categories—organic, non-organic, and combined—were elaborated upon. It was argued that separating failure-to-thrive cases is unhelpful as components of organic and non-organic FTT may be involved in one case. Equally, it was argued that each case must be assessed individually and diagnosis needs to be made on rigorous analysis to avoid misinterpretation of presenting problems. Characteristics of failure-to-thrive children were outlined and the consequences of the syndrome were briefly discussed. Case studies illustrating different routes leading to FTT were presented.

# 4

# PSYCHOSOCIAL SHORT STATURE: EMOTIONAL STUNTING OF GROWTH

*Better is a dinner of herbs where love is, than a stalled ox and hatred therewith.*
The Holy Bible: *Proverbs*, **xv**, 17

## INTRODUCTION

Children who are described as having psychosocial short stature are those who are exceptionally short and remain stunted for a considerable time, although there may be no obvious organic reasons for this. They are usually diagnosed after two years of age. These children are stunted, with a near normal weight-for-height. Their appearance marks them out as different, their body-build is disproportionate (i.e. with quite short legs and enlarged stomach). Often there is microcephaly, and bone-age is normally delayed. Gohlke *et al.* (1998) found that in children they studied the bone-age was delayed on average by 1.9 years, and severe delay in bone maturation of more than three years was observed in 13% of their patients.

This type of failure to thrive acquired various labels over the years; e.g. it was named 'deprivation-dwarfism' by Silver and Finkelstein (1967), 'psychosocial short stature' by Spinner and Siegel (1987). These terms describe a syndrome of physical abnormalities characterised by extreme short stature, voracious appetite and bizarre eating patterns, serious developmental delays, disturbed behaviour, insecure attachment, and mutually antagonistic mother–child relationship (Skuse *et al.*, 1994; Iwaniec, 1995). This disorder has been known for many years and extensively studied. Some investigators hypothesise the existence of a physiological pathway whereby emotional deprivation affects the neuro-endocrine system regulating growth. Some researchers (Talbot *et al.*, 1947; Patton & Gardner, 1962; Powell *et al.*, 1967; Apley *et al.*, 1971; Green *et al.*, 1987; Blizzard & Bulatovic, 1993) favoured a theory of emotional influence on growth, with secondary hormonal insufficiencies as the main cause of psychosocial short stature.

Whitten (1976), on the other hand, concluded that such children were simply starved, and therefore did not grow.

In recent years there has been a considerable debate about whether psychosocial short stature is the extension of earlier failure to thrive and whether it is in any way qualitatively different as the child gets older and more mobile. The point of separation between FTT and psychosocial short stature differs amongst researchers and clinicians; some have set an age limit arbitrarily; others have used clinical presentation and findings, including various hormonal studies to differentiate one from the other. The range for the point of separation has been between 18 months and 4 years.

To start with, this dichotomy occurred, according to MacMillan (1984), because children under the age of 2 are difficult to measure in length, but relatively easy to measure if one looks at weight. A child under the age of 2 is more likely to be noticed and recognised as being abnormal if it is underweight, as opposed to only being of short stature.

Growth failure, as a rule, begins in infancy during the first few months of a child's life, but stunting of growth can occur much later, even at 6 or 8 years of age. All psychosocial short-stature children are severely emotionally abused, rejected, and unloved. The late commencement of growth failure is also often associated with sexual abuse and acute emotional trauma.

It has been recognised that in virtually all cases the relationship between the child and the primary care-giver (which is usually the mother) is seriously disturbed. Additionally, these children are often physically abused and emotionally maltreated and come into a category of suffering significant harm. How bad the relationship can get between mother and child in cases of psychosocial short stature can be illustrated by the following observations.

An Israeli friend of the author, while on a working trip to the Child Treatment Research Unit, accompanied the present writer on a first home visit. The child was referred by the paediatrician because of severe growth failure which lasted for nearly 2½ years. He was hospitalised four times, improved while in hospital, but rapidly lost weight when discharged home. Nothing was done to resolve this problem in spite of the mother's open hostility and negative attitudes towards the child.

During the home visit the author's colleague became so distressed watching the mother–child interaction, the mother's response to the child, and the child's fear and apprehension when she approached him, that she left the house unable to bear the child's distress any longer. The last straw for the visitor was when the mother was asked to hold Mark's hand and to sit him on her lap. She held his hand at arm's length but said she could not sit him on her lap as it would be unpleasant for her to do so. 'He will only become stiff and rigid, so why bother', she said, and promptly told him off for staring at her.

The visitor subsequently recorded her impressions:

> I do not remember seeing a more distressing picture in my long years of working with children and families, and also being unable to cope with it emotionally and professionally. What was worse was that the child was one of twins. In a million years I would never have guessed. He was half the size in weight and three-quarters in height in comparison with his brother. He hardly reached his brother's shoulder. It was not only their size that stood out but their emotional presentation and interaction with their mother which was strikingly different. Mark looked pale with dark shadows under his eyes. His thin face showed sadness, depression, withdrawal, and lack of connection with any member of the family. He sat staring into space, motionless. His brother, on the other hand, was bouncy, rosy-cheeked, smiling, and laughing and completely at ease in his mother's company. He asked questions, interrupting our discussion quite frequently, asking to be given different things, such as crisps. The mother responded to him patiently and appropriately.
>
> During the 1½ hours she never once looked in Mark's direction spontaneously or asked him whether he wanted crisps as well. He did not get any. He never moved from where he was sitting until he was told to do so. He responded automatically. When he looked at her she asked him not to stare at her; when he started to cry she screamed at him and threatened to send him to the bedroom. When she was told that child-protection services might need to be contacted she said we could take him with us now as he brings her nothing but misery and disappointments. She said that she told the doctor in hospital about her difficulties with him, but he said that he would grow out of it.

It is believed that prolonged and severe emotional abuse and rejection produce a high and continuous level of stress in children which affects the rate of linear growth and functioning of the secretion of growth hormones. In spite of eating a huge amount of food (if they have the opportunity) they remain extremely small for their age. Although the precise mechanism of growth-hormone arrest is not clear, it can be assumed that emotional factors play an important role. Once a child is removed from an abusive environment its growth and development quickly accelerate, but when returned to it a marked deterioration becomes evident and behaviour worsens. Observations were made that when such children were in hospital their endocrine function normalised and growth hormones were secreted again, but the growth hormones ceased to function when these children returned to emotionally insulting homes (Spinner & Siegel, 1987; Skuse et al., 1996). Interestingly, it is not just a simple matter of merely replacing the growth hormone. Various investigative studies have shown that even if these children are treated with replacement therapy there is no increase in growth or resolution of other endocrine abnormalities until the child is removed from the stressful and abusive environment (Goldson, 1987). Indeed, some researchers have suggested that diagnoses of psychosocial short stature can only be made on the basis of removal from the stressful environment and subsequent increase in growth velocity.

Emotional upheaval in these children tends to demonstrate itself in bizarre eating patterns, disturbed toileting which goes far beyond enuresis or encopresis, destructiveness, aggressive defiance, non-compliance, and

*Growth retardation*
Child's height and weight and
head circumference below
expected norms

*Physical appearance*
Small, thin, enlarged stomach
Disproportionate body-build

*Characteristic features*
(a) bizarre eating behaviour,
    excessive eating, an obsessive
    preoccupation with food,
    hoarding food, begging food
    from strangers, eating non-food
    items, searching for food during
    night, and scavenging food
    from waste-bins, voracious
    eating, gorging and vomiting

(b) some eat very little—starved
    appearance, characterised by
    poor appetite, chronic
    nutritional deficiencies

(c) attachment disorder, mutually
    antagonistic relationship, active
    rejection, hostile or extremely
    poor mother–child interaction
    and relationship, addressing
    mother as 'Miss', 'Lady'
    (elective mutism), lack of proper
    stranger anxiety, insecure or
    disoriented avoidant
    attachment style

*School attainments*
IQ below average, poor learning
performance, difficulty in
concentrating, poor relationships
with peers, disliked by peers and
teachers, disruptive, manipulative

*Developmental retardation*
Language
Social
Motor
Intellectual
Cognitive
Emotional
Toilet-training

*Behaviour*
Bizarre eating pattern
(over-eating), soiling, wetting,
smearing, defiance, demanding,
destructiveness, whining,
fire-setting, attention-seeking,
screaming, aggression, short
attention span, poor sleeping,
head-banging, rocking,
scratching, cutting

*Psychological description*
Withdrawal, expressionless face,
detachment, depression, sadness,
minimal or no smiling,
diminished vocalisation, refusal to
speak to mother, staring blankly
at people or objects,
unresponsiveness, lack of
cuddliness, lack of confidence,
low self-esteem, eager to be
helpful and useful, craving for
attention and affection,
over-reaction when given praise
or attention, stubbornness

**Figure 4.1** Profile of psychosocial short stature: emotional stunting of growth
*Source:* Iwaniec, D. (1995) *The Emotionally Abused and Neglected Child.* Chichester:
John Wiley & Sons Ltd

self-harming behaviour. Relationships of such children with parents or carers are marked by hostility and active rejection: because these children are unloved and unwanted, and because they are reared in an emotional vacuum, their cognitive, language, emotional, and social development is seriously retarded. When at school they are unable to concentrate and apply themselves to any work for longer than a few minutes. They tend to be disruptive and attention-seeking. Their school attainments, therefore, are very poor. Additionally, they are disliked by peers and as a consequence are isolated in the classroom, playground, and in the community.

In such cases serious attachment disorders are evident and the relationships are mutually antagonistic. If the child is unloved s/he will eventually become unloving, not only to people who hurt him or her but also to anybody who potentially presents a threat and a challenge.

Problem profile of psychosocial short-stature children is shown in Figure 4.1.

## SYMPTOMS OF PSYCHOSOCIAL DWARFISM

Skuse *et al.* (1994) suggest that the symptoms can be considered under four main headings.

### 1. Disorders of biological rhythms

Sleep is disrupted, with frequent waking and wandering around the house in search of food. Appetite is disturbed, with an apparent inability to achieve satiation, and normal hunger rhythms are lost. This may result in stealing food and gorging, which is a characteristic of these cases. The growth-hormone releases are diminished, as is pulse-amplitude, thus the cumulated 24-hour circulating levels of the hormone are severely curtailed.

### 2. Disorders of self-regulation

Manifests itself in deviant patterns of defecation, urination, and attention; this behaviour sometimes becomes aggressive and hostile, such as the deliberate urination over others' possessions.

### 3. Disorders of mood

Show themselves in depression and low self-esteem.

### 4. Disorders of social relationships

The quality of relationships is almost always poor with everybody. The children are disliked by parents, siblings, peers, and schoolteachers.

## Hyperphagic and Anorexic Children

Children of short stature may be divided into two groups: hyperphagic and anorexic.

Hyperphagic children are those who present excessive and bizarre eating behaviour such as: having a high hunger drive; preoccupation with food and eating; drinking excessively, even from toilet-bowls or puddles in the street; hoarding food; searching for food during the night; eating non-food items; scavenging food from waste-bins; eating other people's left-overs; eating voraciously, and gorging. Additionally, they are poor sleepers, present disturbed toileting behaviour (smearing faeces over their belongings and urinating in inappropriate places, e.g. over the bed or in the corners of the room), are destructive, and have short attention spans, and have poor social relationships in most cases.

Anorexic children are very poor eaters, have little appetite, show faddiness, and refuse to eat. When pressed to eat they heave, store food in their mouths, and chew and swallow with difficulty. They tend to be anxious, apprehensive, withdrawn, passive, and unable to stand up for themselves. Relationships with other family members are poor and marked by fear and apprehension. While at school they tend to be excessively quiet and uninvolved, unable to concentrate, and are often bullied by other children.

### *Hyperphagic Case Illustration*

#### *Chris's Case*

Chris was adopted by a middle-class, childless couple when he was 2 years old. Prior to adoption he spent one and a half years in two different foster-homes. He was an attractive boy, developmentally within the lower average, active and curious. Both parents were pleased in securing adoption and having a child they longed to have. When Chris was 4 years old the mother became unexpectedly pregnant, which surprised the couple as they were told they could not have any children. She gave birth to a girl and a year later to a boy.

Since the birth of the first child attention was switched from Chris and their interaction became limited to care and control, and only occasionally was he played with. After the birth of the second child the relationship worsened sharply, not only between the mother and Chris, but also with the father. The more distant and preoccupied they became with the babies the more attention-seeking, disruptive, and demanding Chris became. They increasingly found him hard work, unrewarding, and difficult to enjoy. At the same time they invested energy and affection in their younger children, leaving little time and attention for Chris. Most of the little activities and treats from their early life together were gradually eliminated. He could not come to the parents' bed anymore, his father would not play football with him in the garden or the park, he was not read a story at night, but above all he was not cuddled and was not given attention, praise, and encouragement.

He became a very lonely and confused child. His weight dropped from the 75th to 2nd percentile within a few months and he became stunted in height. He started wandering around the house at night, making bizarre animal noises and searching for food. On many occasions he would take packets of cereals, jars of jam, and bread and hide them under his bed or behind the books on the shelves. His eating behaviour changed dramatically from being fussy and taking a rather long time to eat to becoming greedy, eating fast, and gulping food without chewing. He consumed large amounts and was constantly asking for more. His hunger drive became so excessive that he began to beg people for food in the neighbourhood and at school. Because of his wasted appearance and increasingly disturbed behaviour, the school became concerned about Chris. He started eating left-overs in the school canteen, took other children's food from their bags, and became extremely attention-seeking and disruptive in the classroom. His school-work deteriorated and he was unable to concentrate.

Chris, who was fully toilet-trained day and night by the age of three years, started wetting the bed and soiling three to four times a week. He would sit on the settee at home or at the table in school urinating, leaving puddles on the floor. Soiling became very acute and unmanageable, the faeces would go through his trousers, and his socks and even shoe-laces were soiled.

As Chris's behaviour worsened, the parents became more rejective, hostile, and uncompromising. They felt embarrassed and, as they said, they were let down by Chris and requested to have a break from him, so that 'he gets the necessary treatment for his incontinence and disturbed behaviour'. They stated that they did not love him, but attributed this to Chris's changed behaviour, not theirs. However, they stated that they had a moral obligation to care for him.

Chris was admitted to hospital for observation and testing, although nobody believed that there was anything wrong with him. What he needed was attention, care, affection, and acceptance. Chris was in hospital for three weeks. Within that time he put on weight (over a stone), he never soiled or wet himself, and his eating behaviour improved within a week. He interacted well with nurses, but in a possessive and attention-seeking way. He was jealous when they played or attended to other children, and he tended to be aggressive towards these children, but only when the nurses or doctors interacted with them and not with him.

Chris returned home and within days his disturbed behaviour returned as well. In three weeks he lost 5.5 kg (12 lb. 2 oz.). Parental rejection was so strong and Chris's pain and disturbance so high that the only solution available was to place him in a different home, to give him another chance. Chris was fostered out but never recovered from the emotional rejection. He was killed while joy-riding when he was 16 years old.

## Anorexic Case Illustration

### Gavin's Case

Gavin was diagnosed as having *peloric stenosis* at the age of 2 months, and was operated on two weeks later. He recovered well physically, but his eating behaviour did not improve. He refused to suck, cried while being fed, stretched out, turned his head away from the bottle, vomited frequently, and had diarrhoea. The mother, assuming that there was no longer anything wrong with Gavin, became more persistent and forceful at feeding him, and, not being successful, she became more frustrated and angry. The feeding interactions fluctuated between forceful feeding, screaming, shouting, and even shaking him, to abandoning feeding as soon as he refused to take feeds. Gavin's weight at birth at the 25th percentile dropped to well under the 2nd percentile and was dipping further down as time went on. He remained under the 2nd percentile for five years. There was a slight improvement when solids were introduced but it did not last long. The relationship between the mother and Gavin was getting more problematic, causing concern for the father and the health visitor involved with the family. There were days when he spent most of the time in the cot upstairs, away from everybody, and he was never picked up by the mother unless it was absolutely necessary. Gavin–mother attachment was weak, showing characteristics of anxious avoidant pattern, and the mother's emotional bond to Gavin was, at best, ambivalent and getting more hostile as time went on.

Within two years of his life he was admitted to hospital five times for failure to thrive, but more accurately for failure to accept food from his mother. He would take feeds from his father, from the health visitor, from the next-door neighbour, and from his 5-year-old brother, but not from his mother. Gavin would cry or scream at the sight of his mother and at the sight of food she prepared for him. On two occasions he was admitted to hospital via Emergency as he became so dehydrated that the health visitor feared for his life. On both occasions he had had hardly any food for three days as his father was away on business. The mother became very depressed and completely switched off from Gavin, leaving him to be cared for by his little brother. The marital relationship, which was problematic for a considerable time, deteriorated further as the father and his family blamed Gavin's mother for his poor growth and health. As Gavin looked very much like his father he was a constant reminder to the mother of her now much-hated husband, so she blamed Gavin for causing so much unhappiness and hurt for her.

Each time Gavin was in hospital his weight increased rapidly and he became more alert and responsive. He started to smile and even initiated interaction— behaviour not seen at home. He ate reasonably well, though eating-time was longer than average. On returning home his appetite quickly vanished, and he became withdrawn, unresponsive, and emotionally flat. He would lie in bed motionless for hours, not sleeping, staring into space. His movements were slow, showing lack of energy and enthusiasm. His mood was typical of a depressed child, unloved and treated in a frightening way by his mother, or being ignored and isolated.

Gavin's weight and height remained under the 2nd percentile for five years and never crossed the 9th percentile until he went to live with his father. Chronic long-lasting under-nutrition, depressed appetite, and lack of interest in food were exacerbated in Gavin's case by permanent stress and emotional abuse. When Gavin was 5 years old his parents separated and he went to live with the father and his partner. It took several months for Gavin to settle and to feel reasonably at ease. With extensive help provided for Gavin from his step-mother, father, and the therapist, he began to function and behave in a more alert way, and his growth accelerated beyond recognition. At 6 years and 2 months he reached the 50th percentile in height and above the 25th percentile in weight.

Gavin's school adaptation and performance were rather poor. He found it difficult to concentrate and to learn. He was statemented for special education. His cognitive development was retarded, as was his emotional and social behaviour. After two years he was moved to the main school-stream on his father's insistence, but little progress was made, and he remained at the bottom of the class. He left school without any qualification, a poor ability to read and write, and found it difficult to maintain any employment.

## GROWTH-HORMONE DEFICIENCIES

Gohlke *et al.* (1998), on the basis of their study, note that some children with psychosocial short stature who have been treated with growth-hormone do show an adequate initial response, but this is not maintained, and consequently the child does not grow at the required rate for a child with growth-hormone deficiency. They recommended that psychosocial short stature should be considered in every patient that presents 'idiopathic' growth-hormone deficiency or ineffectiveness of growth-hormone treatment with isolated or multiple pituitary hormone deficiencies. Symptoms such as abnormal eating habits, hyperphagia, global developmental delay, disturbed behaviour, enuresis and encopresis should be investigated as well as the possibility of sexual and physical abuse.

It was suggested that the most important indicator is excessive over-eating (hyperphagia) and this sign accurately predicts the reversibility of growth-hormone insufficiency. Gohlke *et al.* (1998) state that failure to respond to growth-hormone treatment in a child with growth-hormone deficiency may be another presenting sign of psychosocial short stature. These researchers recommended that all children suspected of having growth-hormone deficiency should have a detailed history taken for hyperphagia, polydipsia, hoarding food, and scavenging food, as these are characteristic symptoms that predict reversibility of growth-hormone deficiency and subsequent catch-up growth. A long time ago MacCarthy and Booth (1970) suggested that an identifying characteristic of psychosocial short stature was the rapid reversal of all abnormal physical signs, with growth acceleration when the child was removed from the adverse setting and given no treatment other than normal hospital care.

These children are clearly at risk of gross significant harm on a short- and long-term basis, and require urgent attention to prevent escalation of further harm. The 20-year follow-up study reported by Iwaniec (2000) found that those individuals classified as of psychosocial short stature who remained at home had very poor outcomes on a personal, education, employment, and emotional level, while those who were removed from an abusive situation did much better in every aspect of life.

Gohlke *et al.* (1998) reported that many health and social services professionals are reluctant to take any action concerning the removal of a child from home as damaging to the child. This is worrying since the very fact that they remain in the emotionally insulting environment is the most damaging developmentally, especially affecting emotional and cognitive areas. Additionally, being under continuous stress and emotional pain affects children's emotional and cognitive development, and leads to serious behavioural problems. The evidence of harm is very clear, and alarm-bells are ringing quite loudly to prompt the taking of appropriate action.

## MANIFESTATION OF DISTURBED BEHAVIOUR

Short-stature children present very disturbed behaviour in several areas which (when identified) should guide the making of appropriate diagnosis and intervention strategies. Some of the most easily observable behaviours are described below.

### Bizarre Eating

Some of the eating behaviour was already described in the previous pages of this chapter, but it is worthwhile to expand further on some character-istic features and to give a few brief examples from clinical practice and research.

Psychosocial short-stature children, primarily those falling into the over-eating group (hyperphagic), show an obsessive preoccupation with food. This tends to emerge at an older toddler stage (although an early feeding history is that of under-eating, typically characteristic for many failure-to-thrive chil-dren). As a rule most parents, when asked at what point over-eating and an excessive interest in food started, would say when a child became comfort-able, mobile, and more independent. Preoccupation with food is manifested not only by eating more than expected, but by constantly talking about food, asking for food, and making enquiries as to what and when they are going to eat. The first thing a little boy of four would ask (as soon as he came to the nursery) was, 'What's for lunch?'. He would follow the nursery nurse, repeating the question until she told him, and then he would engage in play activities. The same pattern of behaviour is often observed and described by the nurses in the hospitals, especially during the first few days. The impres-sion is that these children fear that food may be withdrawn from them, they may be denied food, so they seek reassurance that they will be fed.

Distorted behaviour around food is expressed by hoarding food in most peculiar places. A girl of seven years used to make little parcels with pretty ribbon bows and neatly store them on the shelves where her toys and books were kept. The parcels contained bread, sausages, chips, and even mashed potatoes. Food is often hidden under the bed, under pillows, in cupboards, under furniture, and in various drawers.

Begging food from strangers is quite common in severe cases: some children may stop a complete stranger on the street, in the park, or by the house gate, and ask for biscuits, fruit, or drinks, saying that he or she is hungry. This is particularly difficult for the parents to cope with, as they feel they may be judged as neglectful or starving the child. Such parents tend to get very angry, which often leads to punishing the child by withdrawing the next meal to teach a lesson.

Bizarre eating is demonstrated by eating non-food items, such as cotton wool, soil, pieces of paper, cat or dog food from the bowls standing on the floor (one boy ate all the fabric from the inside of his continental quilt), drinking from the toilet bowls, from puddles in the street, or the water coming out from the drain pipes. Getting up at night in search of food is very common, and such children tend to go through cupboards, fridges, and pantries, and will eat whatever they can find, in enormous quantities. Nigel, who was 5 years old, used to get up at three or four o'clock in the morning, and often ate five to six cans of baked beans, with a whole loaf of sliced bread and a packet of margarine or pot of jam, and drank two litres of milk. Once the parents became aware of his nocturnal eating habits they closed the doors or cupboards or put the food away out of the child's reach. Seldom do those strategies work, as the child will hoard food during the day and eat it at night. Many of these children tend to scavenge food from rubbish-bins both at home and in public places. Nursery, hospital, and school staff have reported that they take food from other children's plates or eat left-overs. Teachers reported that these children steal food, from other children's lunch-boxes, and parents often complain that they steal food, leaving other members of the family with nothing to eat for breakfast. These children tend to eat quickly and voraciously, hardly chewing the food (to the point of gorging and vomiting). It is not uncommon to find that these children do not eat with the rest of the family: instead they might be given food sitting on the floor away from the table, excluded from normal family interaction at meal-times. This in itself is rejective and dismissive parental behaviour which is questionable and requires attention.

## Disturbed Toileting

The majority of psychosocial short-stature children show very disturbed toileting behaviour which manifests itself in urinating all over the bed, furniture, personal belongings, or defecating into pants, corners of the room, or under the table, as well as smearing faeces on walls, toys, and other people's belongings. Tipping the contents from the potty all over the room is not unusual, and hiding dirty pants in the most unlikely places are common features among these children. This type of behaviour indicates a high level of emotional turmoil and distress, and appears to be aggressive retaliation directed at the primary care-givers to start with, and then extending itself to other people, like teachers. This kind of behaviour is very offensive to everybody, and it can lead to peer rejection if it occurs at school. Such children are perceived by school-mates as disgusting and dirty. Because of the smell they usually become isolated in the classroom (as nobody wants to sit next to them), and in the playground as they are not considered rewarding to play with; thus opportunities to make friends and to engage in social activities, such as swimming and school trips, are eliminated. They react to peer rejection either by being aggressive and disruptive or by being withdrawn, detached, and isolated. They tend to play on their own away from other children or remain in the classroom looking very distressed and depressed. There are times when teachers have to send them away from the classroom or send them home because of severe soiling and other children's refusal to be near them.

At home these children are often punished for soiling and wetting in a cruel way, e.g. forcing a child into a bath of cold water to teach it a lesson, making a child wear badly soiled clothes the next day, or not changing wet or soiled bedding. They are called nasty names, are deprived of treats, and more often than not are hit, slapped, and pushed away. At school they are bullied both physically and verbally.

## Destructiveness

Most of these children suffer from extremely low self-esteem and depression. They feel that they are unworthy to have anything, that they are bad and therefore do not deserve to have anything belonging to them. Some of them stated as adults that tearing their clothing and breaking toys were done as self-punishment. Others remember tearing bed-clothes to pieces, pulling down wallpaper, splashing paint on the walls, setting fire to curtains, or starting fires in the rooms, as outbursts of anger and helpless despair were experienced at home and at school.

## Behavioural Problems Including Self-Harming Behaviour

There are several ways that these children want to attract other people's attention to their unhappiness, hurt, and confusion. This usually manifests itself in severe head-banging against the furniture, walls, floor, and other objects, when the child is distressed or angry. These reactions tend to be triggered off when food is withdrawn as a punishment; when the child is locked up and isolated from the rest of the family; when it is denied a treat for a minor misbehaviour; or when it is unfairly punished. Some of these children bite, cut, or scratch themselves to the point of bleeding and this tends to occur when they are frustrated or cruelly criticised, blamed, and degraded, and also when they are unable to do or get what they want. Because they suffer from extremely low self-esteem they may punish themselves for their misdemeanours or express hurt and pain visibly to get some care and attention. Some children will injure themselves by putting a hand or a foot into a fire, or burn personal belongings.

These children are characterised by high levels of either over-activity or passivity. Many of them, due to a lack of energy and depression, are withdrawn and lethargic, while others run from one activity to another, unable to concentrate and maintain on-task behaviour. These children are described by parents as moody and unpredictable in their reactions. Once they are in a bad mood it can go on for many hours. They tend to present as either temperamentally difficult or slow to warm up, which can make their daily care demanding or unrewarding. Additionally, they are poor sleepers, with frequent waking and wandering around the house.

## Developmental Retardation

Psychosocial short-stature children show significant developmental delays in language, and in social and cognitive development. Their motor skills can be impaired as well; they frequently lose balance and bump into furniture or fall down, and they have poor verbal skills and poor practical reasoning abilities and skills in problem-solving. All of them have short attention spans, and find difficulty in concentrating and absorbing information. Their receptive and expressive skills are, as a rule, impaired.

## Psychological Description and Mother–Child Relationship

The most characteristic feature in social behaviour of short-stature children is antagonistic and disturbed interaction with the parents (usually the mother) and, to a lesser degree, other members of the family. The child seems to be an outsider in family activities, never fully involved in family life. It is quite common to see such a child standing or sitting a few metres away from the rest of the family, and nobody takes any notice of him or her. It seems that their life goes by without being a part of family interactions. Interaction is marked by dismissal or indifference: parents avoid the child, and at times its mere presence creates a heavy atmosphere of tension and anxiety. The cases of Chris and Gavin demonstrate these dilemmas very clearly. Quite recently the author was told by a mother that her best time was when her son goes to the nursery; when he came back, her stomach churned and her heart sank.

Extreme defiance and stubbornness are prevalent, and these children seem to be oblivious to requests and commands which, in turn, brings about hostile parental reactions. Parents tend to revert to quite cruel and harsh discipline to exert control and authority which they do not use with their other children when they misbehave. Disciplining may involve getting rid of a child's favourite toy or pet; locking the child up in a bedroom, dark cupboard, or shed for many hours; tying a child to a bed; making a child stand for a prolonged period in one spot; forcing a child to keep hands on its head to stop it taking or touching things, usually food; smacking; and shouting. However, the most common way of punishing a child is withdrawal of food and drink; making a hungry child watch others eat; sending the child to bed early without being fed; taking food away if the child eats in a messy way; or denying pudding or a treat. It is not unusual to see that the child is left out when treats are given to other children. There is always some justification given as to why this child is not given treats while others are. These may include observations of disobedience, cheek, or destructiveness, but often turn out to be of small importance.

Sibling–child relationships in many instances are hostile or indifferent: siblings usually ignore the child, do not include it in their activities, blame the child if something goes wrong, and behave towards it in the same way as the parents. Because parents seldom take the side of the target child, it is smacked, pushed, and toys are frequently snatched from it. It is not unusual to see that the child is being bruised by its siblings (even the younger ones).

It is not an uncommon feature in severe short-stature cases that a child will not speak to the mother, will not answer her questions, and seems to dismiss any attempts at contact she tries to make with him or her. Some children do not address their mothers as 'Mum' or 'Mummy' but refer to them as they would a teacher at school or nurse in the nursery. They sometimes call them 'Miss', 'Mrs', or 'that Lady'. Mutual dislike becomes more acute as the child gets older and the battle of wills intensifies. As an already fragile relationship and a sense of belonging deteriorates, the child becomes an intruder in the family. The attachment disorders are evident and they tend to attach themselves indiscriminately to strangers who give them some attention and show interest in their needs. It has been observed that some of them call strange women 'Mummy' and go willingly, without any protests, with strangers and seldom show separation-anxiety.

The following passage demonstrates vividly the distortion of the mother–child relationship (Iwaniec, 1995).

## *An Example of Psychosocial Short Stature: 'John'*

(Iwaniec, 1995, 45)

John will not speak to me (I know he can—he speaks to other people). I heard him swearing at me when I put him into his room. When I asked him to repeat what he said, he would not—even a swear word from him is better than nothing. He would not answer my questions—he would just stare at me. He refers to me as 'Miss' or 'this Lady'—he never calls me 'Mum'. He would position himself in a provoking way, for me to see him. He makes this awful noise, in a high-pitched, squeaking voice, which drives me mad. I just cannot stand him, I cannot bear having him near me—he deliberately behaves like that to hurt me—so for his own good I put him into his room, for his safety and my sanity, so that I do not have to look at him. I cannot allow him to annoy me so much. And yet, I worry so much about him—even though I do not like him. I keep wondering where I went wrong, what has happened. I get on so well with my two other children. I feel so guilty and ashamed and desperately unhappy. People like my family do not believe me that he is, and has always been, so difficult to care for and to enjoy. I went through hell trying to feed him when he was a baby. My whole life revolved around feeding John and coping with his crying and screaming. I tried to defeat him but he has defeated me instead. He does not want me and I do not want him. One of us has to go. He does not fit into this family: I feel that someone has dumped him on me and forgotten to take him away again.

**Table 4.1** Characteristics of psychosocial short-stature children

The following check-list may help in identifying children of psychosocial short stature.

| Characteristics | Yes | No | Do not know |
|---|---|---|---|
| Child is very small for its age | | | |
| Child stunted in growth for several months | | | |
| Child's weight and height below 3rd percentile for considerable time (minimum 6 months) | | | |
| Bizarre eating behaviour | | | |
| Excessive hunger-drive | | | |
| Voracious eating habits, eating quickly and gorging to the point of vomiting | | | |
| Eating huge amounts of food | | | |
| Wandering around the house at night in search of food | | | |
| Hoarding food | | | |
| Eating non-food items, e.g. cotton wool, pieces of paper | | | |
| Drinking from drainpipes, toilet bowls, puddles in the street | | | |
| Eating from dog or cat dishes | | | |
| Begging food from strangers | | | |
| Eating left-overs when in public places | | | |
| Scavenging food from waste-bins | | | |
| Constantly asking for food | | | |
| Stealing food from other children at school | | | |
| Having a poor appetite | | | |
| No interest in food | | | |
| Exceptionally long time spent eating | | | |
| Heaving and vomiting when pressed to eat | | | |
| Consuming small amounts | | | |

**Table 4.1** (*Cont.*)

| | | | |
|---|---|---|---|
| Soiling | | | |
| Smearing | | | |
| Wetting bed | | | |
| Wetting pants during daytime | | | |
| Urinating over personal and other people's belongings | | | |
| Defecating in inappropriate places | | | |
| Lying awake and motionless in bed for long periods | | | |
| Self-harming behaviour, including: | | | |
| • head-banging | | | |
| • cutting, scratching and self-biting | | | |
| • rocking | | | |
| • burning | | | |
| Severe non-compliance and stubborn defiance | | | |
| Reluctance to communicate with the mother | | | |
| Destructiveness (tearing cloths, breaking toys, pulling off wallpaper, destroying things) | | | |
| Fire-setting and burning things | | | |
| Short attention span | | | |
| Poor ability to concentrate and to complete tasks | | | |
| Disruptive behaviour when in the company of other children (including classroom) | | | |
| Attention-seeking | | | |
| Withdrawn, lethargic, passive behaviour | | | |
| Depression | | | |
| Irritability | | | |
| Hyperactivity | | | |
| Poor relationships with siblings and peers | | | |

(*Cont.*)

**Table 4.1** (*Cont.*)

| | | | |
|---|---|---|---|
| Attachment disorders | | | |
| Rejection by the primary care-giver | | | |
| Negative parental attitudes (dislike, rebukes, belittling, screaming and shouting, dismissiveness of child's attempts to please a care-giver) | | | |
| Physical abuse | | | |
| Possibilities of sexual abuse | | | |
| Emotional abuse | | | |
| Developmental delays: | | | |
| • motor | | | |
| • language | | | |
| • cognitive | | | |
| • social | | | |
| • emotional | | | |
| Acceleration of growth in terms of weight and height when removed from home, e.g. hospital, short-term care | | | |
| Deterioration of growth and behaviour when returned home | | | |
| Age of identification: | | | |
| • toddler | | | |
| • early childhood | | | |
| • middle childhood | | | |
| Being unappealing to other people | | | |
| Eagerness to be helpful and useful (teachers, nurses) | | | |
| Shortness | | | |
| Thinness | | | |
| Playing alone | | | |
| Weight-for-height normal or greater | | | |

## 20-YEAR FOLLOW-UP STUDY

The author recently completed a 20-year follow-up study of 31 subjects who failed to thrive as children. Fifteen out of 31 were classified as of psychosocial short stature, eight falling into the hyperphagic group and seven into the anorexic group.

The long-term outcomes varied amongst them and appeared to be determined by two factors: *the onset and length of psychosocial short stature*, and *type of intervention*. Children with a long history of failure to grow and who remained at home had disappointing outcomes. Six subjects out of these 15 were removed from neglectful and abusive homes. They achieved better outcomes than the nine remaining at home. Two subjects who were adopted at three and five years respectively have done well both professionally and personally, had better educational attainments, more secure employment, and were taller than their parents. Children who were fostered (three subjects) at the ages of four, five, and seven had lower educational achievements and were not so successful in securing good and permanent employment, as did one subject who was accommodated with his father at the age of 11 years.

Nine out of the 15 who remained at home (three on the At-Risk Register on and off for a long time) developed serious anti-social habits, such as delinquent behaviour, running away from home, glue-sniffing, drug abuse, and destructive behaviour. Seven of them were 'statemented' for special education. While at school they had difficulties with concentration, and were reported to be disruptive and attention-seeking. They had no playmates at school or in the community, and generally were not popular or liked by their peers and their teachers.

Six subjects had, on average, three to four episodes of short-term foster-care lasting between four and eight months. During their stays with the foster-parents their weight and height accelerated, bizarre eating or poor appetite normalised, and disturbed toileting and destructive behaviour improved. On returning home the growth and development slowed down and behaviour worsened.

All the subjects reported being badly treated as children by parents and sometimes by siblings. They reported being deprived of food, often isolated from the rest of the family, locked up in bedrooms for a long time, and persistently criticised and rebuked; furthermore, there was little affection and attention shown to them by the members of the family. Withdrawal of food as punishment for any misbehaviour was common and frequent, which begs the question as to whether these children are offered adequate food. What parents say and what actually happens might not be a true story and caution is needed when carrying out assessment. Taking into consideration the very poor relationship of the child within the family—often open rejection, and insecure attachment—and the remarkable recovery when cared for by other people, but deterioration on returning home, should keep us alert to the possibility of severe maltreatment and abuse. The following statements indicate the seriousness of parental behaviours generally and effects on the children, and specifically on a child's actual nutritional intake. What parents told the author during the assessment stage and what she was related 20 years later by those subjects differs sharply and is of concern:

- I was sent to bed without having tea at least three or four times a week if I was lucky.
- I was so hungry I could not sleep.
- No amount of crying and screaming and saying that I was hungry would do any good; the door was locked and that was that.
- If I did eat quickly and made a mess, she would take my plate away from me, and ask me to get up from the table. I had to sit still and watch the others eat.
- Of course I have hidden food, even under the carpet—wouldn't you if you were hungry all the time?
- I felt so miserable that I often cried myself to sleep.
- I did break things and smashed my toys and scratched myself until blood started to run. I don't know why, I guess I was hurting inside—I guess I wanted to let my Mum know I wanted someone to see how unhappy I was. No one took any notice of me anyway.
- Often I had to sit on the floor to eat while all of them sat at the table.
- I was so hungry at times that I could not sleep. I would go downstairs when everyone was asleep to find something to eat.
- Treats were not for me—I was told I did not deserve them. Others were given crisps or sweets, I was seldom given any.
- Well, I was a burden to them all—I was told often enough that I was stupid, sick, and good for nothing.
- Whenever I brought home something I made at school she would not even look at it. I was so hurt.
- I got so angry at times that I would break everything I could put my hands on.

The above few statements made by the ex-short-stature subjects are based on their memories and interpretations of experiences from their childhood.

However, there were some unexpected and positive outcomes in four cases. Two subjects who were adopted at the ages of 4 and 5 years respectively received higher education and were in successful jobs and had stable marital relationships. One of them had a 2-year-old son, thriving and well cared for.

The other two, in spite of extremely poor relationships with their mothers as children and the consequent reception into care of one of them (the other went to live with his father), gradually rebuilt their contacts with their natural families. It needs to be said that they received considerable therapeutic help. Once they established their own families and had children themselves, the relationship with their mothers warmed up, and attitudes were reappraised with the arrival of the child.

## Other Findings

The most worrying and long-lasting defect appears to be in the cognitive area in 40% of the cases. School attainments in those cases were poor or very poor. Six subjects had not passed any exams such as GCSE, and seven were moved to special education due to their slowness in learning and maladjusted behaviour. It is important to point out that six of these children remained at home with the parents, where difficulties were noticeable all the time, such as lack of stimulation, lack of interest in the child, and prevailing insecure attachment to the family members. Five subjects are semi-literate and four have considerable difficulties with reading and numeracy in spite of finishing secondary education.

Difficulties with maintaining employment are apparent where the ability to read and act upon written information and instructions is necessary. Six subjects had had between seven and ten different jobs since they left school. These findings are in line with other shorter-term follow-up studies, indicating that children who fail to thrive exhibit significant deficit in cognitive development, and that the problems can prevail if active intervention does not take place to remedy early deficit (Oates & Yu, 1971; Drotar & Sturm, 1988; Achenbach *et al.*, 1993).

## SUMMARY

Psychosocial short-stature children present serious and urgent problems to be dealt with as soon as they are identified. They are in danger of being physically and sexually abused, and they are, as a rule, emotionally abused and rejected. These children are exceptionally small for their age as a result of persistent stress, which affects growth-hormone function. In spite of excessive appetite they remain stunted in growth and their general development is retarded (in particular in cognitive and emotional areas). The long-term outcomes are very poor if constructive and decisive intervention does not take place early in the child's life. Children presenting a bizarre eating pattern, disturbed toileting, attachment disorders, and self-harming and destructive behaviour, when removed from their stressful homes, rapidly put on weight, begin to grow in length, and their behaviour calms down, but when returned to their homes they lose weight, become stunted in growth, and their behaviour worsens. The environment in which they live and the care they receive are highly inadequate. They are simply suffering significant harm.

# 5

# FEEDING/EATING BEHAVIOUR OF CHILDREN WHO FAIL TO THRIVE, AND PARENTAL FEEDING STYLES

*...as the proverb says, 'One man may lead a horse to the water, but twenty cannot make him drink'.*

Samuel Johnson, 1763

## INTRODUCTION

As we have seen in the previous chapters, failure to thrive in children is directly linked to under-nutrition (and under-nutrition is considered a major aetiological factor for these children's growth failure). The eating/feeding behaviour of the children and the way parents interact and manage the process of feeding therefore has to be explored, as well as the actual intake of food and possible associated difficulties. We know from the substantial literature available on the subject that feeding difficulties are often present, such as oral-motor dysfunction or other minor neurological problems, and that parental feeding behaviour fluctuates between tension, anxiety, worry, frustration, and anger, to misinterpretation of their children's signals of hunger or satiation, lack of understanding of children's nutritional needs, attitudes towards food, and neglect. Equally, we know that parental feeding interaction plays an important role in the way children react to parental feeding style and subsequent intake of food. Parental worry, tension, and anxiety regarding a child's poor growth is known to exacerbate difficulties already experienced in feeding the child, so a bad situation tends to get worse if some sort of intervention does not take place. It has been observed in a number of studies that changes of interaction, positioning, and provision of a more conducive feeding environment produce good outcomes for the child. For example, when a child is being fed by another person, oral-motor problems subside due to the reduction of anxiety and a more comfortable feeding style (Iwaniec *et al.*, 1985a; Iwaniec, 1991; Hobbs & Hanks, 1996; Hampton, 1996).

Let us look first of all at some studies and how knowledge and understanding regarding eating behaviour, feeding difficulties, and intake of food have developed over the years and how these general eating problems are linked to failure to thrive in children.

The prevalence of feeding problems among pre-school children was found to be remarkably high during investigations into the matter: Minde and Minde (1986) discovered (by reviewing the available epidemiological data) that between 12% and 34% was a norm. The problems associated with eating fall into two categories: *refusal to eat* (which often leads to growth failure), and *excessive faddiness*.

Studies exploring eating behaviour among babies and young children (Harris, 1988; Harris & Booth, 1992) suggested that there appears to be a sensitive period between 4 and 6 months of age, during which infants will accept any new taste. They argued that if babies tasted something on several occasions, a preference may be induced that can last into later childhood. Since solids are introduced around the age of 4 months it might be useful to start experimenting with different tastes so that babies can get used to them very early on. Harris suggested that delay in introduction to a wide range of different tastes until after 6 months is likely to meet with food refusal (especially by babies who are temperamentally difficult).

It has been known for many years that there may be specifically sensitive times to introduce different textures of food into a child's diet. It is said that, if children are not exposed to solids that require chewing by about 6 to 7 months of age, they tend to be resistant to accepting such new textures in later childhood (Illingworth & Lister, 1964). Feeding problems can result in refusing to accept lumpy foods, spitting out, and occasionally vomiting. The lack of experience of chewing firm solids may be associated, by a year or so of age, with immature and restricted tongue movements. Consequently, firm solids will not be masticated well enough for ease of swallowing. Attempts to swallow will then lead to gagging, which is believed to be a powerful aversive stimulus for the child, after which refusal to ingest anything but liquids or puréed food may follow. Early experimentation with a variety of textures, therefore, seems to be of crucial importance for the development of good oral-motor skills. Contrary to conventional wisdom, a significant number of young children who present feeding or weight problems are fed for a prolonged time by naso-gastric tube. Infants fed by this means are not exposed to concurrent oral stimulation and so there is a dramatic reduction in the amount of sensory input and exercise of the mouth. A healthy and otherwise normal infant receives, as a rule, substantial and continuous oral stimulation through food, sucking fingers or dummies, or other objects. When such oral stimulation is reduced or withdrawn because of naso-gastric tube feeds, the oral cavity can become hypersensitive and excessively irritable. There may be an associated loss of sucking and swallowing skills, depending on the timing and duration of the artificially provided food.

## FOOD-FADDINESS

Young children show excessive faddiness regarding food. They indicate a strong preference for familiar taste and texture and persistently refuse to try new things. Their fear of new tastes and textures has been termed 'neophobia', and it generally emerges in the second year of life (Birch, 1990). Most parents deal with a child's refusal to eat new foods appropriately by being firm, encouraging, and patient. It needs to be remembered, however, that neophobia is a perfectly normal part of any child's adaptation to the environment in which they live, and in many ways such exposure enhances the chance of the child's survival. Rejection of new foods is usually a transitory phenomenon which can be eliminated by repeated exposure and appropriate parental management of the child's eating behaviour (*see* Chapter 12 for further discussion on eating management).

## FORCE-FEEDING

Children who are difficult to feed are often exposed to force-feeding, not only by their parents or carers, but also by hospital staff. There is overwhelming evidence that force-feeding does not produce the desired outcome; instead it leads to food-avoidance behaviour and at times to food phobia. Additionally, parent–child interaction and relationships will suffer because of increased anxiety and stress in both parties. The child who is force-fed begins to associate eating/feeding time with painful and frightening experiences, and comes to regard feeding time and food generally as something to avoid. If such experiences are repeated time and time again with force and determination the child will avoid the source of force-feeding—the feeder. Several children who were referred to the present writer for treatment were hospitalised because they stopped taking feeds from their mothers as a result of force-feeding. The treatment process and the length of intervention is extensive and difficult as many problems need to be tackled, not only related to food intake but also to breakdown in the relationship between mother and child.

## EATING PROBLEMS AND FAILURE TO THRIVE

Although eating disorders in children are not always associated with growth failure, the majority of children who present feeding problems at an early age tend to fail to thrive. Many projects investigating children who fail to thrive explore eating behaviour, intake of food, parental behaviour, attitudes, and child-rearing methods. Let us look at findings regarding the eating patterns among failure-to-thrive children and issues emerging from research and clinical work that need to be tackled to resolve or prevent these problems.

Pollitt and Eichler (1976) have studied eating, sleeping, toileting, auto-erotic, and self-harming behaviours of pre-school failure-to-thrive children. Their behaviour was compared to a control group of children growing normally for their chronological age: the latter met all the same criteria except for weight and height, which were required to be on or above the 25th percentile. Relevant information was obtained by studying the histories of feeding: dietary intake over 24 hours was recorded, and the average intake from all records was the measure used for comparison. Direct observation and open-ended interviews were used on the child's eating habits, response to food and moods during eating, the quality of sucking as an infant, and the presence or absence of behaviour such as polydipsia, hiding food, or eating non-food substances. The findings of this well-designed and comprehensive study revealed difficulties in feeding, such as: poor appetite; poor sucking; crying during feeding; vomiting after each feeding; and refusal to switch from liquids to solids. Significant differences (p < 0.02) were found between the groups in a number of difficulties presented as infants, as well as in the meal patterns and content of meals. It was found that meals were more skimpy. The total calorific intake was statistically different (t = 1.02, df = 13, p–05) on one-tail test. The index children showed a poorer response to food than their counterparts. Hyperphagia was found in 4 out of 19 index children and none in the contrast group. In conclusion, it was found that there is some support for the view that the observed behavioural abnormalities among failure-to-thrive children might stem partly from conflicts in the interpersonal relationship with the child's primary care-giver. Their hypothesis, however, did not exclude the possibility that the alterations in behaviour might also be related to neuro-hormonal disturbances.

Iwaniec's (1983) study of non-organic failure-to-thrive children and two control groups' eating behaviour showed striking differences of both organic and non-organic failure-to-thrive groups and normally growing children. Differences between the organic and non-organic group were not statistically significant, but comparison with the normative group showed a high statistical difference in eating behaviour, intake of food, and parent–child interaction during feeding (p >0.01). Feeding time appeared to be a period of heightened stress for about 70% of the mothers. These children showed remarkably similar feeding problems: an inability, reluctance, or refusal to suck (taking up to two hours to take 3–4 oz. of milk); falling asleep every few minutes; crying while being fed; vomiting; stretching out; turning head; rapidly moving hands; looking distressed; and having diarrhoea. This pattern of behaviour was consistent with the majority of babies while they were on liquids. Although most mothers found it very tiring and extremely anxiety-provoking, they described the real onset of acute feeding difficulties as dating from the time when solids were introduced. The children persistently refused to take solids, vomiting and diarrhoea increased, and screaming while being fed was persistent in duration and intensity. Regurgitating and heaving were common, especially with lumpy foods; the children also showed a tendency to store food in their mouths, and a reluctance, unwillingness, or perhaps inability to chew and swallow. Even small pieces of vegetables and bread caused heaving and vomiting.

The period of refusal to take solids and liquids altogether ranged from two to six days in eight children (complete food-avoidance behaviour) aged from 11 months to $2\frac{1}{2}$ years. Refusal to take food at all, from anybody, was found in only three cases, but refusal to take food from the mother alone was found in five cases. These children would accept some feeds from the father, health visitor, and neighbours (in fact from anybody but the mother). The events prior to complete refusal to take food could not be specified in every case, but in three cases it would appear to be connected with excessive pressures put on the child to eat: such pressures might involve force-feeding, anger expressed by screaming and shouting, smacking, keeping the child in the high-chair until the food was consumed, and the creation of a heightened anxiety level. Those episodes were, in turn, associated with pressures put on the mothers, either by health professionals concerned about the child's prolonged failure to thrive, or by families and neighbours worried about and critical of the children's physical appearance and deteriorating mother–child relationships.

It needs to be stressed that 40% of children did not have a history of feeding difficulties but had histories of under-feeding and under-eating. The reasons for being under-fed ranged from deliberate reduction of food and limitation of range of food (because of parental attitudes to food and weight [as demonstrated in Previn's case, *see* page 48]), to unawareness of how or when to feed, what to feed, and the amount of food required (as shown in Rose's case, *see* page 48), and sheer neglect and rejection (as demonstrated by Kevin's case, *see* page 46).

There can never be certainty as to how much children eat and how they are being dealt with regarding their consumption of food. There may also be certain grey areas regarding other activities. What carers tell us about a child's food consumption, or what they have recorded concerning this, is not always true. Information may be notoriously inaccurate for a variety of reasons, not the least because carers do not wish to be seen as neglectful or uncaring. Again, observations made when parents or carers know that they are going to be judged must be interpreted with caution, as the interaction and the approach to the child will differ in quality, either more anxious and negative than usual, or much better and less angry than when not observed: a typical 'observer effect'.

When we look at other studies, they report remarkably similar feeding behaviour, although interpretations of feeding difficulties vary amongst researchers. Findings will very much depend on the severity and duration of failure to thrive. Children referred early on or identified in the community will present less severe eating problems and less problematic mother–child interaction, simply because full interactional distortion has, as yet, not taken place. As time goes on (especially if eating is exacerbated by oral-motor dysfunction), difficulties may intensify, bringing about serious food-avoidance behaviour and other interactional problems.

Most researchers state that difficulties emerge during the first year of life, so they could be identified early on and dealt with to prevent further deterioration in eating and associated interactional and attachment problems. For example, Raynor and Rudolf (1996) reported that a concerning number of mothers described difficulties in feeding their infants starting in the first three months of life. They argued that their findings suggest either some degree of early oral-motor dysfunction, which is considered as a causal factor (Ramsay, Gisel and Boutry, 1993), or that there were difficulties in mother–infant attachment from early infancy. A large proportion of the children studied were described as having an adverse response to food. Behaviours included: repeatedly turning the head away; spitting food out; and vomiting. Heptinstall *et al.* (1987) reported similar observations when they compared eating behaviour and dietary intake of children who failed to thrive and those growing normally. Although no significant differences were found in calorific or protein intake between the two groups, the non-organic failure-to-thrive families were observed to be functioning less satisfactorily at meal-times, with children showing negative attitudes to food.

Some studies show contrasting results, however. For example, Chatoor *et al.* (1997) comment that not all children who fail to thrive have feeding disorders. Mathisen *et al.* (1989) found that in their sample non-organic failure-to-thrive children were eager to accept offered food and mothers did not describe their non-organic FTT children as more fussy or difficult during meal-times. Both non-organic failure to thrive and comparison infants were described as active, happy, adaptable to new foods and tastes, and moderately regular in their hunger demands. In fact, most of the non-organic FTT mothers described meal-times as the easiest time of the day (Wolke *et al.*, 1990). However, in this study the signals sent by non-organic FTT children were observed as relatively ambiguous and difficult to interpret (such as when they were hungry, when they wanted more food, wanted to eat slower or faster, or wanted to stop eating (Mathisen *et al.*, 1989). Non-organic failure-to-thrive children tended to resort to crying in order to draw attention to their needs, whereas comparison infants used more sophisticated systems incorporating gesture, vocalisations, and body and facial postures. The authors state that 'it is difficult to determine the direction of this response' but felt that 'an infant's lack of communication skills is likely to be exacerbated by unresponsive maternal interaction' and mothers of failure-to-thrive infants were observed 'to engage in less verbal and non-verbal dialogue with their infants while feeding them'. They found a marked difference in the clarity with which infants communicated their needs at meal-times. Index infants were less adept,

Table 5.1 Interactional styles and characteristic behaviours of carers and children

| Carer's feeding style | Behaviour of carers | Reaction of children |
|---|---|---|
| Forceful, impatient and angry | Rushing child to eat, getting easily frustrated and angry, screaming, shaking, smacking, frequent force-feeding, anxious | Refusal to eat, crying, choking, vomiting, stretching out, fearful and apprehensive, uneasy when in the carer's company. Little intake of food |
| Unconcerned and neglectful | Failure to respond to child's signal of hunger and distress. Fed irregularly and in a haphazard way. Not appropriate food given. Seldom picked up when fed | Lethargic, withdrawn, sleep a lot. Little movement, seldom heard. Looking detached and sad. Little intake of food |
| Not persistent, passive | React to stress with high anxiety. Tend to get depressed and helpless. Low self-esteem. Give up easily, unable to cope and to exert authority | Strong-willed, persistent, irritable, getting their own way, manipulating, miserable. Persistent refusal to eat, to swallow and chew. Little intake of food |
| Determined and coaxing | Preoccupied with feeding. Generally resourceful, patient, try different ways to manage, try different food. Anxious about child's poor growth | Long feeding periods, faddiness, spitting, storing food in mouth, heaving, refusal to chew. Stubborn and difficult to distract. Little intake of food |
| Preoccupied with weight, restrictive of food intake | Restricting intake of food, putting child on low-calorie diet. Diluting formula to prevent weight acceleration. Anxious about excessive weight gain | Children appear to be always hungry, looking thin and undernourished. There are no eating problems as such. Food is simply not available. Little intake of food |

*Source:* Iwaniec, D. (1995) *The Emotionally Abused and Neglected Child.* Chichester: John Wiley & Sons Ltd

which seemed to contribute to less successful interaction in acquiring adequate nutritional ingestion. They also seemed less able to indicate that they wished to feed faster or slower or that they were still hungry. The contexts in which they were fed and the mother's style of feeding seemed to add to these difficulties.

## FEEDING BEHAVIOURS AND CHILD CHARACTERISTICS

Poorer cognitive function and school grades, behavioural differences, neurological soft signs, and poor motor performance have all been reported in children who are protein-energy malnourished (Grantham-McGregor et al., 2000). Children who are protein-energy deficient also reportedly form poor relationships and have poorer attention spans (Grantham-McGregor, 1995). Children who have been placed into more prosperous homes have been shown to improve greatly in their development, demonstrating that the subsequent quality of the child's environment can mediate the long-term effects of this type of malnourishment (Winick, 1976; Colombo et al., 1992). Behaviours that are associated with malnourishment include fist-clenching and apathy towards the care-giver: however, failure-to-thrive children can exhibit additional abnormal behaviours that are not solely attributable to malnourishment.

If an infant has suffered nutritional deficits while still in the womb, it is important for that infant to be able to obtain the required nutrition through feeding (Steward, 2001). However, the necessary feeding behaviours must be present for this to occur: if they are not, then this will interfere with normal growth and development. Negative behaviours that can militate against sufficient calorific intake include: refusing or rejecting the nipple; spitting up; not sucking; drowsiness; and/or jerky movements. In fact, the more negative behaviour displayed, the fewer calories per kilogram are ingested (Steward, 2001). It is possible that these difficult feeding behaviours are so subtle that they go unrecognised by the mother and there is the danger that the infant's behaviour will be misinterpreted as lack of hunger or lack of interest. The child is then at greater risk of developing failure-to-thrive problems.

Infantile anorexia is characterised by food refusal and failure to thrive, and was originally termed separation disorder. Chatoor et al. (1997) proposed that infantile anorexia occurs as a result of conflictual interactions which arise because characteristics in the child clash with the vulnerabilities of the mother, resulting in negative responses. The behaviour of the child can affect the interaction between mother and infant during feeding. If the feeding interaction between mother and infant is not synchronous, then the nutritional intake of the child can be compromised and contribute to faltering growth. Anxiety is then provoked in the mother when the child refuses to feed and is oppositional. Oppositional behaviours involved in food refusal include: refusing to open the mouth; arching the back; attempting to climb out of the high-chair; and throwing feeding utensils. The onset of food refusal most commonly occurs between the ages of 9 and 18 months during the transitional period from milk to solids and from dependent feeding to autonomous self-feeding. Chatoor has described the characteristics of infantile anorexics as emotionally intense, distractible, unstoppable, or stubborn, and dependent. She has proposed that these infants find it more difficult to focus on the physiological signals indicating hunger and satiety, and suggests that the toddlers ensure their needs are met and control their parents' attention through food refusal, being aware of the inability of parents to set boundaries.

Douglas and Bryon's (1996) research focused them more towards child-related factors and away from parent- or family-related factors when it came to the development of eating difficulties in young children. They reported a higher incidence of behavioural problems (tantrums, poor concentration, etc.) and sleeping problems (regular waking, sleeping in parents' bed, etc.) among children with severe eating difficulties.

Another study by Chatoor et al. (2000) found that the mothers of children with infantile anorexia reported that their children had more difficult temperaments, had irregular sleeping and feeding patterns, and had more negative moods than children who were healthy eaters. These mothers also perceived their children to be more demanding of attention and more wilful. The authors also examined picky eaters and reported that although the temperaments of picky eaters and infantile anorexics were similar, the children with infantile anorexia displayed the shared characteristics in greater extremes. However, the authors questioned whether the perceptions of the mothers of infantile anorexics were objective, and suggested that observational methods should be employed where possible. It was found that the mother's ratings of the child's temperament and maternal-attachment representations had a direct impact on conflict during the feeding interaction. Specifically, child characteristics such as 'irregular', 'sober', and 'difficult' were positively related to feeding difficulty. Maternal-attachment representations and drives for thinness were also significantly related to feeding conflict. The mothers of the children with infantile anorexia were more likely to have insecure attachment representations and to experience conflict during feeding than the mothers of healthy eaters. Chatoor et al. (2000) reported that a diagnostic category (i.e. infantile anorexic, picky eater, healthy eater) significantly predicted conflict during feeding, i.e. children with infantile anorexia showed the most intense conflict. It was also found that maternal representation and toddler temperament were significantly predictive of conflict even when the effects of diagnostic category were accounted for. The authors suggested that picky eating characterises a sub-clinical form of infantile anorexia, but that picky eaters experienced less feeding conflict and were not malnourished: they postulated that perhaps a decreased level of conflict acts as a protective mechanism to prevent full-blown infantile anorexia, and suggested it might be useful to consider intervention aimed at reducing feeding conflict.

Mathisen et al. (1989) reported that in their study failure-to-thrive infants were fed more quickly than the comparison infants, and it has previously been reported that the infants of mothers who quickly terminate interactions are at high risk of failing to thrive. Drotar et al. (1990) found that the mothers of children with non-organic failure to thrive ended feeding with their children more arbitrarily compared to the mothers of normally thriving children. They found that mothers of non-organic failure-to-thrive children fed them in a shorter time compared with mothers of healthy children.

Raynor and Rudolf (1996) found that in their sample of 63 children, all diagnosed with non-organic failure to thrive, 58% of mothers said that feeding difficulties started before the baby was three months old. Douglas and Bryon (1996) also reported that over half of the infants they studied experienced significant distress during feeding and that 62% of mothers reported that feeding difficulties started before the infant was three months old. Raynor and Rudolf (1996) put this down to either early oral-motor dysfunction or difficulties with mother–infant attachment. Sixty per cent of mothers in Raynor and Rudolf's study reported that their children had adverse responses to food (turning the head away, spitting out food, and vomiting), and the mothers attempted to deal with this behaviour by trying another type of meal, playing games, and bribery. However, Foy et al. (1997) emphasised that force-feeding should be avoided because it involves an emotional component (anger, stress, anxiety) to the feeding interaction which is mostly negative. The mothers in Raynor and Rudolf's study also reported that difficult behaviour was not just confined to meal-times but was evident at other times as well. It might be that the difficult temperament of a child impairs the mother's ability to nurture it. Psycho-motor delay was apparent in this group of children; however, the authors pointed out that the size of the family and ordinal position might also have influenced development.

Hawdon et al. (2000) studied a group of infants admitted to neo-natal intensive care, of which over half the parents at six months reported feeding problems with their children, even the parents of those children who had originally been assessed as being normal feeders. The authors suggest that this might be because feeding difficulties are more prevalent than was first supposed, or it may reflect the extreme anxiety that parents suffer regarding the feeding and growth of their baby, whom they consider vulnerable (Skuse, 1993; Ramsay & Gisel, 1996). Those infants who had been assessed as disorganised or dysfunctional feeders were far more likely to be affected by vomiting and coughing during feeds and to show an intolerance of lumpy food than were children who fed normally.

## Oral-Motor Difficulties

Oral-motor dysfunction can be minor and subtle and occur in otherwise healthy children; however, it can result in significant feeding difficulties (Skuse, 1993). Oral-motor dysfunction includes hypotonic lips, incompetence in removing food from a spoon, tongue thrust or persistent tongue protrusion, and a weak or unsustained suck. A child who is premature or developmentally delayed will have a structurally weak oral-motor mechanism and consequently a weak suck and swallow. Reflux or recurrent vomiting is common in children who are experiencing difficulty feeding, and if eating is associated with discomfort or pain, conditioned dysphagia can result (Foy *et al.*, 1997). Selley and Boxall (1986) stated that a possible cause of failure to thrive was incoordination of feeding mechanisms. Heptinstall *et al.* (1987) found that in a population of inner-city children with chronic growth retardation almost half had some sort of oral-motor dysfunction. Oral-motor problems can be subtle and not easily recognised, not only by the mother of the child but by the health workers as well. Previous research surrounding non-organic failure to thrive has centred on the mother supplying sufficient nutrition, and intervention has concentrated on family dysfunction. Consequently, the ability of the child (or lack of it) to actually ingest food largely has been neglected (Reilly *et al.*, 1999).

It is possible that oral impairment directly affects adequate food intake and leads to a subsequent diagnosis of non-organic failure to thrive. This would then mean that if oral impairment is present, the term 'non-organic failure to thrive' should be reconsidered. Ramsay, Gisel and Boutry (1993) examined 60 infants aged from 1 to 42 months. Of the sample of 60, 22 infants were diagnosed with organic failure to thrive and 38 were diagnosed with non-organic failure to thrive. The authors found that a high percentage of infants in both groups had a history of abnormal duration of feeding time, poor appetite, delayed texture tolerance, and difficult feeding behaviour. There were no significant differences between the two groups on any of the aforementioned variables; however, it was noted that the onset of feeding difficulties in both groups was early and subsequently became persistent. Six of the infants identified with non-organic failure to thrive showed no deviant feeding behaviour. Two of the case-infants had no feeding-skills disorder (compared to one infant in the comparison group), and it was found that four of the case infants were inappropriately positioned for their age during feeding, and/or were presented with food textures inappropriate for their age (compared to two infants in the comparison group). There were no differences between organic and non-organic failure-to-thrive infants regarding early feeding problems. The authors suggest that this might indicate a common cause that varies in severity. It was also found that none of the children diagnosed with non-organic failure to thrive had diagnosable neurological disorders. However, the histories of nearly half of these children pointed towards some neurological involvement. The authors suggested that an organic cause cannot be ruled out for these children, and postulated that an underlying factor of the feeding-related symptoms might be neuro-physiological, the expression of which is varying degrees of oral sensori-motor impairment.

*Feeding-skills disorder* (FSD) was the label created to encompass the abnormal feeding-related symptoms observed in infancy (abnormal duration of feeding time, poor appetite, delayed texture tolerance, and difficult feeding behaviour). FSD at birth or shortly after was observed in twice as many of the infants in the non-organic group as in the organic group. The authors proposed that the origin of FSD is neuro-physiological (rather than experiential or environmental) because in the non-organic group the two peak periods of feeding impairment coincided with the beginning and end of the reflexive phase of ingestion. Their conclusions supported previous claims that non-organic failure-to-thrive children are minimally neurologically abnormal (Accardo, 1982; Mathisen et al., 1989). Feeding skills change as the infant grows and develops and the types of food needed to provide sufficient nutrition change. This advancement and development of feeding skills is achieved through developmental changes in the central nervous system in addition to learning through experience. If feeding problems exist early on in the life of the infant it is likely that they will impede the development of advanced feeding skills. It has been suggested that non-organic FTT is no longer an accurate depiction of the growth-faltering observed in many infants. They suggest that because the underlying cause might be neurological, non-organic FTT should be renamed *growth failure secondary to feeding-skills disorder*. However, this does not take into account the environmental and maternal factors which can influence growth-faltering. It is well known that children cared for by different people take more food, eat quicker, and after a few days present fewer feeding/eating problems. Interaction and the manner in which children are fed mediates neurological problems (Iwaniec, 2000). Therefore, it would appear that attempts to create a sick model are unhelpful, but that an awareness of the importance of oral-motor difficulties may help to inform palliative strategies.

Douglas and Bryon (1996) studied 201 children aged from 4 to 100 months over a five-year period. These children all had severe eating difficulties. In order to assess the possible presence of oral-motor difficulties, a speech and language therapist rated the incidence of speech delay among the children. Nineteen per cent of the children showed mild speech delay (single words at 2–3 years) and 10% demonstrated severe delay (no words before 3 years). Eighteen per cent of the children were too young to be assessed. The incidence of speech delay among these infants is higher than would be expected in the general population of under-fives (from 3.1% to 10%, Richman et al., 1982; Butler & Golding, 1986). The authors suggest that this could be indicative of oral-motor immaturity or general developmental delay. Among many of the children there was evidence of a general disinclination to experience oral stimulation. Of 82 families interviewed, one-third of the children never sucked their fingers or thumbs, one-quarter refused to have their teeth brushed, and just over one-fifth of children were resistant to the oral exploration of objects. This study suggests that oral-motor dysfunction affects other areas of child development such as language and communication skills.

Mathisen et al. (1989) investigated oral-motor dysfunction and contextual factors during the feeding of one-year-old infants with non-organic FTT. They found that the index infants (those with non-organic failure to thrive) without exception were fed in the main living area, which was a noisy and distracting environment in which to be fed. In contrast, the comparison infants (healthily thriving infants) were all fed in the kitchen or dining areas. Significantly, more comparison infants than case infants were fed in a high-chair, and it took significantly longer to feed the comparison infants than the case infants. When the mothers were interviewed about the ability of their child to communicate their needs at meal-times, it emerged that comparison infants used various means of communicating (such as gestures, vocalisation, and body and facial postures), but the failure-to-thrive infants indicated their needs by crying. Observation of the interaction between the mothers and the case infants showed that there was less verbal and non-verbal dialogue with the infants while feeding them, and it was thought that the case child's poor communication skills might be due to impoverished maternal interaction. As we can see, omission of parental attention is evident, which, one can argue, may contribute to poorer developmental attainments.

A significantly greater number of the case infants had hypotonic lips than the comparison infants. Case infants showed a significant aversive response to facial touch and being touched on the limbs and trunk. The mother might misinterpret this dislike of being touched as rejection, and subsequently emotionally withdraw. Consequently, this might turn feeding from a social occasion to a perfunctory task. When being fed puréed food, the case infants had significantly poorer quality of oral-motor functioning and a significantly higher rate of abnormal features for puréed and solid food. Semi-solid food posed no significant problems for either group and there were no significant differences between groups. When the mothers in this study were asked whether they considered their child to have a feeding difficulty there was no significant difference between the responses of the two groups. In fact the mothers of the case infants described meal-times as the easiest part of the day. When the behaviour of the infants was observed using structured and standardised play procedures, it was noted that the case infants were more 'difficult', had a poorer attention span, and ate less of the food that was proffered.

## Parental Attitudes

Increasing concerns over the last few years regarding animal welfare, the environment, and healthy eating have led to an increased number of people who exclude meat, and sometimes dairy products, from their diet. If this dietary behaviour is inappropriately enforced on an infant and vital nutrients are not compensated for, failure to thrive can result.

In a study by McCann et al. (1994), the mothers of 26 children with non-organic FTT were identified in order to determine whether disturbed eating habits and attitudes towards body shape, weight, and food were more prevalent among these mothers than mothers in the general population. It was established that none of the mothers with failing-to-thrive children had a clinical eating disorder: however, they did restrict food intake to change weight or shape significantly more often than did the mothers in the comparison group. Fifty per cent of the mothers of the failing-to-thrive children reported that they limited the amount of 'sweet foods' that they allowed their children to have, and 30% of mothers limited foods they considered unhealthy and possibly fattening. This was despite the fact that the reason for their child's referral to the paediatrician was poor weight gain. The authors suggested two alternative reasons to explain why mothers did not attempt to increase their child's nutritional intake, despite poor weight gain. First, the mothers believed sweet and fattening foods to be unhealthy (and should therefore be restricted), and, second, their high level of dietary control led them to limit the amount and type of food they allowed their children to have.

After referral to a paediatrician, over half the parents (54%) in this study increased the frequency and quantity of food they gave their children. Mothers of 'finicky eaters' reported that clarification of the feeding difficulty in conjunction with the support and advice they received resulted in improved feeding behaviour. The authors acknowledged that the relationship they found was not causal. However, they suggested that parents of children who failed to thrive should also be assessed, and their eating habits and attitudes addressed if necessary.

Another study conducted by Pugliese *et al.* in 1987 found that the health beliefs of parents were involved in the non-organic failure-to-thrive cases they examined. The parents who expressed concerns about obesity in their children because of their own personal experience of obesity were likely to restrict their children's diet by diluting the formula with water, restricting snacks, sweets, and high-calorific food. Concerns of parents about the potential risk of cardio-vascular disease in their children led to them being fed restricted diets low in saturated fats, red meat, and full-fat dairy products. In this study it was the case that one parent felt that a healthy diet for her child consisted of mostly fruit, vegetables, whole grains, and some lean meat and low-fat milk. Parents were conscious of the beneficial effects of breast-milk as a sole source of nutrition for infants, and extended this to include older children. Therefore they fed the children breast-milk until they were nearly two years old. Delaying the introduction of solids into a child's diet and prolonging dependence on breast-milk has been associated with delayed growth. All of the children examined in this study were diagnosed with non-organic FTT due to insufficient calorific intake. This was directly related to their parents' belief that they were providing their child with a healthy diet in order to try to prevent obesity and cardio-vascular disease. Although the intention of the parents was not to deprive the child, only to give them a healthy diet, they were still reluctant to change their child's diet despite being presented with evidence of failure to thrive. It was more important to the parents to avoid obesity than to eat potentially harmful food.

Saarilehto *et al.* (2001) also found that reported eating problems in young children were associated with parental eating habits and attitudes. A child was at increased risk of problems concerned with eating if the mother did not take pleasure in eating and snacked even though not hungry. However, mechanisms of this are unclear. A study by Stein *et al.* (1995) investigated the attitudes towards eating of 30 mothers of children with feeding difficulties. The results indicated that the mothers of children with eating difficulties had significantly more disturbed attitudes towards eating and eating habits than a matched control group of mothers whose children did not present with any eating difficulties. It was concluded that the disturbed eating habits and attitudes towards eating displayed by the mothers are specifically associated with feeding difficulties in children.

## WEANING AND TRANSITION

During the weaning period, feeding changes for infants in several ways. They progress from milk to solids, they go from sucking to chewing and biting, and they start to feed independently rather than be fed by the mother. It was demonstrated by many researchers that there were wide variations in the degree of self-feeding and being fed among children aged 12–14 months. During the transition period from dependent feeding to autonomous eating, mother and infant need to co-operate, and this is reliant on effective communication between mother and child.

When the child is being fed by the care-giver it is important to be aware of the components that are involved in this interaction: the offers of food by the mother, and the child's responses to these offers. Insufficient intake of food can be the result of either the mother not offering enough food or the child being offered sufficient food but rejecting it. This distinction is not always recognised and either leads to perceptions that the failure-to-thrive child is maltreated in some way or that the child is failing to thrive simply because of some neurologically determined feeding problems.

Abnormal meal-duration can be a sign of early feeding problems, and anything above 45 minutes has been suggested as an appropriate cut-off point (Ramsay *et al.*, 1993). There is inconsistent evidence regarding the relationship between the length of meal-times and feeding behaviour. Longer meal-times might be the result of the child eating more; feeding might be slower and less effective; and the degree to which the mother is feeding the child or allowing self-feeding may also be significant. Food intake is much more efficient when the mother is feeding the child than when the child is self-feeding, so, when examining issues such as low food intake, it is important to take into account whether the child is being fed by the mother or is self-feeding. The authors developed a coding system that particularly distinguishes between feeding behaviour when being fed by the mother and feeding behaviour when self-feeding. This allows a distinction to be made between children who are not offered sufficient food in the first place and children who are but do not accept it.

It is often the case that children who fail to thrive are experiencing difficulties with the transition from tube-feeding to oral feeding. It has been reported that the use of endo-tracheal tubes and feeding-tubes can contribute to sucking difficulties, and feeding problems are most common among those who have severe respiratory disease (Palmer *et al.*, 1993). In cases where it is impossible to avoid such things, it has been suggested that preventive measures, including oral desensitisation, non-nutritive sucking, and reduction of environmental over-stimulation, be introduced. In a study by Foy *et al.* (1997), 19 infants who were making this transition from tube-feeding to oral feeding were studied. Their ages ranged from 9 to 51 months and all infants were refusing oral feeds. The intervention strategy used by the authors to treat this severe feeding refusal and to encourage infants to feed orally was performed by occupational therapists. The therapy involved ignoring negative behaviour of the child during feeding (e.g. coughing, gagging, resisting food) and praising appropriate behaviour (such as opening the mouth or accepting food). This consistent approach to oral feeding combined with a steady reduction of tube-feeding resulted in 12 of the 19 infants taking all their calories by mouth at the follow-up clinic.

Iwaniec and Herbert (1982) reported a case study of a 2½-year-old girl who, after a successful hernia operation (where it was thought feeding and weight gain would improve), stopped taking feeds altogether and had to be tube-fed for two months. She had gained weight but lost the oral skills in eating which had to be taught step by step (*see* page 229 on treatment programme of Emma, Chapter 12).

## SUMMARY

Eating/feeding behaviour of children who fail to thrive was discussed, exploring various difficulties of eating during infancy, the toddler stage, and early childhood. Factors such as food-faddiness, force-feeding, food refusal, oral-motor dysfunction, and weaning have been described and supported by relevant research literature. Additionally, associations between feeding behaviour and a child's individual characteristics were explored. Parental attitudes regarding healthy eating and restrictions of food, which may contribute to poor growth, were brought to the reader's attention.

# 6

# PARENT–CHILD INTERACTION IN FAILURE-TO-THRIVE CASES

*The joys of parents are secret, and so are their griefs and fears.*

Francis Bacon, 1625

## INTRODUCTION

It is important for diagnostic and treatment purposes to investigate how caregivers interact with their FTT children generally and particularly during the act of feeding. It is recognised that mother–child interaction during feeding may be problematic. What is far from being clear, however, is whether poor intake of food is the result of inappropriate mother–child interaction, or if persisting feeding difficulties lead to problematic interactions and consequent failure to thrive. This uncertainty is not surprising for many reasons, one of which is the difficulty in establishing what feeding style is being adopted, and what is the mother–child interaction over a given period. Occasional observations are of questionable use, as parental behaviour is always affected by the presence of observers. As a rule only one child in a family fails to thrive, so we need to examine what is different about that particular child, the quality of care it receives, the problems that it presents, and how its parents react and manage its refusal to eat. There may also be further child-rearing problems, so it is important to establish what these are, what causes them, and how they are perceived by the parents.

In the majority of FTT cases, parental reactions to feeding difficulties and consequent poor weight gain and development will cause considerable concern and worry, as discussed in Chapter 5. When these difficulties persist, heightened anxiety is observed in some parents, quite often creating a sense of helplessness and low self-efficacy. Other parents get very frustrated with poor results of feeding, so interaction with their children tends to become more angry and anxiety-provoking. There are also those who do not pay much attention or hardly notice that their child eats very little, and is very thin, small, and lethargic.

The extent and quality of interaction differ substantially amongst failure-to-thrive children and their parents, as do the reasons for mutual contacts and pleasures deriving from those interactions. Most parents want the best for their children, and parents of FTT children are not different. There are some, nevertheless, who do not know how to facilitate appropriate growth and development: their lifestyle is not conducive to sensitive and responsive care-provision; and environmental stresses might also contribute to an impoverished or unrewarding parent–child relationship.

A nurturing environment in terms of caring consists not only of good physical care but also emotional availability. The timing and manner in which care-givers respond to their infants' various needs is of immense importance as it lays the foundation for the way children will perceive the world around them. If children's needs are going to be met in a sensitive way they will build trust in their carers' availability, e.g. to alleviate distress and provide social companionship, to make them feel wanted and involved in social and emotional interaction.

The importance of the nurturing environment and provision of social interaction and emotional availability was demonstrated by the early studies of hospitalised children (see Chapter 2). It was found that these children, cared for by many people, soon became lethargic, withdrawn, apathetic, and sickly, and failed to thrive in spite of the adequate physical care they received. It was thought that the reason for a child's poor growth, withdrawn behaviour, and poor speed of recovery was due to the lack of parental availability to serve as a safe haven when in a strange environment.

The researchers of those early studies of failure to thrive conducted in the children's own homes assumed (on the basis of observed symptoms in these children, both physical and developmental—which were so similar to those seen in the hospitalised children) that the same forces were at work. But, whereas with hospitalised children the mothers were not able physically to spend much time with their children, in cases of non-organic failure to thrive in the home, the mothers were thought to be unable or unwilling to provide emotional care and sensitive parenting. Recent studies disregarded those early assumptions and recognised that growth-faltering is far less associated with maternal psychopathology and more with feeding/eating abnormalities or difficulties, which can lead to tense interactions and disturbances in parent–child relationships.

It is thought that there are also problems in the way parents are receiving, interpreting, and responding to a child's various communication signals on the one hand, and participating and stimulating mutual communication with the child on the other. It is believed that there are problems in the attachment process which influence how mother and child interact and feel about each other (Dawson, 1992). There may be many inter-related factors (fully discussed in the next chapter) which can interfere or disrupt the formation of a strong and secure attachment, such as emotional problems, health, and economic difficulties which can preoccupy the parents and disturb development of emotional bonding. These include: depression (which is often accompanied by high levels of anxiety); chronic anger; and feelings of inadequacy (Hathaway, 1989); problems in marital and extended family relationships (Drotar & Malone, 1982); loss of a loved person (Benoit *et al.*, 1989); alcohol and substance abuse; and family violence (Iwaniec, 2002).

## PARENTAL RESPONSIVENESS

The interactions between parents and children (particularly the early ones involving communication between mother and baby) are of crucial significance in a child's development. What a baby needs is close, confident, and caring physical and emotional contact with the parents or carers in order to be healthy and to develop vigorously. The absence of such continuing nurturance and physical intimacy can bring about anxiety in a child, fretting, and disruption of biological functions. One of the indices of basic trust and security in an infant is stable feeding behaviour. In order for eating to be nutritionally beneficial and enjoyable it requires conditions that denote a relatively benign and calm state of psychosomatic harmony. If the eating time is fraught and tense, the intake of food will be insufficient, difficult, and stressful, resulting in poor physical growth and psychomotor development.

Parental responsiveness is a complex and many-sided phenomenon, but there are at least three different elements that make for what one might assess to be sensitive responsiveness: these are tendencies to react promptly, consistently, and appropriately in response to crying and other communications and actions. Mothers who are responsive, available, and comforting generate a soothing, predictable environment for the child: maternal sensitivity to a child's signal of distress produces securely attached children, and in interaction with their children such mothers show synchrony, involvement, interest, and warmth—there is a sense of harmony between child and mother, with well-timed reciprocal interactions and communication of feelings. Positively involved mothers tend to show a great deal of interest and fascination in their babies, recognise their needs, and respond to communication signals.

## PARENT–CHILD COMMUNICATION

It is believed by many that communication and all forms of social interaction provide the basis for the development of attachment. Important communication abilities are present from birth. Both crying and being at peace are signals that tell the carers when a baby is distressed or happy.

When human babies are born they are unable to care for themselves, so they have to rely on their care-givers in order to survive. In pursuit of these goals the human baby is seen to be active rather than passive. Although babies lack the actual wording to tell their parents what these needs are, they have several sophisticated ways of communicating. These range from obvious vocalisations (such as crying, which can vary in pitch) to signify different needs, to more subtle factors such as maintaining or breaking eye-contact with the mother during an interaction (Messer, 1999). In this way, with a responsive parent the infant can potentially alter its environment to meet these needs. In the initial interactions with others the mother is likely to play a central role. Interpretation of a baby's crying is important for both mother and child. A crying baby can be particularly annoying to some people, and at times can trigger irritation and anger leading to abuse. In others the noise can activate acute anxiety, frustration, and a sense of help-lessness if it is difficult to pacify. Different types of crying can be identified, such as those associated with hunger, pain, tiredness, discomfort, and so on. A sensitive mother who is well tuned to her child's communication signals can, as a rule, distinguish between different tones of crying telling her what help and assistance the child needs. Crying attracts the attention of carers to take appropriate action to remove the causes of crying. On the other hand, peaceful sleeping, or just looking around and cooing, tells carers that the child is relaxed and satisfied. Again, smiling and cooing are powerful signals in-forming adults that the child enjoys interaction with them and seeks their presence.

A child's communication with adults increases with age: it will begin to understand what is wanted from him or her, and what care-givers mean by using different tones of voice or facial expressions. During the first six months of a child's life, carers and babies tend to engage in social interaction which concerns them only. Adults tend to imitate a child's voice, and make affectionate noises to elicit a response from the baby. After six months babies become more aware of their surroundings, and begin to recognise people as familiar figures and show joy at seeing them. At about nine months there are important developments in communication. Babies point to the things and objects they want to have or are curious about, using babbling and words such as 'dada', 'mama'. If care-giver–child interaction is positive and encouraging, and if the child feels at ease in the presence of the carer, communication (both verbal and non-verbal) will rapidly develop.

During the second year the child increasingly begins to understand adult speech and can respond to simple commands. Vocabulary gradually grows, using more words and putting some together. At about 18 months there is rapid expansion in language and ability to communicate more clearly, widely, and precisely. At this stage children also begin to play more independently: they can concentrate better and pick up some messages from adult conversa-tions. Children between 2 and 2½ years are capable of understanding simple verbal messages and can hold simple conversations, answer questions, or ask for what they want and convey what they want to do.

Apart from the use of language, children of all ages can understand and use non-verbal signalling. They often attach more importance to non-verbal communication than speech as they may be trying to provide the answers they think the adults want to hear, rather than trying to say what they themselves think and feel. Children who are maltreated will use non-verbal communication more often to express pain, anxiety, and fear because of emotional confusion and deeply felt insecurity in their relationship with carers. The communication of failure-to-thrive toddlers with their carers and their social interaction with them is somewhat qualitatively different to their thriving siblings or to the normative control groups: probably because they may be undernourished they will have less energy for robust activities. It could also be that siblings and parents perceive them as preferring to be left alone. So, the way children communicate and respond to their carers is influenced by their feeling of security or lack of it, trust in adults, responsiveness when in need of comfort, or alleviation of stress, and their experiences in social interaction with people around them. If these experiences have been positive over time, the child will feel at ease, and ready to engage in social behaviour with peers and adults outside the family. However, if early social interaction with the primary care-givers has been anxiety-provoking, confusing, painful or very limited, the child will be apprehensive, fearful, resistant, and incompetent to engage constructively and positively with others. To illustrate serious interactional problems, let us look at the case of Jimmy and Mark.

### The Case of Jimmy and Mark

The case is an example of twins identified as Jimmy and Mark. Jimmy was a chubby, rosy-cheeked, boisterous 2-year-old, who appeared to be a happy, mischievous boy, who ran, played, talked, and laughed. He went to his mother for help and comfort, and cuddled up spontaneously to her; he responded readily to her attention and affection; she smiled at him, provided comfort, showed concern, picked him up, sat him on her lap, played with him, answered his questions, watched his movements, showed pleasure in his achievements, corrected him in an encouraging way, and warned him when he was in danger. Her voice was soft when she talked to him.

On the edge of the room, like a stranger, stood his twin brother, Mark, his posture rigid, staring fixedly. He was a sad, lethargic-looking child, very small and extremely thin; his pale face threw into relief the dark shadows under his eyes; he remained in one spot, as if at attention; he gazed unswervingly at his mother, who took no notice of him. When asked to call Mark over to her she looked in his direction: as she did so her face hardened and her eyes became angry; she addressed him with a peremptory command; and when he hesitated she showed irritation and shouted at him.

Observations of his interaction with the mother confirmed that she never smiled at him, never picked him up, never sat him on her lap, never played with him, never showed satisfaction when he did something praiseworthy, and never encouraged him in the pursuit of new activities. She told him off for minor misdemeanours, and persistently criticised and shamed him. The only physical contact came about when she fed, bathed, or dressed him, and at such times her handling was rough, and she seldom spoke to him. When she approached him he appeared to be frightened, and occasionally burst into tears. He never came to her for comfort or help, and she never approached him, except to carry out the bare essentials of care and control. Living standards in the household were high, and both children were meticulously clean, well dressed, and materially well provided for. However, Jimmy and Mark did not play together, but Jimmy frequently pushed his brother and smacked him. The ensuing cries of Mark were usually ignored by his mother. Looking at Mark and Jimmy, it was hard to believe that they were twins who were the same weight at birth. At the point when the case was referred to the social services (some two years after the birth of the twins) it was impossible to see that they were exactly the same age, or indeed were twins at all.

## MOTHER–CHILD EARLY INTERACTION

In order to understand the synchrony between mother and child and the way early connectedness develops and influences growth of interaction and relationship, let us look at how a baby interacts with the environment.

It can be observed that a short time after birth a baby begins to make sense of the world around it and to work out what is predictable from interactions with the environment. Interacting with objects, for example, involves short and intense exploration. Interaction with people, however, requires more attention and gives pleasure since there is much more cognitive and affective information to be gained, and this information may change rapidly and frequently. The baby is unable to maintain a high level of concentration for a long time, so a cyclical pattern of attention and inattention is used. As Brazelton (1981), and Brazelton *et al.* (1974) note:

> [while] interacting with a person all parts of the infant's body move in cyclical patterns, outward to the person (attention) and back towards his body (non-attention).

The ebb-and-flow of attention occurs several times per minute. Without an economical homeostatic model he might easily be overwhelmed by the many cues flowing from another human in a short period of time.

As the infant in the interaction with a person approaches the peak of his attention cycle, he slowly reaches out and coos, his eyes dilate, his head moves backward, and his face brightens. He then appears to reach a limit and begins to turn away. This begins the cycle of non-attention in which the infant seems to recover or readjust. When in synchrony, his mother increases her interaction in intensity and frequency as he approaches the peak of his attention cycle, then reduces her interaction as he shifts to non-attention.

Mother and infant seem to become synchronous when they develop well-balanced attention/non-attention cycles so that the attention is not overloaded. However, problems can occur when mothers misinterpret their baby's signals. For example, some mothers will put the baby down when he or she breaks eye-contact, thus stopping the interaction. They believe that the baby has signalled that it wants the interaction to end and not merely that it needs a 'breather'. Alternatively, some mothers will not let the baby look away, but instead will move and follow its gaze. An infant who is constantly bombarded by an insensitive mother will quickly establish a pattern of prolonged non-attention and brief periods of attention (Brazelton, 1981).

The cyclical nature of this interaction is well demonstrated by Field's study. Field (1984) watched how a mother spontaneously interacted with her three-month-old baby. During play, the mother looked at the baby 70% of the time and the baby spent 70% of the time looking at the mother. When the mother was asked to stimulate the baby and get his attention, her activity increased from 70% to 80%. However, the baby's gazing at the mother went down to 50% of the time. The baby was taking his attention off his mother because he was being overloaded. When asked to mimic her baby the mother slowed her pace and her activity went from 70% to 50%. The baby began to look at her more often. Mothers of high-risk infants in Field's study spontaneously spent not 70% but nearly 85% of their time stimulating their babies. These infants looked at their mothers only about 45% of the time. When Field asked the mother to stimulate the baby, her activity went to nearly 100% and the baby's looking at the mother went from 45% to 35% of each minute. However, when she asked the mother to mimic the baby, to move at the baby's pace, the baby's gazing at the mother increased to 70%.

This may help to explain why some mothers of failure-to-thrive infants who are desperate to get their children to react to them may experience such negative results. The truth of the matter may be that the harder they try to get the child's attention, the more they overload the child's system and the more the child may withdraw. The mothers may simply be trying too hard. It may be possible, for example, that if the mother suffers from depression just after the birth, she may be less responsive to her child's signals and unable to tune in to the child's interactional needs. The child may not receive enough stimulation from the mother, and may withdraw from the interaction. If the mother later recovers from depression and wants to get the child to interact with her, it will be doubly difficult since the harder she tries, the more the child will withdraw. Perhaps if the mother mimicked the child's behaviour, then the interaction would move at a more mutually beneficial pace that both partners would enjoy. It is also possible that, when the mother insists, a baby takes a bottle and sucks at the speed she thinks is right, she might be overloading the child's system. The child's reaction tends to be one of anxiety, fighting back, pushing the bottle away, stretching, often vomiting, and crying.

## THE INFLUENCE OF THE CHILD'S TEMPERAMENTAL CHARACTERISTICS ON THE PARENT–CHILD INTERACTION

It has to be stressed that in any interaction there is a two-way process: in this context the infant and the care-giver will both contribute to the interaction and influence each other's behaviours. The infant's behaviour will be influenced by its own characteristics as well as prior experiences. The child and the carer shape up each other's behaviour as each child has an individual way of responding to his environment, an idiosyncratic pattern of behaviour which is not totally determined by the way the child is brought up, or where, or by whom. The New York longitudinal study, conducted by Thomas *et al.* (1968) on 136 infants, increased our understanding of such individual differences in temperament: it demonstrated that certain children with so-called 'difficult temperaments' (which are evident soon after birth) produced problems for parents such that they were unable (or found it extremely exhausting) to cope with the child and its rearing. Such infants were resistant to child-rearing. In many of the fraught confrontations that arose, parent–child interactions led to distressing and deviant outcomes. Seventy per cent of the children classified as 'difficult' developed serious behaviour problems.

Thomas, Chess and Birch found three distinguished clusters of temperamental characteristics which were grouped under the terms of 'difficult babies', 'easy babies', and those who were 'slow to warm up'. The *difficult child* showed irregularity in biological functioning, a predominance of negative-withdrawal responses to new stimuli, slowness in adapting to changes in the environment, a high frequency of expression of negative moods, and a predominance of intense reactions. The *easy child*, on the other hand, was positive in moods, highly regular, low or mild in the intensity of his reactions, rapidly adaptable, and usually positive in his approach to new situations. In short, his temperamental organisation was such that it usually made his early care very easy. The child is rewarding to his mother and vice versa. The third temperamental type—the *slow to warm up*—combined negative responses of mild intensity to new stimuli with slow adaptability after repeated contact. An infant with such characteristics differs from the difficult child, in that he withdraws from anything new quietly rather than loudly. In addition, he does not exhibit the intense reactions, frequent negative moods, and irregularity of biological functions of the difficult child. Iwaniec (1983) found interesting differences between non-organic FTT children and the two control groups: 40% of the sample was classified as temperamentally difficult, 30% as slow to warm up, and 30% as easy children. Many of the failure-to-thrive children were predisposed to difficulties from the word go, and their management, not surprisingly, was difficult from early on in their lives. Given vulnerable parents as well, the stage is set for unrewarding, and indeed aversive, parent–child interactions.

It can be seen that different temperaments may influence the interaction with the care-giver, and possibly care given to the child. Derivan (1982) suggests that FTT children are hard to handle from birth and that their temperaments could be classified as 'difficult'. It is also possible that infants who fail to thrive do not provide satisfactory cues to initiate or maintain positive contacts. For example, Wolke et al. (1990) found that FTT infants had more ambiguous signals, such as when they were hungry, whether they wanted to eat slower or faster, etc. When this 'difficult' temperament is coupled with a mother who has difficulties interpreting her infant's signals, then poor interactions will result. However, research has shown that infants described as difficult during their early days can become happy, easy toddlers when given sensitive mothering. In the same way, insensitive or rejecting mothering can turn placid newborns into anxious, moody, demanding, or awkward toddlers (Bowlby, 1988a). It may also be possible that there is a mismatch between a child's temperament and its parent's expectations. For example, the 'slow-to-warm-up' child may never reach the required level of stimulation before an impatient parent breaks off the interaction.

As Dowdney et al. (1985) note, parenting 'skills' are thought to include sensitivity to children's cues and a

> responsiveness to the differing needs at different developmental stages: in social problem-solving; coping skills; in knowing how to talk and play with children; and in the use of disciplinary techniques that are effective in the triple sense of bringing about the desired child-behaviour, doing so in a way that results in harmony and increasing the child's self-control.

In an ideal situation there will be synchrony between the mother and her infant. Each will respond to the other, and in this way the interaction will be mutually enjoyable and positive. Both mother and infant must correctly interpret and respond to each other's signals in a sensitive way, each influencing the behaviour of the other. In accordance with Schnierla's model of an optimal range of arousal or stimulation (Stern, 1985), the baby is always peripherally monitoring the mother. If she does not provide enough stimulation the baby does not centre his attention on her. If she provides too much, on the other hand, the baby will turn away.

The process of interaction can be as follows:

mother unresponsive to child's cues (may be influenced by factors
such as depression);
↓
child actively seeks to start interaction;
↓
mother does not respond;
↓
child does not receive positive reinforcement for making effort;
↓
child increases behaviour to start interaction;
↓
mother again fails to respond;
↓
and
↓
child withdraws.

In the same way the mother can be conditioned to the child's behaviour:

lack of synchrony between infant and mother;
↓
child sends ambiguous cues;
↓
mother responds by taking part in interaction;
↓
child's attention peaks and then begins period of inattention (normal cycle);
↓
mother misinterprets signal, and tries to continue interaction with child;
↓
child withdraws from interaction, and experiences stimulation overload;
↓
mother feels rejected, gains negative reinforcement from child's withdrawal;
↓
and
↓
mother withdraws from interaction.

As Stern (1985) postulates:

the interaction is a two-way street. If there is something wrong with the baby
so that it cannot put its stimulation into the system, then the infant-elicited
maternal behaviours will not appear. As a result, the stimulation within the
system remains low because the baby is not a good elicitor.

Many mothers whose children are failing to thrive are unable to engage their children in satisfying attention/non-attention cycles (Derivan, 1982). This might become a chronic problem in time and might influence the pattern of feeding in a negative way which, in turn, might affect the intake of food leading to poor weight gain and disturbed development. Failure to establish psychosomatic harmony in the feeding/eating behaviour early in a child's life would appear to be symptomatic in failure-to-thrive children and their mothers.

It is important to note that we all influence our environments by the way in which we act. For example, in social interchanges the behaviour of one person exerts some degree of control over the actions of others (Rausch, 1965). If a child exhibits hostile responses, this is likely to elicit unfriendly reactions from other children, whereas a child who is friendly will receive more cordial responses. Difficult children tend to create, through their actions, a hostile environment, whereas children who display friendly interpersonal modes of response tend to generate an amicable social milieu (Iwaniec, 1983). In the same way, babies and children who are hard to feed and to care for may create an anxious or hostile response from their parents. Taking into account that many children who fail to thrive have been labelled as 'difficult' from birth, this perhaps encourages care-givers to interact with them in a particular way. Qualitative differences in mother–child interaction and the corresponding effect have been found in several studies (Pollitt & Eichler, 1976; Powell *et al.*, 1987; Skuse, 1988; Iwaniec, 1991; Hanks & Hobbs, 1993; Raynor & Rudolf, 1996).

## PILOT STUDY

The author conducted a pilot study on parent–child interaction with eight failure-to-thrive children, using their 14 siblings as a control group. The children were recruited from the GP files. The age range of FTT was between 11 months and 3 years, and the control siblings were between 9 months and $5\frac{1}{2}$ years. The aim of the pilot study was to compare the quality of interaction in terms of maternal responsiveness to the signalled needs of children; frequency of signalling; responsiveness to those signals; parental sensitivity in dealing with distress; parental initiation of interaction with their children; the length of time spent involved with the child when dealing with the specific task; and the emotional tone (negative or positive) when dealing with different children. Additionally, parental thoughts and ideas regarding failure-to-thrive problems were discussed and examined in order to understand parental perceptions, observations, and interpretation from their point of view. The data were collected by the use of direct observation, using strict protocol to record positive and negative parental responses and children's reactions. Two sessions in each family were video-taped, played back, and then the content examined with the parents in order to elicit parental understanding and interpretation regarding their different responses to different children. Parent–child and child–parent reactive and proactive behaviour checklists (Iwaniec *et al.*, 1985a) were used to measure the frequency and nature of parental involvement with their children, and apprehension or easiness of children when approaching or reacting to their parents' interaction with them. Semi-structured interviews were conducted to examine parental attitudes towards each child and to take the social history.

The results of this detailed study clearly indicated that interaction of parents with their FTT children was more anxious and based on necessity to intervene or to react rather than on willingness and pleasure in doing so. All mothers stated that constant battles with feeding and other aspects of caring did not give them a sense of a job well done or a sense of satisfaction. Three out of eight mothers felt that their rapport with the FTT child was significantly different to that with their other children, stating that the child was far more difficult to care for and enjoy, and that they had less positive feedback from it. Two children were described as spiteful, deliberately disrupting other children's play or breaking their toys; reluctant to answer questions; ignoring requests; and being attention-seeking. Mothers of the three youngest FTT children reported preoccupations with their children's poor weight, with feeding, with worrying about their child's health, and with thinking that there was something physically wrong.

Observation of interaction with four failure-to-thrive children showed excessive interference and faulty interpretation of the cues presented by the children. For example, a baby's irritability and uneasiness were interpreted as indicative of being hungry (in spite of having been fed half an hour previously with a good intake of food and milk) and not as a child's need for a nappy-change. In another case, a response to a child's five minutes of crying was rocking, giving toys, and singing (instead of feeding, as the child was fed four hours previously with apparently little intake of food). In six cases the mothers responded to their FTT children's signals of distress less frequently, and it took them twice as long to attend to the failure-to-thrive child in comparison to its siblings. The manner, in terms of tone of voice, show of concern, firmness in dealing with each child, actual action taken, and the suitability of that action, was somewhat different between failure-to-thrive children and their siblings. In response to FTT children, the mothers were less attentive, less vocal when soothing or dealing with them, more confused in reading their distress, less sensitive when resolving conflict between children, and had less eye-contact and physical closeness than with their other children.

Four out of eight felt that their FTT children preferred to be left alone, and three perceived them as odd and difficult to understand. However, three mothers did not see much difference between their FTT and other children in terms of the way they felt about them and the number of child-rearing problems they presented. Five failure-to-thrive children were more apprehensive and unsure of themselves when interacting with others: these toddlers appeared to be more nervous or hesitant to initiate contact. They also seemed to be more withdrawn and unconnected with their siblings and their activities: the siblings' reactions to them mirrored parental reactions. The mothers spent twice as much time answering siblings' questions, helping them if they were in difficulties, and warning them if they were in danger of harming themselves, than they did with FTT children.

It would appear that mothers and failure-to-thrive children interact less frequently in contrast to their siblings. The interaction was associated with responses to a problem and seldom initiated as a need for stimulation or personal desire to do things with the child. In cases where frequency of interaction was higher it tended to be of interfering quality influenced by ill-judged interpretations of the child's signals. These mothers were not emotionally demonstrative generally to all their children: they were more reserved, less sensitive, and generally less engaged in their children's activities. They tended to perceive FTT children as less rewarding to be with, more anxiety-provoking in terms of their growth and development, less affectionate, as more passive, and as indifferent to their caregiving activities. Interestingly, the history of these mothers' interaction with their mothers as children showed a remarkably similar pattern. They felt their mothers were rather distant and not always ready to engage with them.

Half of them stated that the struggle to feed their FTT children was considerable, and they believed that failure-to-thrive children did not need much food and did not like eating. Additionally, they tended to associate their smallness and thinness to genetic factors, connecting them with different members of the family, e.g. grandparents, uncles, aunts, and so on. It can be seen that the combination of limited involvement, or over-involvement, faulty perceptions, and inaccurate interpretations of the children's signals can lead to less effective and pleasurable parent–child interaction. When these mothers were asked what they thought about the presenting problem and what was their diagnosis of failure to thrive, they saw it as something very specific to a failure-to-thrive child, e.g. being over-sensitive, slow in feeding, slow in reaction to their contact with them, more miserable and difficult to care for, and unsatisfactory in many ways. Five mothers stated that they might have contributed to feeding difficulties as they rushed their children to eat, instead of taking time and going at their speed. Four felt that problems became worse when solids were introduced and when they became more forceful. Interestingly, they observed better and quicker intake of food when being fed by a grandmother, friend, or neighbour (who were perceived as having more patience, as being more positive, and as feeding the children without fussing or getting anxious).

The following perceptions and interpretations were given which fell into the anxious, worrying type, or the angry or dismissive one:

- 'There must be something wrong with her, she might be ill or something';
- 'He is not a great eater, does not need much food';
- 'Children do not starve themselves, he will eat when really hungry';
- 'She is doing it on purpose, just to be difficult';
- 'There is nothing wrong with him. I do not know what the fuss is all about';
- 'She is just small, that's all. I have no time to fuss, she is just stubborn and awkward';
- 'It is best for him to be put somewhere away from me, so we do not irritate each other';
- 'It is difficult to like being with a child who causes you so much misery.'

Parental reactions to experienced difficulties are worth mentioning as they have to be addressed during therapeutic intervention. These are a few of them:

- 'I feel embarrassed and guilty when people remark about his thin and miserable appearance';
- 'I know they think I am deliberately starving him, and not looking after him properly';
- 'People talk about me, and stare at both of us when we are out';
- 'When I take her to the health centre and she has not gained weight they ask me questions which suggest that I am a bad mother, that I neglect her and tell me how to feed and handle her, which does not work. They are quick to criticise but do not really help';
- 'I am petrified to see the health visitor or the doctor, as they may think that I have not done what they asked me to do. It simply does not work. Why don't they try?';
- 'I often go out when I know that the health visitor is coming. It will only upset me. She may even send a social worker to see whether I am cruel to her';
- 'I am so worried about her that I cannot sleep or enjoy myself. I constantly think what to cook and how to make her eat so she gains some weight'.

In comparison to their other children they were hard work, and a constant worry. A statement of one mother summarises it all:

> Rick is a constant worry to me. He looks as though I starve him, he behaves as though I neglect him, he reacts to me as though he does not trust me, or is frightened of me. I have never hit him or been cruel to him. I fight over him with my family as they think I do not pay enough attention to him. I argue with my GP and health visitor regarding his health as I think there must be something not quite right with him. I do whatever they want me to do and I get more anxious, more disillusioned, and more angry, which I know does not help Rick. Quite often we are both in such a state that I am not surprised that he can't eat. If I could relax more and not worry so much about his weight, and not feel a failure and be sure that others would not judge me as a bad mother, we both would be better off. He puts pressure on me and I put pressure on him. We are both failing to thrive.

## WHAT CAN GO WRONG?

Let us look at what tends to go wrong. As has been noted, there are two partners in the interaction, and in the early days it usually involves a mother and child. We have also seen how the synchronous relationship can be successful and mutually satisfying for both players in the interaction. It is important to examine what happens when one partner fails to keep his or her side of the bargain and does not behave as expected. When the mother under-stimulates she does not meet the baby's expectation for interaction. Brazelton (1981), in his experimental work with the mother–child dyad, observed that when mothers were asked to maintain still-face for three minutes after three weeks of normal interaction, the infant became aware that this normal expectation was not being fulfilled. The child attempted to elicit a response, followed by waiting periods. The extent and urgency of the attempt to elicit a response was quite impressive. After repeated failure to get his mother back on track, he withdrew and seemed to expect no response. It is striking that in failure-to-thrive infants the withdrawal is seen, in the extreme, as wariness and aversion. However, after repeated reassuring contact with care-givers (especially when they learn the baby's rhythms), the non-thriving infant begins to interact and becomes more responsive. Brazelton noted that a baby can develop 'an appetite', a greediness that allows him/her to feel at ease to go from one person to another without fear. He further proposed that if the scaling responsiveness is encouraged this would later lead into deepening attachment to one or two care-givers which is closely followed by a rapid gain in weight. He argued that in order to develop a psycho-physiological mechanism for gaining weight, the infant must first be given rewarding emotional experiences. How those rewarding emotional experiences contribute to the development of secure attachment and an affectionate relationship will be discussed in the next chapter.

## SUMMARY

The importance of anxiety-free and positive interactions during the acts of feeding and other areas of a child's and parents' mutual contacts and activities were discussed. The ways children learn to respond to parental overtures and stimulation, and what determines development of effective communication was explored, as well as the effects of individual characteristics of children and parents. The way both sides of the dyad interact together and influence each other was emphasised. A pilot study measuring the level, quality, and nature of parents' and FTT children's interactions in comparison to the siblings was presented.

# CHILD–PARENT ATTACHMENT BEHAVIOUR OF CHILDREN WHO FAIL TO THRIVE AND PARENTAL RESPONSIVENESS

*Children begin by loving their parents; after a time they judge them; rarely, if ever, do they forgive them.*

Oscar Wilde, 1893

## INTRODUCTION

To understand better how children develop an affectionate bond with their parents or what stands in the way to distort such development, a discussion of attachment behaviour is necessary. As a considerable number of children who fail to thrive are insecurely attached to their mothers, we need to understand why this is the case so that preventive strategies can be designed to help the child and the parents (who are often bereft of hope).

Ainsworth (1982) postulated that there is some basic behavioural system that has evolved in social species that leads individuals to seek to maintain proximity even when conditions are not satisfactory. Findings that infants become attached even to abusive parents strongly suggest that the system is not driven by simple associations such as meeting basic human needs, but also by genetic predisposition.

Ethologists believe that humans are predisposed to make strong emotional bonds with particular individuals throughout their lives: during infancy, children bond to their care-givers who offer them protection, comfort, and assistance. These bonds are likely to persist for the rest of that individual's life, and later during adolescence and adulthood are complemented by other relationships such as those with sexual partners (Bowlby, 1988a). Many studies have examined how these attachments develop throughout life and, more specifically, how an individual's early experiences with care-givers may influence later attachments.

Bowlby (1973) proposed that the need for security is the prime motivator and this derives from a child's appraisal of an attachment-figure's availability. He further argued that, apart from the physical attachment-figure's availability, the infant must believe that the attachment-figure will be available when needed at times of distress. If security is felt, there is trust, and intimacy is possible so the care-giver can be allowed to separate from the child without undue stress, when it is known that such separation is only temporary. Bowlby (1973) made a point that even ready accessibility to a care-giver is not enough to establish security for the child. Apart from the physical presence of a primary care-giver there must be emotional presence as well. The need for a baby to have emotionally responsive parents when feeling hungry, or tired, when experiencing frightening and confusing events, or when a child is uncertain about the location or behaviour of its parents, is of primary importance. The emotional availability and sensitivity of the parents is at the core of development of secure attachment of the child to his/her parents. (*See* Chapter 11 for further discussion.)

## PARENTAL SENSITIVITY AND FORMATION OF ATTACHMENT

Early studies on attachment (Bowlby, 1973; Ainsworth *et al.*, 1978) defined parental sensitivity as parental ability to perceive and interpret children's attachment signals correctly and to respond to those signals promptly and appropriately. They proposed that early difficulties, lack of parental responsiveness to many of a baby's needs, inconsistency, and insensitivity could lead to feelings of insecurity in children, whereas persistent sensitive responsiveness would build secure bonds between children and parents. Bowlby (1973) also suggested that the parents' childhood attachment experiences would influence the way they respond and relate to their children. Parents who were neglected, both physically and emotionally, or rejected would be prone to neglect or reject their children as well.

The causal role of parental sensitivity in the formation of attachment security is now firmly accepted (De Wolff & Van Ijzendoorn, 1997). The validity of this statement is based on a causal analysis of 66 studies consisting of 4,000 families as well as on intervention studies directed at parental sensitivity. It was found that the correlational studies on parental sensitivity and infant attachment security showed a consistent association, indicating that more sensitive parents have more secure children. The results of the intervention studies also support the correlation evidence in showing that enhancing parental sensitivity by a means of help and treatment leads to more secure children.

The extent and quality of sensitive responsiveness of the parent to the child will determine either secure or insecure attachment (Isabela *et al.*, 1989).

Ainsworth & Wittig (1969) indicated that there were different forms of attachment to a parent. Rather than measure the amount of attachment, Ainsworth observed the organisation of attachment behaviour. In laboratory conditions, observations were made of the ways children interact with their care-givers, and how they behave when they are separated and reunited with them. These were used to identify three different patterns of attachment behaviour: secure; anxious/resistant; and anxious/avoidant, which will be further described below.

## 1 Secure attachment

Individuals are confident that their care-giver(s) will be available, responsive, and helpful should they encounter adverse or frightening situations. The care-giver(s) is/are seen as readily available, sensitive to the child's signals, and responsive when the child seeks protection, comfort, or assistance. This security builds confidence in the child, encourages exploration and competence, and is thought to be consistent with healthy development. These infants use the attachment-figure as a secure base from which to explore.

## 2 Anxious/resistant attachment or resistant insecure

Children are uncertain that their care-giver(s) will be available, responsive, or helpful when needed. The care-giver(s) is/are less predictable with responses, being available and helpful on some occasions but not on others. The pattern is also promoted by separations from the care-giver and threats of abandonment used as a means of control. The child tends to be clingy and anxious about exploring the world and may suffer from separation-anxiety (Bowlby, 1988a). These infants fail to move away from the attachment-figure and show little exploration. They are also highly distressed by separations and are difficult to settle after reunion (Rutter, 1995b). Neglected children tend to be anxiously attached to their care-givers.

## 3 Anxious/avoidant attachment or avoidant insecure

Individuals expect to be rejected by their care-giver(s) when they seek support or care. The care-giver(s) constantly rebuff(s) the child when approached for care or protection, and as a result these children will attempt to live their lives without the love and support of others. If this pattern persists, these children may later be prone to a variety of personality disorders, from compulsively self-sufficient individuals to persistently delinquent ones (Bowlby, 1988a). These children explore with little reference to the attachment-figure and seem to show ignoring or avoidant behaviour on reunion (Rutter, 1995a).

During the last decade a fourth category of disorganised/disorientated pattern has been identified by Main and Solomon (1986). The behaviour of these children did not easily fit into any of the other categories: for example, children with a known history of abuse and neglect may be classified as secure, although their behaviour outside of the 'Strange Situation' test (*see* below) may indicate abnormalities (Rutter, 1995a). These children show inconsistent behaviour, confusion, and indecision. They tend to freeze or show stereotyped behaviour such as rocking. This behaviour is thought to result from an extremely unpredictable care-giver's interactive behaviour. Conflict behaviour results because the source of security for the infant is also a source of fear. Many children who fail to thrive fall into the disoriented/disorganised attachment style.

## ATTACHMENT AND FAILURE TO THRIVE

Social interaction and attachment behaviour of failure-to-thrive children to their mothers has been studied by many researchers over the years using observational measures and *Strange Situation Protocols*. They found differences in parental responsiveness, sensitivity, demonstration of affect, and perceived attribution of the child. Let us look at some of the studies.

Kotelchuck *et al.* (1981) observed infant behaviour with the mother, with the mother and a stranger, with the stranger alone, and with the mother alone upon her return. The researchers used failure-to-thrive infants as an experimental group and a control group of infants hospitalised for various medical reasons. They found that both groups of infants demonstrated attachment–separation protest and stranger anxiety, and both groups similarly explored the room and played with toys in the same way.

However, the failure-to-thrive group reacted to being left with a stranger in qualitatively different ways during separation from their mothers. The experimental group of infants showed less distress when left with the stranger in terms of crying or verbal protestation, and recovered from the mother's departure more quickly than the control group. It was observed that failure-to-thrive infants appeared to have a flat effect and low frequency of initiated verbalisation. This research indicated manifestation of insecure attachment style of FTT children to their mothers and concluded that failure-to-thrive children were cognitively aware of social events, but effectively inappropriate.

Gordon and Jameson (1979) studied 12 failure-to-thrive hospitalised children and a control group also drawn from the hospital population. Using *Strange Situation Protocols*, the results showed that 50% of FTT infants were insecurely attached while only 10% of controls were classified as insecure. The experimental group showed lower affective response, fretting during separation compared to the control children who would cry as well as fret. The samples of both groups were drawn from the hospital population; therefore the environment and conditions were the same at testing for all children and results should be seen as valid.

Ward *et al.*'s second study (2000) provided further evidence for the co-occurrence of atypical patterns of attachment and failure to thrive. They studied 83 children with FTT and 130 normally growing comparison children using Ainsworth's *Strange Situation* at ages 11 to 32 months. These subjects came from all social and economic backgrounds. Children who failed to thrive were significantly less likely to show secure attachment and more likely to show anxious, disorganised/disorientated attachment styles than the normally growing comparison. Only 34% of failure-to-thrive children were secure, while 46% showed disorganised attachments. In contrast, 66% of the comparison children were secure and 16% were disorganised. In addition, a sub-sample of 59 mothers (23 failure to thrive and 36 comparison) were interviewed with the *Adult Attachment Interview (AAI)*. Mothers of FTT children were more than twice as likely as the comparison (65% versus 22%) to use discourse indicating unresolved loss or trauma. Similarly, mothers of FTT children were less likely to show autonomous (secure) discourse than mothers of well-nourished children (13% versus 58%). Interestingly, they did not find differences in infant or adult attachment classification between organic and non-organic failure-to-thrive groups, which supports abandonment of such division. Ward and her colleagues' findings support other studies in this area that disturbed patterns of attachment are common amongst failure-to-thrive children, regardless of the aetiology of growth failure. This further confirms that failure to thrive is closely associated with disturbed interaction and relationship. These findings strongly suggest that evaluation and treatment of FTT should address psychological/social, as well as medical, problems in these families.

Children who are failing to thrive are more likely to show insecure attachment. Dawson (1992) describes three studies in support of this:

1. Among children from families with a wide range of income, children who failed to thrive (organic or non-organic) had higher rates of insecure attachment than controls (64% versus 36%) (Ward *et al.*, 1993);
2. Among children who failed to thrive, who were abused and neglected by their parents and referred to protective services, 92% of children were insecurely attached compared to 33% of controls (Crittenden, 1987);
3. In Santiago, Chile, chronically undernourished children had a higher prevalence of insecure attachment (93%) than did controls (50%); and
4. Iwaniec's (1983) study showed significant differences between failure-to-thrive children and two control groups—FTT children being insecurely attached in 70% of cases in comparison to 40% in the first and 25% in the second control group.

Let us look at a few cases to illustrate different types of attachment behaviour and the possible explanation as to why this is the case.

## Robbie's Case

Robbie was aged 2 years 8 months when the present writer first met him. He had to be asked several times whether the stated age was right as he was very small and thin, and looked very unhealthy. His language consisted of many unconnected words and his social behaviour was immature. However, the interaction with his mother was striking. During the visit, which lasted for about an hour and a half, Robbie kept away from his mother, but positioned himself in front of her at 2–3 metres distance, looking intensely and persistently into her face. If she moved, he moved, but was constantly trying to have her in his vision. The only time the mother looked in his direction was when she criticised him or when she was making complaints about his difficult behaviour. The mother's facial expression was hard and her eyes were angry. She said that he was stubborn and destructive; that he broke toys, tore wallpaper, and cut his clothes; that he deliberately wet his bed; that he wandered around the house at night looking for food; and that when he was given food he would not eat it. She described an event of alleged food refusal. At 6pm he was given three fish fingers, some mashed potatoes and some peas. He only ate a small corner of one fish finger, so he was put to bed, but awoke at 10pm to finish his meal. The mother went to bed at 10.30pm, leaving Robbie with her partner to finish the meal. At 12.30am she was woken up by the partner screaming in exasperation as Robbie had still not eaten the meal, and that there must be something wrong with the child and he was washing his hands of Robbie.

As a result of prolonged emotional and physical maltreatment Robbie showed extremely disturbed behaviour at the nursery; because of his short concentration span he was not included in the story-reading as he disrupted other children's listening. He showed no ability for social play with other children, was aggressive, disruptive, and lacked impulse control. He tried to climb out of an upstairs window and set fire to his bedroom.

Interaction between the mother and Robbie was extremely antagonistic. She found him unrewarding, believing that he deliberately behaved in a defiant attention-seeking manner, so she spent as little time as possible with him and when she did, her approach was harsh or silent. She claimed that he did not love her but would attach himself to strangers and call them Mummy. She felt there was no point showing him affection. He did not want it. After six missed appointments in hospital he was eventually admitted and diagnosed as suffering from severe failure to thrive of long duration. His weight and height were well below the 3rd percentile. Both parents were tall—the mother was 5ft 7in and the father 6ft 1in. When in hospital Robbie made remarkable progress in terms of both his physical growth and social behaviour. In the first few days he responded to warmth, encouragement, and routine in a very confused way, either being extremely attention-seeking, following nurses and doctors around constantly asking whether this was his home now and what was for dinner, or being uncommunicative and apprehensive. He tended to attack other children, slapping them across the face for no apparent reason. During the second week he calmed down, became more stable and responsive, and his preoccupation with food was substantially reduced. Within 10 days he put on 9 lb. in weight. His mother and her partner seldom visited. The mother said that she felt embarrassed because he would prefer to be with nurses and other staff rather than with her. On his return home Robbie lost weight rapidly and his behaviour worsened. The same pattern was witnessed when he went to a foster-home and when he was discharged back home.

Robbie's attachment to his mother was avoidant as a result of highly insensitive and rejecting parenting of long duration. Robbie's behaviour reflected his unhappiness and confusion. He had developed a negative self-image as being unworthy to be loved or to have anything belonging to him.

*Problems identified in this case were both historical and current:*

1. The mother had a history of being rejected by her mother, and had little experience of being nurtured in a caring, warm, and sensitive way;
2. Lack of parenting skills and understanding of children's basic developmental needs;
3. Robbie's prematurity and associated problems, such as difficulty in feeding and generally managing the child;
4. Misinterpretation of Robbie's signals of distress, and hostile responsiveness over a long time, resulting in insecure attachment;
5. Maternal immaturity and lack of insight into Robbie's unhappiness and distress;
6. Rejecting parenting resulting in a painful relationship and hostile interaction between Robbie and his mother;
7. Serious emotional problems presented by Robbie at home and in the nursery;
8. Developmental delays in all areas;
9. Stunting of growth due to emotional abuse; and
10. Maternal lack of co-operation with helping agencies and professionals and refusal to carry out instructions and advice.

## Jane's Case

Jane was born prematurely to a 17-year-old mother, who had spent all her childhood in care. She deliberately got pregnant as she wanted to have someone who would belong to her and who would love her. She tried very hard to provide good care for her daughter with extensive help from the community centre, but found it difficult to understand Jane's signals of distress and the need to respond appropriately and quickly to Jane's needs. Quite often Jane was given cold milk straight from the fridge or stale milk when the mother came back from town and Jane was crying with hunger. Jane's refusal to take feeds was interpreted by her mother as not being hungry, so she rocked her, tapped, sang, or put the dummy into her mouth to stop her crying. Not only was Jane not putting on weight but she was losing it. She became irritable, unsettled, and generally distressed, while her mother became more anxious, helpless, and disillusioned with her romantic notion of having a perfect child who would give only pleasure. Her child care became unpredictable. When she was in a better mood and felt more energetic she would interact well with Jane, and would change, bathe, and feed her, but when Jane cried or was restless she would just become anxious, lock herself in a bathroom, put the radio on in order not to hear her cry, and smoke cigarettes. The mother refused to co-operate with social services and the health visitor as she felt they would take her daughter away. She claimed that the community centre did not tell her anything she did not know, and that the health visitor expected her to do impossible things, which she tried to do but the advice given was not working in practice. She loved her daughter when she was good, i.e. sleeping, feeding, and when being quiet, but was neglectful and unresponsive when she was crying, keeping her awake at night, or when she was irritable.

Jane was assessed as ambivalently attached to her mother because of unpredictable maternal behaviour. Sometimes the mother responded to her needs in a nurturing and sensitive manner, but at other times left her unattended and distressed. Lack of constancy in emotional availability was not conducive to building trust and secure feelings so that comfort and satisfaction would be provided when needed.

*This case demonstrates:*

1. A serious lack of parenting skills;
2. Maternal immaturity and poor insight;
3. Unawareness of children's basic developmental needs and lack of knowledge of how to facilitate meeting these needs;
4. Insecure attachment stemming from insensitivity and inconsistency in responding to Jane's needs; and
5. Inability to take advice and work co-operatively with professionals.

## Nicola's Case

Nicola was diagnosed as failing to thrive at $4^1/_2$ months. Both parents were concerned about her poor weight gain and were extremely worried about their inability to feed her and about the limited intake of food that Nicola took at each feed. They described feeding time as a battle of wills with Nicola screaming, pushing the bottle away, stretching, and eventually vomiting, and the mother becoming worried, anxious, and depressed. They tried various ways to hold and feed her as well as giving her different milk formulas but with little effect. They followed instructions and advice given by the health visitor and the family doctor, but there was no improvement. The mother was told by her GP that she must try harder and not to feel sorry for herself. She was also told that there was no point in referring Nicola to the paediatrician as he felt there was nothing wrong with her. In despair the mother started force-feeding her, which resulted in more vomiting and in panic reactions whenever she was approached to be fed. The mother became totally demoralised and depressed, worrying that Nicola might die and that there was nobody who was willing to help her and her daughter. The situation became so serious that the father approached the author for help. Nicola was eventually admitted to hospital for medical investigation, where she was diagnosed as having malabsorption problems. Prior to admission to hospital the interaction between the mother and the child became anxious, frightened, and at times angry, and eventually very passive due to maternal depression and loss of self-confidence. Nicola's attachment to her mother seemed to be disoriented and confused at times of great stress such as force-feeding and constant battles associated with feeding, while obviously she was in pain. Nicola's experience of the world around her was anxiety-provoking,

> painful, and did not serve as a secure base where relief and comfort would be provided when in distress or pain. Her attachment to her mother and father was of disoriented type as the quality of their nurturing differed, being harshing and pain-inducing when feeding her and warm and sensitive with other care-giving tasks.

*The following problems were identified:*

1. Lack of medical diagnosis when the problems began to emerge, creating serious problems of mother–child interaction;
2. Disoriented/disorganised attachment behaviour;
3. Maternal depression;
4. Loss of self-confidence by the mother; inadequate intake of food; and
5. Anxious-avoidant interaction during feeding time.

It is important to state that the above problems could have been avoided if appropriate early diagnosis had been made, as both parents were caring and committed to their daughter's well-being.

Ainsworth (1982) suggested how early interactions between mother and baby may produce significant influences on later patterns of attachment. During the first three months after birth, babies who failed to respond to maternal initiations of face-to-face interaction and/or to terminate it once it had begun were more likely to be anxiously attached by the end of their first year. Their mothers tended to be those who maintained neutral or matter-of-fact expression while feeding their children. Mothers whose babies became securely attached were conspicuous for gradual pacing of their behaviour in face-to-face interaction. They were responsive to the attention/non-attention cycles of their infants and paced themselves accordingly.

Close physical contact is an important factor in the communication between a mother and her infant. Ainsworth (1982) found that there was a relationship between maternal holding and the eventual nature of the infant's attachment. Securely attached and anxious/resistant infants tended to respond more positively to close bodily contact and to its cessation compared to anxious/avoidant babies. Mothers who had been relatively tender and careful when holding their babies during the first three months tended to have infants who were securely attached to them at one year. However, mothers who had handled the baby ineptly tended to have anxiously attached children later on. It was not that these mothers held their babies for any less time than the mothers of the other groups; rather the type of holding was qualitatively different, being less tender and more interfering. The mothers of the anxious/avoidant babies also *all* showed a marked aversion to close bodily contact, whereas none of the mothers of the securely and anxiously attached babies did. This was mirrored in the behaviour of their infants: when aged between 9 and 12 months, the anxious/avoidant babies almost never 'sank in', moulding their bodies to the mother's body when held.

Ainsworth (1982) suggests that the way a mother holds her infant may have great consequences for their later interactions. Tender, careful holding in any one quarter significantly influenced positive infant response to being held in later quarters, whereas the reverse was not the case. On the other hand, from the second quarter on, positive infant response to holding did increase maternal affectionate behaviour whereas the reverse was not the case. These two findings together suggest a 'virtuous' spiral. Mothers who are tender and careful early on, gearing their behaviour to the baby's cues, tend to evoke a positive response in the baby which carries over into later quarters. This positive response evokes maternal affectionate behaviour which in turn reinforces positive infant response and so on. First-quarter maternal ineptness seemed to begin a vicious spiral: it was associated with negative infant response to holding later on, but from the second quarter on there was as much evidence for infant negative response being the cause of maternal ineptness as for its being the effect.

Some observations have been made on children who fail to thrive and how they react to close personal contact: they have been described as centring around two extremes, the spastic and rigid babies on the one hand, and the 'floppy' babies, i.e. those with an extreme decrease in muscle tone, 'who practically fall through your hands', at the other. Barbero (1982) concluded that regardless of which extreme they present, the failure-to-thrive children tend to be almost immobile. Mathisen et al. (1989) found in their sample of non-organic failure-to-thrive children, that several of the case infants seemed hypersensitive to tactile stimuli. As Mathisen et al. (1989) note, Crickmay (1955) has described hypersensitivity as 'a distinctive behaviour which normally disappears at 7 to 8 months of age', and Evans-Morris and Klein (1987) regarded it as a sign of neurological impairment.

> When there are already tensions between mother and infant about feeding, an adverse response to a mother's touch could be misinterpreted as a sign of rejection; she might respond by emotional withdrawal resulting in the observed tendency for feeding to be a functional rather than a social occasion for the case infants.

Equally, Iwaniec (1995) and Hanks and Hobbs (1993) observed maternal lack of interest showing itself in the way they held and interacted with their FTT babies while feeding. The head of a baby was not supported, the posture was uncomfortable, and there was very little eye-contact with the baby. These mothers seldom spoke or showed tenderness to the child. There were obvious absences of synchrony which would promote emotional tuning in to each other if they had been present.

The type of attachment which is shown between an infant and its primary care-giver is important because it is shaped by daily interaction and may affect the child's behaviour, not only in the short term but also potentially in the long term. Long-term behavioural consequences of ambivalent or avoidant attachment may include aggressive behaviour in older children, severe feeding problems and cognitive and learning deficits (Hufton & Oates, 1977). For example, Bowlby (1988a) describes one study which examined how mothers interacted with their 2$\frac{1}{2}$-year-old infants who were attempting a task they could not manage without a little help. Mothers of secure toddlers helped their children to focus on the task, did not interfere, and responded with the required help when needed. The mothers of insecure infants were more unpredictable, being less sensitive to toddlers' states of mind, and either giving no support or else interfering when the children did not really need help.

## ADULTS' ATTACHMENT STYLES

It is thought that early attachments will influence later relationships, not only with the mother but also with other individuals. As Rutter (1995a) notes,

> Hazan and Shaver (1987) have provided a useful review of the features of adult relationships that are thought to reflect insecure attachment. These include both a lack of self disclosure; undue jealousy in close relationships; feelings of loneliness even when involved in relationships; reluctance to commitment in relationships; difficulty in making relationships in a new setting and a tendency to view partners as insufficiently attentive. ... Thus, strong claims have been made about the ways in which insecurity in a person's attachment relationship with parents in early childhood influences their relationships in adult life (Main, 1991; Main & Hesse, 1990; Main et al., 1985).

These propositions might partly explain why some mothers of FTT children are classified as having an insecure/unresolved attachment pattern. Benoit, Zeanah and Barton (1989) reported that only one of 23 mothers of 1–8-months-old infants hospitalised for failure to thrive was judged secure/autonomous. Schuengel et al.'s (1999) observation of 85 mothers and their 10–11-month-old FTT infants in their own homes found that mothers presented unresolved/insecure attachment patterns. They exhibited frightened/frightening behaviour during routine feeding, changing, and other care-giving activities. Unresolved mothers whose alternative attachment category was secure did not exhibit frightened/frightening behaviour. This might suggest that an underlying secure/autonomous attachment organisation might act as a buffer between unresolved aspects of a mother's mental state and her behaviour towards her infant. The life history of unresolved mothers has been described as continuously difficult, lacking stability and security, and devoid of any meaningful and sustainable relationship throughout their lives.

It could be said, therefore, that they had no life chances and did not get help to resolve their early insecure experiences.

## WHY SHOULD THESE PROBLEMS OCCUR?

There has been much debate as to why problems in interactions between mothers and their infants may result in failure to thrive. It is not always clear how this defect arises or why it takes the form it does, and what are the factors or parenting styles that might weaken mother–child attachment. Derivan (1982) suggested that failure to thrive and child abuse are associated with the disorders of parenting and other life stresses. Let us look first at dismissing and rejecting mothers.

### Dismissing and Rejecting Mothers

Clinical evidence suggests that a proportion of failure-to-thrive children have experienced dismissing and rejective parenting. This is without much doubt the case of psychosocial short-stature children. Patrick *et al.* (1994) found that between 15 and 23% of people show dismissing patterns of attachment, and that these patterns are distinctive of those who feel anxious in the presence of strong feelings, either in themselves or in other people. Experiences of insensitivity, rejection, interference, and being ignored are associated with insecure attachment. A carer who feels agitated, distressed, or hostile towards her child causes the child particular difficulties, as was demonstrated in Robbie's and Jane's cases. The ways in which the mothers had attempted to deal with their children's feelings and their own agitation was to try to control the children's affective states. Hollburn-Cobb (1996) suggested that the mother might attempt to define how her baby 'ought' to feel or what such feelings mean in a way that suited *her* needs rather than her child's.

Dismissing mothers are reported to have an excessive and unobjective preoccupation with their own attachment relationships or experiences (Crittenden, 1992). This might show as fearful preoccupation and a sense of being overwhelmed by traumatic experiences when dealing with the child, as shown in Jane's case, or it might be more subtle and presented as uncritical or unconvincingly analytical.

Dismissing mothers do not recognise or respect their children's independence. They tend to define their babies' experience in a manner that is often abrupt, impatient, and aggressive. Insensitive mothers fail to read their infants' signals, tending to interact according to their own thoughts, feelings, needs and wants. Cassidy and Berlin (1994) note that the immediate, proximate function of behaviour associated with resistant attachment is to re-cruit more care and attention and this may come out in the form of compulsive care-giving (as shown so clearly in Nicola's case), but here out of desperation and wrong advice. Parents of resistantly attached children were found to be prone to intrude, control, and over-stimulate their children in ways that bore little relation to the child's actual needs, as in the case of Jane, playing with her instead of feeding her properly with the right food.

Dismissing mothers like Robbie's tend to be less emotionally supportive and helpful and tend to be cold and controlling. This seems to be consistent with Robbie's mother's description of her own experience of being pushed to become independent as a child. Such mothers were found by Belsky and Cassidy (1994) as least responsive and affectionate with their children, proba-bly because they had insensitive care in their own infancy. The mother's state of mind seems to indicate an attempt to limit the influence of attachment rela-tionships. There is a claim to strength, normality, and independence. There is an over-reliance upon 'felt security', and this is achieved by an over-reliance on the self and under-reliance on other people. This is the reason why help is often not accepted, as they feel they can manage themselves. There is evidence of poor insight and poorly developed critical self-evaluation.

Mothers classified as dismissing were found in Van Ijzendoorn's (1995) meta-analysis to be disproportionately likely to have children classified as avoidant or resistant. As the children became adults, such individuals ex-perienced increased unease and nervousness about entering into close rela-tionships at times when greater intimacy is expected, such as marriage or parenthood. However, changes in attachment style are possible if the right conditions occur (Rutter, 1995b; Clarke & Clarke, 1999; Iwaniec & Sneddon, 2001). Let us look at the attachment style of FTT children measured at the assessment stage in childhood and then 20 years later, as adults.

### Comparison of Attachment Style in Childhood with Attachment as Adults—20-Year Follow-up Study (Iwaniec & Sneddon, 2001)

The attachment style of 44 children who failed to thrive, aged between 8 months and 6 years, was measured using *Strange Situation Protocol*, and cases were followed up for 20 years. Adult Attachment Style Classification (Hazan & Shaver, 1987) was used to measure attachment of the former failure-to-thrive patients, and scores were compared to their childhood style of at-tachment behaviour. There was attrition of 13 of the former participants in the sample, either because they could not be traced or were unwilling to par-ticipate. The remaining sample consisted of 16 males and 15 females, with a mean age of 21.6 years (range 20–28).

Comparison of childhood and adult attachment classifications produced some interesting results. There were differences observed in the style of

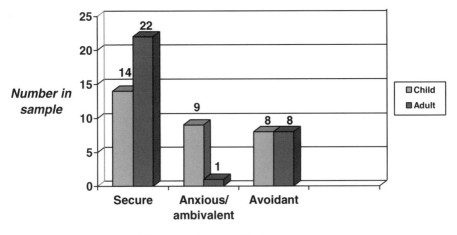

**Figure 7.1** Numbers of individuals in the sample who were classified as either secure, anxious/ambivalent or avoidant as children and adults

attachments of the children who failed to thrive. In total, 14 of the 31 children were classified as secure, nine as anxious/ambivalent, and eight as avoidant. The picture is slightly different when we look at the attachment classifications of these individuals as adults.

There was an increase in secure attachment from 14 individuals in childhood to 22 in adulthood. There was a marked decrease of anxious/ambivalent style from nine children to only one in adulthood. The number of clients falling into the avoidant category remained the same (eight) for both children and adults. Analysis of Chi Square shows that there is a significant relationship between the type of attachment observed in the children using the *Strange Situation Test* and the subsequent classification of the adults using the Attachment Style Classification questionnaire (Kendall's Tau b, p = 0.046).

It is of interest to point out which individuals became securely attached as adults when previously they had shown insecure patterns of attachment. A summary of the changes can be seen in Table 7.1.

- The majority of children who had been classified as secure were also *seen* as secure in adulthood (13 individuals). Most children classified as secure were younger children at the time of referral. All these children were wanted pregnancies. Eleven were classified as temperamentally easy (Carey Temperamental Test), and only two were slow to warm up. Easy babies are thought to be predisposed to be more placid, positive in moods, easy to instruct, not intensive in reactions, and happy.
- Only one person who was secure in childhood was avoidant as an adult. This participant had several traumatic events throughout childhood,

**Table 7.1** Numbers of individuals in the sample whose attachment changed or stayed the same between childhood and adulthood

| Change from Child to Adult Classification | Frequency | Percentage of total sample |
|---|---|---|
| *No change from child to adult* Child anxious/ambivalent to adult anxious/ambivalent | 1 | 3.2 |
| Child avoidant to adult avoidant | 5 | 16.1 |
| Child secure to adult secure | 13 | 41.9 |
| *Change in insecurity from child to adult* Child anxious/ambivalent to adult avoidant | 2 | 6.5 |
| Child secure to adult anxious/ambivalent | 0 | 0 |
| Child secure to adult avoidant | 1 | 3.2 |
| *Change in security from child to adult* Child anxious/ambivalent to adult secure | 6 | 19.4 |
| Child avoidant to adult anxious/ambivalent | 0 | 0 |
| Child avoidant to adult secure | 3 | 9.7 |

including her father's suicide. Although she had remained in the home throughout the intervention, there was inconsistent improvement in the emotional environment experienced there. This client has also been diagnosed as suffering from mental illness.

- Most of the sample who had been avoidant as children were also avoidant as adults (five out of eight individuals).
- Three previously avoidant individuals were classified as secure adults. In two of these cases the children were removed from the home environment and placed in long-term foster-homes in which they remained all the time. In the third case there was a dramatic change in home circumstances when the mother left the children's father and established a very positive relationship with a new partner. In essence each of these children experienced a new and much emotionally improved environment, either by being physically removed to a foster-home or by the home atmosphere changing dramatically.
- There is more variation in the group that had been anxious/ambivalent as children. Only one individual was classified as anxious/ambivalent as both child and adult. Two individuals showed a change from being anxious/ambivalent children to avoidant as adults.
- However, the majority of people showed a change from being anxious/ambivalent children to secure adults (six individuals). One of these

children was adopted at a very early age and three children were fostered out long term. One child remained in the home environment and showed improvement when her mother's new partner moved in (as above). The other two children remained in the home environment throughout intervention.

Twenty years had passed between the initial measurement of the child's style of attachment and the Adult Attachment Style Classification. As Fahlberg (1994) notes, 'A child's developmental progress is the result of the individual's unique intermix of genetic endowment, temperament, and life experiences.'

Many things had happened in the lives of these individuals during the last 20 years. Each person was classified as suffering from non-organic FTT and then received treatment and intervention. They also had their own particular life experiences which are bound to influence their development and attachment patterns. As children, many of them suffered from developmental delays and behavioural problems. Human interaction and social behaviour are complex: how we interact with others affects how they interact with us and vice versa. This contributes greatly to the way people feel about themselves and the way they build and maintain relationships with others.

In the light of this, how predictive should the childhood behaviour of this sample of non-organic failure-to-thrive individuals be of their adult attachments? If there are changes, to what should we attribute them? There are several possibilities, including:

- natural changes in attachment patterns;
- intervention;
- change in quality of parenting;
- temperamental factors and cognitive abilities; and
- other unidentified factors.

Intervention with failure-to-thrive children and their families, using various services and therapeutic methods, proved to be beneficial and effective in eliminating or reducing stress levels which directly or indirectly affected parental reactions towards the failure-to-thrive child and consequently the child's reaction to the care-giver. We could argue that responding to people's immediate needs and dealing with crises (ranging from housing, economics, child care, etc., through to personal factors) provided necessary help and support for the parents and consequently the child, as is demonstrated in Section III of this book (*see* page 187). There is substantial evidence from various research projects on failure to thrive (Drotar, 1991; Hanks & Hobbs, 1993; Hampton, 1996) that when support for struggling families is provided, they tend to overcome major difficulties and children begin to grow and develop appropriately for their developmental age. Equally, relationships between parents and children improved to satisfactory levels. There is ample evidence that intervention and treatment provided for those families and children over a period of time improved the quality and quantity of relationships and interactions between parents and infants (*see* Chapter 12). Interventions such as obtaining Care Orders where there was no improvement at home and placing children in caring and stable foster-homes, and in two cases having then adopted, proved to be stabilising and wholly helpful strategies. It needs to be noted that these children stayed in one foster-home all the time they were in care and had extensive contacts after leaving care. Those individuals were able to develop secure attachments both with their foster or adoptive parents and later with their romantic partners. It can be argued that early and appropriate intervention can help to provide bases for developing secure and meaningful attachment and trust to parents and other significant people (such as daily minders, nursery nurses, and foster or adoptive parents). Help was also provided by paediatricians, health visitors, and GPs, but major interventions were of a psychosocial nature.

Clarke and Clarke (1992, 1999) argued convincingly that probabilities for developmental changes, both positive and negative, are influenced by biological trajectory, the social environment trajectory, interactions and transactions, and chance events. The life-path of each individual is the result of combined interaction of all four influences emerging during development. There is ample evidence to suggest that people's early experiences, even if they are of an extremely damaging nature, can be overcome if radical remedial action takes place and emotional stability and security is provided (Rutter, 1995a; Clarke & Clarke, 1999; Messer, 1999). The results of this study support the above-mentioned findings and suggest that attachment style is not static and changes are probable. These changes appear to be influenced by many factors.

Some theorists of development have suggested that over the course of adulthood there is a natural process of re-evaluating relationships with others in response to key life events or changes in circumstances (Diehl *et al.*, 1998). For example, by becoming a parent for the first time, a person may reach a new or deeper understanding of their relationship with their own parents. This may result in a more integrated understanding of self and others, the outcome of which may be a different evaluation of their attachment relationships, a changed evaluation of their family of origin, or both. With this idea in mind it would be worthwhile to present two of the cases as possible examples of how change in attachment styles can occur.

The first individual, 'Sebastian', was severely emotionally abused by his mother until the age of 11, and had little contact and no relationship with her until his own child was born when he was 22 years old. He was able to reappraise the complexity of his relationship with his mother over the years, and becoming a parent himself enabled him to understand difficulties with child-rearing:

I never thought I would want to see or have anything to do with my mother again. She was always hitting and screaming at me. I was much happier when I went to live with my father and his new wife. Now that I have a baby I know how tough it is to cope when she cries or does not want to eat. I must have been a difficult child to look after and she found it hard to look after me. Mind you I would never hit my baby, but I understand my mother, she must have been under a lot of pressure. What is gone is gone; she helps a lot now.

The second individual, 'Peter', was sexually abused by his stepfather from toddler age until he was five years of age. He gradually recovered from those damaging experiences and rebuilt his trust in people after his mother left her husband and provided a healing environment in which emotional recovery was possible: his attachment style changed from anxious/avoidant to secure. At the time of referral (six years of age), the stepfather was no longer in contact with the child, but Peter suffered from severe behavioural and developmental problems and was very emotionally disturbed. After the stepfather left, mother and child undertook therapy: Peter was very bright at school and once the environment became caring and predictable, he began to relax, communicate, show affection, and to feel comfortable in the company of other men and peers. Major improvements were seen by the time he attended secondary school. He established a close romantic relationship, got married at 22 years of age, and became a loving father at 23 years of age.

Intergenerational aspects of attachment are of interest since the mothers of non-organic FTT children are also more likely to exhibit insecure patterns of attachment. For example, Benoit *et al.* (1989) compared the attachment behaviour of 25 mother–child pairs of failure-to-thrive children with the same number of normally growing infants while in hospital. Results showed that 96% of mothers of failure-to-thrive infants were insecure with respect to attachment (Adult Attachment Interview) compared to 60% of the control-group mothers. Lack of resolution of mourning over the loss of a loved one was found in 52% of FTT mothers compared to 32% of mothers of the control group.

The optimistic findings of this longitudinal study confirmed that people are able to change if they are provided with the right help, are able to reappraise their experiences, and if life events create an opportunity for getting emotional security and a strong belief of being wanted, loved, and appreciated.

## SUMMARY

This chapter examined different styles of attachment behaviour of children who fail to thrive and argued that maternal sensitivity in responding to the child's signals of distress and needs determine the level of security and quality of relationships between parents and children. Case studies were presented to illustrate different attachment patterns and parental behaviour which might have contributed to the development of particular child–parent attachments. Additionally, Adult Attachment Style Classification was explored briefly and parental-attachment attributes were linked as examples to the case studies presented in the chapter. Finally, the findings of the author's 20-year follow-up study were discussed examining the stability of an internal working model in a sample of individuals who had failed to thrive as children, by comparing each individual's adult attachment style with their childhood attachment to their mother. Several cases showed changes from *insecure* to *secure* attachment styles. Possible reasons for *positive* and *negative* changes and *no change* were discussed.

# 8

# FABRICATED OR INDUCED ILLNESSES AND FAILURE TO THRIVE

*Fancy is the friend of woe.*

William Mason, 1756

## INTRODUCTION

As has been discussed in the previous chapters, there are many reasons why children fail to thrive. The range, as we have seen, is quite extensive and varied. However, there are some children who fail to thrive because their parents (usually the mother) fabricate illness in the child or induce illness in order to get attention and sympathy from the medical profession, and by doing so expose a child to unnecessary painful and repeated medical treatments. For example, it might be claimed (falsely) that a child is allergic to certain foods, and special diets and treatments therefore sought. Some would induce illness, such as giving a child laxatives to produce diarrhoea, or giving it medication to induce vomiting or a high temperature or other symptoms requiring medical investigation.

Such parental behaviour was first coined by Meadow in 1977 as *Münchausen*[1] *Syndrome by Proxy* (MSbP), describing the trial of the 'duped doctor', 'harmed child', and fabricating parents. The term *Münchausen Syndrome* was introduced in 1951 by Dr Asher, who described a psychiatric disorder wherein adults invented false stories of illness or induced actual illness in themselves. Their untruthful medical histories resulted in

---

[1] Hieronymus Karl Freiherr von Münchausen of Bodenwerder (1720–97) was celebrated for his relations of his extraordinary experiences in the Russian service, and in action against the Turks. His stories were much relished by his circle, and his acquaintance, Rudolf Erich Raspe (1737–94), wrote a slim volume of improbable narrations loosely based on the Baron's tales, published in London in 1785. Subsequent editions, embroidered by various hacks, were entitled *Gulliver Reviv'd: the Singular Travels, Campaigns, Voyages, and Sporting Adventures of Baron Munnikhousen, commonly pronounced Munchausen; as he relates them over a bottle when surrounded by his friends* (1786), and many later editions and continuations appeared, several embellished with weird and wonderful illustrations.

needless medical investigations and treatment. The persistent and repetitive nature of falsified complaints has been noted by Dr Asher in the following way:

> They persisted, they fooled us, they used up scarce resources, and doctors had few skills to help them.

Dr Asher's humorous title of the syndrome (which is far from being amusing) is based on the eighteenth-century mercenary, Baron von Münchausen, who was well known for his embellished tales of his travels, which were both fantastic and unbelievable (*see* footnote 1). The last few years have shown considerable interest and enhancement in knowledge on the subject, but also created a lot of controversy about definition, classification, and the dividing line as to when it is a genuine illness and when it is fabrication.

The fabrication or induction of illness in children by parents (or *in loco parentis*) is referred to by a number of different labels, most commonly *Münchausen Syndrome by Proxy* (Meadow, 1977), *Factitious Illness by Proxy* (Bools, 1996), or *Illness Induction Syndrome* (Gray & Bentovim, 1996). In the United States the term *Paediatric Condition Falsification* is being adopted by the American Professional Society on the Abuse of Children (APSAC). This term is also used by some as if it were a psychiatric diagnosis. The American Psychiatric Association's Diagnostic and Statistical Manual (DSM-IV) has proposed using the term *factitious disorder by proxy* for a psychiatric diagnosis applicable to the fabricator. In the International Classification of Diseases—10C World Health Organisation (1991)—no separate category was allocated and it was put under the child-abuse category.

The controversy over definition has not been resolved and has been the subject of considerable debate between professionals of many disciplines. These differences and debates about whose terms are better or more appropriate are of some concern as they may result in a loss of emphasis on the well-being and safety of the child. The key issue, however, is not what term to use to describe this type of abuse, but the harm that fabricated or induced illness may have on the child's health and safety, and consideration of how best to protect children from such abuse. The meeting of the Royal College of Paediatrics and Child Health (2002) argued that fabrication or illness induction includes all forms of parental activities such as delusion, excessive anxiety, masquerade hysteria, doctor shopping, doctor addicts, mothering to death, seekers of personal help and attention or financial gain, and those who fail to give needed treatment, as well as those who treat unnecessarily. Additionally, they argue that accepting the term 'Fabricated or Induced Illness' (FII) embraces the wide spectrum of physical injury and emotional harm.

In contrast, the term *Münchausen Syndrome by Proxy* is only valid when a person who has Münchausen Syndrome him/herself uses others, particularly children, to manifest the disorder. It is argued that even when one parent has

Münchausen Syndrome it may be the other parent who is harming the child, as described in Dominic's case. The most useful definition and points for identification from the clinical practice point of view is that of Bools *et al.* (1992), who refer to:

1. illness in the child which is fabricated by a parent, or someone *in loco parentis*;
2. the child being presented for medical assessment and care, usually persistently, often resulting in multiple medical procedures;
3. the perpetrator denying the aetiology of the child's illness; and
4. acute symptoms and signs of illness decreasing when the child is separated from the perpetrator.

Presentation of the cases varies from lying about the child's symptoms (such as claiming that a child has hallucinations when it does not), or actively inducing symptoms in the child (such as feeding the child laxatives to cause diarrhoea and weight loss, or overdosing with salt to cause convulsions). Apart from fabrication of signs and symptoms there could be falsification of hospital charts and records and specimens of bodily fluids such as urine. This may also include falsification of letters and documents.

Baldwin (1996) describes a possible scenario. As a rule the parent presents the 'sick' child to a doctor and lies about what has happened. The child is then subjected to unnecessary and sometimes painful medical investigations and treatment. To the outsider the perpetrator may appear to be the perfect care-giver, spending most of the time at the child's bedside, taking part in its care, and often refusing to let anyone else take his or her place. The perpetrator seems to thrive in the hospital environment, offering help to the nursing staff and maintaining a constant presence. However, at the same time, these apparently caring people may be poisoning, suffocating, and otherwise maltreating their children in order to keep them sick. This is well demonstrated in the case below.

### Harry's Case

Harry, a 4-year-old, was admitted to hospital in a semi-conscious state for observation. His mother appeared to be very worried about her son, and stayed in hospital most of the time, looking after him and assisting the nurses in their duties on the ward. The blood-test revealed the presence of pain-killing and anti-depressant substances. It was claimed that he could have taken it from his mother's drawer as she kept them there.

Harry looked very thin and small for his age, and he was diagnosed as a severe case of failing to thrive, and that he would need urgent attention to improve his growth on returning home. In spite of being in hospital Harry did not improve, slept all the time, and presented as a child suffering from doses of drugs, and in a bad state of health. Further blood-tests revealed a high level of anti-depressants, which raised concerns that something was going wrong and that someone was giving him those drugs in hospital. The mother expressed bewilderment, denied any knowledge of it, and asked the nurse to inform Barry's estranged father to come and see him as he might die.

The father did not come to see them, and the mother showed distress that Harry's father did not bother to come to see his seriously ill son. However, the mother remained attentive, concerned and dedicated to caring for Harry, who was deteriorating rapidly. One nurse was asked to supervise Harry as there was suspicion about malpractice. The mother welcomed this decision and remained with him all the time.

The nurse was called to see someone urgently, left the mother with Harry, but returned after about 10 minutes or so as she had forgotten to take her notebook. As she entered the cubicle unexpectedly she saw the mother hiding a syringe in her pocket after injecting her son with painkillers. Harry was lucky that the nurse (who never expected his mother to harm him) forgot her notebook and returned to the cubicle in time to see what was happening.

The analysis of the mother's history provided many explanations why she was prepared to kill her son and why she neglected him physically and emotionally to the point of severe failure to thrive for a long time. Harry was the result of the mother's affair and obsessional love for a man who was her best friend's husband. She believed that he would leave his wife once she gave birth to their child. That did not happen, and although they did see each other for a while, there was no sign that he would come to live with her and Harry. He showed little commitment to or interest in Harry, and indirectly blamed her for getting pregnant. Gradually she became resentful of Harry, blaming him for ruining her life and the fact that she was losing his father because of him. Harry was seriously neglected physically, and rejected emotionally, as the mother was not able to tune into his needs and did not want to. However, she knew that Harry's father would occasionally come to see him, so she needed to keep Harry with her. Her plan was to get him back and threaten to tell his wife about their affair and that Harry was his son. Contrary to her expectations he said that she could tell his wife if she wanted to and that he would not see her again. He insisted that she must not bother him and that their relationship was finished.

In order to bring him back to her she started poisoning Harry, believing that he would come to see his seriously ill and dying son, and that the tragedy would bring them together again. She was prepared to do anything to get her lover back.

The obsessional, tormenting love for a man, who (to start with) was extremely caring and loving towards her, is not surprising if we look at her childhood history. She was sexually abused for many years by her father in a brutal and commanding way. Her mother was aware of what was happening, but was too afraid to intervene to protect her only child. There was terror and violence if they did not do what he wanted them to do. Harry's father, on the other hand, was gentle and loving, so she saw protection, care, and security when in his company, and in spite of betraying her best friend (and feeling guilty about it) she went on seeking his love and presence at all costs. She described her feelings towards Harry's father as completely overwhelming, never leaving her for even a moment. He was always in her thoughts, wherever she was and whatever she was doing. She was completely possessed by thoughts and feelings towards him, and nothing mattered but to be with him and to have him. She described driving to his house at night and watching movements in the house, telephoning to hear his voice and waking up in the morning always thinking of him. She was not able to free herself, feeling extremely jealous, and holding on to any word or gesture which would indicate that he still loved her and firmly believing that he would come back.

Identification of Münchausen's Syndrome is not easy, and the literature is, at times, contradictory, as demonstrated by Baldwin (1996) in two different versions. However, both versions are valid, as fabricated or induced illness takes different terms and routes. Baldwin (1996), on the basis of the literature review of Münchausen's Syndrome, put forward two versions of indicators, which at first glance might appear to be contradictory, but on closer examination are realistic.

### Version 1 indicators

- Persistent or recurrent illnesses for which a cause cannot be found or which are very unusual.
- Discrepancies between history and clinical findings.
- Symptoms and signs that do not occur when a child is away from the mother.
- Unusual symptoms, signs or hospital course that do not make clinical sense, causing experienced physicians to say they have 'never seen a case like it before'.
- A differential diagnosis consisting of disorders less common than MSbP.
- Persistent failure of a child to tolerate or respond to medical therapy without clear cause.
- A parent less concerned than the physician, sometimes comforting the medical staff.
- Repeated hospitalisations and vigorous medical evaluation of mother and child without definitive diagnoses.
- A parent who is constantly at the child's bedside, excessively praises the staff, becomes overly attached to the staff or becomes highly involved in the care of other patients.
- A parent who welcomes medical tests of her child even when painful.
- Doctor-shopping or hospital peregrination.
- Unusual or unexplained illness or death of previous children.
- Patient has multiple allergies.
- Parents or care-givers are over-attached to the patient.
- In children, one parent (usually the father) is absent during hospitalisation.

### Version 2 indicators

An extended list of MSbP indicators:

- Presentation at hospital.
- Non-presentation for medical attention.
- Over-concern about the child's health in the form of extreme exaggeration of symptoms.

- Not as concerned about the child's health as the medics.
- Co-operation with the medics.
- Non-cooperation with the medics, e.g. seeking alternative medical opinions which counter the diagnosis or conflictual relationships with the medical staff.
- Confession.
- Denial.
- Medical knowledge on the part of the mother.
- Medical ignorance on the part of the medics.
- Symptoms only beginning in the presence of one parent (usually the mother as the absence of the father is also indicative).
- Collusion of father or other family if symptoms start in the presence of more than one person.
- Poor intellectual relationship with the husband.

Rosenberg (1987) demonstrated that there are several groups of fabrications. These include:

1. Verbal fabrication:
    - verbal fabrication of seizures or apnoea;
    - other verbal fabrications;
    - verbal fabrication plus the falsification of specimens or charts.
2. Fabrication associated with:
    - poisoning to produce signs;
    - smothering to produce signs;
    - production of signs by other means.
3. Fabrication associated with feeding, e.g.:
    - withholding nutrients and medicines;
    - making allegations of allergy and withholding of food.
4. Fabrication of psychiatric disorder;
5. Factitious disorder in pregnancy; and
6. Fabrication in the presence of genuine physical illness.

Rosenberg (1987), in her review of 117 cases of MSbP, identified the most common presentations as bleeding, seizures, central nervous system depression, apnoea, diarrhoea, vomiting, fever, and rash. Failure to thrive was associated with MSbP in 14% of cases. The average length of time between the onset of symptoms and diagnosis is 15 months, ranging from a few days to many years.

With regard to failure to thrive and its associated growth problems, fabrications relating to feeding are of particular interest. General dietary restriction, and specific restriction (such as of foods containing iron) have been reported (Bools, 1996). These cases are not a result of misunderstanding dietary needs or pure neglect, but appear to be a result of more deliberate actions of the carers.

Factitious disorders in pregnancy are also interesting from the point of view that the mother is harming both herself and her unborn foetus. Jureidini (1993) presented five cases of factitious disorders in pregnancy which progressed to Münchausen Syndrome by Proxy after birth. These included probably feigned premature labour, factitious bleeding, and bruised abdomen consistent with foetal abuse. Jureidini concludes that obstetric complications are common in the histories of Münchausen Syndrome by Proxy, and pregnancy and childbirth can facilitate the transition from self-focused hostile behaviour of Münchausen Syndrome (MS) to the externally focused Münchausen Syndrome by Proxy (MSbP). This interesting formulation, however, may simplify a more complex phenomenon when one considers the postulated abnormal psychological boundary between mother and child after delivery and into childhood. An interesting question is: to what degree is the foetus perceived by the mother as being separate from herself? And how does this relate to the 'normal' attachment process?

## FABRICATED OR INDUCED ILLNESS AND FAILURE TO THRIVE

Many researchers have shown strong association between fabricated or induced illness and failure to thrive in children. For example, Money and Werlass (1976) and Money *et al.* (1985) postulated that the seeking of care by proxy is the feature that distinguished classic Münchausen Syndrome by Proxy from factitious illness and conditions such as failure to thrive, failure to feed, and allegations of allergy. It can be argued that seeking of care by proxy, although not from the medical profession but from social services, is a common feature in cases where there are psychosocial short-stature children. Such children are undoubtedly abused in a destructive and often sinister way, and the carers persistently claim that there is something medically wrong with the child. Some of the carers may bring the child to the GP's surgery asking for investigation: however, most carers avoid medical contact simply because they do not care what happens to that child.

The relationship between non-organic failure to thrive, mood disturbance in the mother, and active failure to feed adequately, has been widely discussed. Gray and Bentovim (1996) were the first to describe the active withholding of food as a type of Illness Induction Syndrome.

### Dominic's Case

Dominic, an unwanted child, was placed by his father in three different, privately arranged, foster-homes. Each placement did not last long, and each home was very neglectful. A fourth home was found and the fee was increased substantially to keep Dominic there. The health visitor became very concerned about the child's poor development, and questioned the foster-parents' suitability, but no action was taken to investigate the quality of child care. At the age of 5 years Dominic presented as a very thin, small, and withdrawn child, well below the 3rd percentile in weight and height, and his foster-parents claimed that it was due to his allergies to food. They requested admission to hospital and attended the GP's surgery on a regular basis. There were seven admissions to various hospitals, yet many tests did not show any allergies. The foster-parents insisted, however, that when Dominic ate meat, cheese, most fruit, and vegetables, he had acute diarrhoea and tummy ache. The foster-father stayed with him in hospital to keep him company and to make sure, as he said, that he took the necessary medication and to help with establishing an appropriate diet. As the paediatricians did not come up with the diagnosis they were looking for, they went to another hospital to seek a second opinion, portraying themselves as very caring and concerned about Dominic's problematic weight gain and short stature. After exhaustive investigations and a prolonged period of hospitalisation, in yet another hospital, nothing was found to suggest allergies to food. The foster-father became angry and abusive to hospital staff, stating that they were incompetent and did not listen to him. The foster-father wrote letters of complaint to the hospital administration, the Trust manager, and his Member of Parliament. The foster-parents then approached social services to be compensated for the bedding, carpets, settee and chairs that Dominic had, allegedly, ruined by soiling and requested payment for managing his difficult behaviour, which they claimed existed, but no one else witnessed.

Dominic, in spite of negative results from various hospitals, was put on a strict diet consisting of bread, potatoes, tea, and jam. He was not allowed to have school dinners, and was prohibited from taking food from anybody.

Having failed to convince the paediatrician that Dominic was allergic to most foods, the foster-parents turned to psychiatrists and a psychologist claiming that Dominic was not showing affection, was stubborn and disobedient. Again, they requested appointments with different psychiatrists, this time claiming that he was stealing food at home and at school, searching for food at night, and that he was hoarding food in peculiar places. Not knowing the earlier history and being persuaded by the 'concerned carers' that Dominic needed help in terms of emotional development, an attachment work was undertaken, but the foster-parents refused to participate in the therapy. Dominic collapsed at school and was taken to hospital. He was passing blood when going to the toilet, and was extremely withdrawn and ill-looking. This time the foster-parents were not allowed to be with Dominic while in hospital. He did not show any allergies to any food, he put on weight rapidly, and stopped bleeding. Within three weeks he gained $1\frac{1}{2}$ stones in weight and became alert and responsive to people around him. After being discharged from the hospital Dominic was placed with very caring and affectionate foster-carers, and within a year his weight and height reached the 25th percentile and his behaviour improved. He became more sociable, confident, and less frightened. He began to smile as well.

Dominic was starved for a long time. The foster-parents, and in particular the foster-father, fabricated food allergies to justify withdrawal of food and to portray themselves as caring, and seeking help for the child. They also wanted to get sympathy from the doctors for caring for a child who was rejected by the natural parents and wanted approval of their behaviour towards Dominic. However, the most important motive for fabricating and inducing illness would appear to have been financial (in this case). As was eventually discovered, the boy was given laxatives on a regular basis which induced diarrhoea, leading to uncontrollable soiling and spurious claims that such soiling was caused by allergic reactions to food, so that the carers could justify the withdrawal of food, thus leading to starvation. Excessive use of laxatives also induced bleeding and wasting in the child, leading almost to a point of collapse because of starvation. The financial gains were substantial, and it became clear that the foster-parents behaved as they did in order to claim various allowances and compensations from social services as well as extra money from the natural father for all the trouble involved in looking after his problematic child.

Failure to thrive was associated with illness induction and fabrication in 14% of cases reviewed by Rosenberg (1987) and 29% of the sample of Bools *et al.* (1992). Gray and Bentovim (1996) found a higher incidence of 41% of failure to thrive in their study. They reviewed case-histories of these 41 children, who were identified as having had illness induced by the parent, and found four distinct patterns:

## 1 Failure to thrive through the active withholding of food

A sample of 10 children fell into this group (Group 1), aged from 13 months to 9 years, with a mean of 27 months. These children presented as distinct from more commonly seen non-organic failure to thrive. In most of these cases close observation by the ward staff provided evidence of gross, secret withholding of food from a child. The parent was deliberately starving the child and obviously growth failure directly resulted from inadequate amounts of food.

## 2 Allegation of allergy and withholding of food

This group (Group 2) consisted of five children, aged from 19 months to 14 years, mean age 6 years 2 months. The diet of these children was severely restricted, so insufficient food was received for them to grow according to their age. In most cases there was an organic basis to the allergic symptoms, but not to the extent described by the parent. As in Group 1, growth-failure will result from inadequate amounts of food and also from an unbalanced diet. However, the interaction between mother and infant may play a role in this group of children. It is well known that a child will eat less of food that is known to be aversive to the care-giver when presented with that food by that person; however, if the same food is given by someone else, it will be accepted by the child. One can speculate that it is possible that, if those mothers were afraid that their child might be allergic to a particular food, they might show an aversive response to that food during feeding. That might result in the child refusing the food and might also explain why that food was subsequently accepted when offered by someone other than the mother. It might be the mother's fear of her child's refusing the food which results in the self-fulfilling prophecy that the child *does* refuse the food.

### 3 Allegation and fabrication of medical symptoms

This group (Group 3) consisted of 15 children ranging in age from 5 months to 13 years with a mean of 6 years 3 months. The mothers claimed that these children had stopped breathing, were having fits, or failing to concentrate urine.

### 4 Active interference by poisoning or disrupting medical treatment

The fourth group (Group 4) consisted of 11 children ranging in age from 4 weeks to 12 years 3 months, with a mean of 3 years. Unprescribed medication, salt, or laxatives might have been administered to these children, or the parent might have actively interfered with the child's medical treatment, for example, rubbing skin-grafted burns to prevent healing.

Seventeen out of 41 of these children had previously presented with failure to thrive, feeding problems, or food allergies. There were more boys than girls associated with feeding difficulties and failure to thrive (in the first two groups 12 out of 15 children were male). In the other two groups the gender balance was even.

The authors found that there were no specific characteristics of either the child or the family associated with each type of presentation. In 17 children there had been previous failure to thrive, feeding problems, or food allergies. Interestingly, all of the mothers had suffered at least one of the following: privation, child abuse, psychiatric illness, or significant loss or bereavement. Forty per cent of the parents were seen as having serious marital problems. However, it is clear that not all people who present those worries and are concerned about their child's health go on to fabricate illnesses in their children. As always, findings of this kind beg the question 'was there something else in these parents' backgrounds or in the children themselves that made them vulnerable to these sorts of abuse?'. In Gray and Bentovim's study a combined medical/psychosocial team attempted to understand what the family thought about the illness. It was concluded that 'the process of illness induction was initiated by the parents perceiving the child to be ill and using this focus as a way of solving major personal, marital and/or family difficulties'.

## CHARACTERISTICS OF THE FAMILIES WHO FABRICATE OR INDUCE ILLNESS

### The Victim

Fabrication or inducement of illness usually involves young children, often starting during the first year of life, with an average age of diagnosis being just over three years. It is generally agreed that children younger than the age of 6 years are at greatest risk since older children might refuse to collude with their carers. There are no gender differences as far as victimisation is concerned. However, Gray and Bentovim (1996) found that males in their sample were more likely than females to fail to thrive through the active withholding of food or through receipt of a severely restricted diet because of perceived food allergies.

## Siblings

The siblings of the victims are also at risk. Bools *et al.* (1992) found that 39% of siblings had suffered fabricated illnesses, with 11% having died in early childhood from unidentified causes. It is, therefore, absolutely necessary to register siblings of such children as 'at risk' and to monitor those cases very closely until they are old enough to understand what is going on.

## The Carer

The carers of the victims come from all social classes and usually include the natural mothers of the children. However, adoptive mothers and fathers (Anderson & McKane, 1996) have been implicated as well as foster-parents. It was found that the mother would have some medical knowledge, would be interested in diseases, would have undertaken training as a nurse, although would not necessarily have completed it (Rosenberg, 1987). The mothers might have suffered privation, child abuse, psychiatric illness, or significant loss or bereavement, or had a personality disorder (Gray & Bentovim, 1996). It was noted by many researchers that a common theme in the childhood of those mothers was emotional neglect and psychological abandonment. Although mental illness *per se* is rare, the carer is likely to have a personality disorder, Münchausen Syndrome, or somatisation behaviour. Depression and suicidal ideation are also common (Anderson & McKane, 1996).

Baldwin (1996) summarised the characteristics of such a carer, usually the mother, in the following way:

- She appears as the 'perfect parent', nurturing, loving and caring;
- She has had some medical training or has been active in health service affairs, e.g. officer of the hospital league of friends;
- The father is absent for long periods of time or is inconspicuous;
- The mother comes from a higher social background or seems much more intelligent than her husband;
- There are similarities between the medical histories of the mother and child;
- She may have features of Münchausen Syndrome herself;
- She is characterised by severe emotional deprivation;

- She has previously worked with children in some capacity;
- She has a previous history of hysterical illness;
- Both parents have a history of unusual illness, or themselves have suffered physical, emotional, or sexual abuse in childhood;
- Both parents have a history of conduct or eating disorders;
- She has a history of marital discord;
- She denies involvement in deception;
- She has suicidal ideation or attempt before disclosure or after discovery;
- She is lonely and isolated; and
- She has a previous criminal record.

Fathers tend to be passive in the majority of cases, or absent from or peripheral to the family system. However, there have been cases published where the father has been the perpetrator (Single & Henry, 1991; Samuels *et al.*, 1992; Meadow, 1993; Samuels, 2002), as was pointed out in Dominic's case. Most writers refer to the natural mother or father and yet the problems appear in foster-homes as well. Special attention needs to be given to children in care as they can be at particular risk, especially as there may be the possibility of financial gain if the child presents chronic health problems (Mehl *et al.*, 1990).

## Eating Disorders

Several researchers (such as Samuels *et al.*, 1992; Muszkowicz & Bjørnholm, 1998) have observed that perpetrators are likely to have eating and/or weight problems. For example, Warner and Hathaway (1984), writing about factitious allergy affecting 17 children, found that mothers were on diets themselves without any obvious justification. These cases may range from mothers who deliberately restrict certain foods from their children, to the mother (suffering from a serious eating disorder herself) who does not want her children to become fat and who gives her child ipecacuanha to cause failure to thrive (Feldman *et al.*, 1989).

Muszkowicz and Bjørnholm (1998) describe a boy with polydipsia by proxy as part of factitious illness by proxy resulting in severe failure to thrive. They concluded that this was due to a severe disturbance in the parent–child relationship. The mother was herself force-fed as an infant because of food refusal, and later suffered from anorexia nervosa and polydipsia psychogenica. When born and until the age of eight months her son was overweight, but by 13 months he had dropped from the 97th percentile for weight to below the 3rd percentile. There were complaints of vomiting, fever, and growth retardation. By 19 months the child was malnourished, showing deficits in cognitive, linguistic, emotional, and social development. The mother–child interaction was observed to be dominated by conflict, restriction, and mutual rejection, especially during meals. The mother interpreted any cue given by the child as a sign of thirst and hence the child's intake of fluid was much higher than it should have been. Since the case-history reports problems of the mother with her own childhood, this case is also a good example of the inter-generational aspects of these problems.

There have also been cases of the infants of bulimic mothers becoming Münchausen-Syndrome-by-Proxy victims of ipecac administration. Ipecac (or ipecacuanha), an emetic, is a highly effective means of removing poisons from the stomach. Feldman *et al.* (1989) report a case of ipecac administration in a victim of Münchausen Syndrome by Proxy. Initial symptoms were shown at 1.5 weeks after birth with a baby girl admitted to hospital with vomiting, blood-streaked diarrhoea, and hypothermia. There was immediate concern since the child's siblings had all grown poorly after laxative intoxication by their mother. The baby girl would feed for hospital staff but would vomit when fed by bottle or breast by her mother. By 11 months of age the child was suffering from severe FTT. Later, the mother admitted that she herself suffered from anorexia nervosa and had been sexually molested by her stepfather and her stepbrother. She admitted that she did not want her children to become fat and that she had induced failure to thrive in them.

## Interaction

At first glance the parent's close attention to the child may suggest that they are attentive and good care-givers. However, closer examination paints a different picture. These mothers are clinging on to their children rather than interacting with them in a meaningful way. As Bools (1996) notes, 'accompanying the frequent observation that in "classical MSP" the mother remains unusually close (geographically) to her child, is the notion that the mother is psychologically over-involved with, and over-dependent on her child'.

As Gray and Bentovim (1996) observed, the 'children were not allowed to play or to have fun. One mother slept on the ward holding her son (aged 5) tightly in her arms throughout the night. Another mother carried her two-year-old son around for the whole day with him clinging to her, and a father undertook all his son's care and slept next to him during the entire admission. At the same time these children were having their temperature charts and medical tests interfered with, food thrown out, and symptoms exaggerated.' These behaviours were indicative of the abusing parents' highly anxious attachment and extreme ambivalence towards the presenting child(ren)—they were both deeply concerned about and harming them.

As Skau and Mouridsen (1995), in a review of Münchausen Syndrome by Proxy, noted, there has been no large systematic study of family dynamics associated with the diagnosis of MSbP. Research has also failed to explain why one particular child within a family may be abused, while others are not. Griffith (1988) completed two family studies. They reported a high level of family enmeshment where individual personality boundaries were diffuse within the family system. Their study suggested themes of dominance and submission in family relationships with no protective mechanism in place for the non-dominant family members. Multi-generational themes of exploitation (including physical and sexual abuse) were common. Inter-generational family patterns of illness behaviour, especially those involving chronic medical or factitious illness, occurred across at least three generations on the maternal side of the family. A study of the characteristics of four families with MSbP (McGuire & Feldman, 1989) supported previous findings and added other dimensions. In all four families the mother had a marital dysfunction. Medical abuse of other siblings, alcohol and drug abuse by the father, and physical and sexual abuse of the mother by the child's father or her own father were reported in three of the four families. Meadow (1990), who studied 27 young children from 27 different families who were suffocated by their mothers, found that at least 70% of the mothers had had unhappy childhoods and could be considered to have suffered emotional abuse. At least 25% had suffered physical or sexual abuse as children.

## Albert's and Stan's Case

Albert and Stan, ages 5 and 6 respectively, had been persistently referred by the GP to the paediatricians at the mother's request for the treatment of hyperactivity and food allergies. She imposed a rigid diet on the children, claiming that this was the only way she could control their behaviour. After two hospitalisations (to observe the children's behaviour and reactions to various foods) the children were referred to the psychologist for full assessment as nothing was observed to suggest that the children were hyperactive and that the alleged hyperactivity was associated with reaction to many brands of food. Both boys were very thin, small for their age, and their weight fluctuated either just above the 2nd percentile or just under. Their behaviour was timid and often withdrawn.

The psychologist did not find the boys' behaviour to be hyperactive, and the school-teachers reported that their behaviour was normal; in fact they stated that their concentration span was very good. Because the mother did not get satisfaction from the local hospitals she started to shop for sympathetic doctors in the private sector, and searched the internet for doctors willing to see her and the boys. The diet regime became worse, and the school reported both boys being hungry but afraid to eat, because the mother insisted that they should not take anything without her permission. In one year she took them to five different hospitals and three private clinics to seek treatment for a non-existent problem.

The mother, who held a responsible position, was well educated, and had completed a course in counselling and nutrition, insisted that her sons required medical attention and one way or another she would get appropriate assistance and help for her children. Yet it became apparent that she was a very troubled person, in spite of a very polished appearance and the coherent arguments she put forward. The marital relationship was dominated by her in every respect. The husband had little to say, and most decisions were made by the mother. She had no friends, and apart from colleagues at work she had no social contacts.

> When under stress or feeling lonely (which happened frequently) she would go to town to buy a jumper to cheer herself up. She had expensive jumpers, all of them still unwrapped, everywhere in the home. The drawers were full, as were two wardrobes, and she had 537 jumpers stored in the suitcases and boxes in the attic. Altogether she had 731 jumpers. This compulsive and secretive behaviour tended to become more acute when she felt isolated, unwanted, and unloved. She felt that her sons required protection from becoming more hyperactive and that restricting consumption of various foods and drinks, especially those containing sugar, would help. While that sort of restriction would have been acceptable, it did not stop there. She eliminated all meats, breads, and some fruit as well, so in the end there was hardly anything they could eat at all.
>
> After being accommodated with very caring, paternal grandparents (some 60 miles away) they began to grow at a remarkable speed, and there was no sign of hyperactivity or disturbing reactions to foods (as persistently claimed by the mother).

The Royal College of Paediatrics and Child Health puts forward the following recommendations for the paediatricians, cited in Samuels (2002):

- Paediatricians need to recognise that fabrication of symptoms or signs (and sometimes the induction of illness) by carers may be the explanation for a child's illness;
- Fabrication or induced illness by a carer is the preferred terminology for this form of behaviour, which is likely to cause significant harm to a child;
- Paediatricians need to be aware of the very wide range of illness and symptomatology which may result from fabrication or illness induction by a carer;
- Paediatricians need to be aware of the very wide range and severity of harm that may result, ranging from the induction of acute life-threatening illness to the less well-researched harm from verbal fabrication of symptoms (which overlaps with excessive anxiety and misunderstanding by the carer);
- Paediatricians need to recognise that fabrication of symptoms or signs without actual physical injury by the carer does result in harm to the child from unnecessary investigation and treatment;
- Paediatricians need to be aware of the potential for long-term harm as a result of fabrication or illness induction;
- When suspicion of fabricated or induced illness first arises, the paediatrician has a duty to consult widely in an attempt to confirm or refute the suspicions;
- A review of all available health records for the child with careful documentation of all events and the parties involved can be very helpful in establishing whether fabrication or illness induction has taken place;
- When concerns of fabrication or induced illness persist after consultation and review, the risk of significant harm becomes a priority and requires assessment within the framework of child protection;

- Covert video surveillance is required when life-threatening induced illness is suspected and satisfactory evidence cannot be obtained in any other way. It should only be considered by a child-protection strategy meeting and can only be instituted by the policy authority according to their guidelines;
- Paediatricians who suspect fabrication or induced illness need to retain a central role throughout the continuing assessment and enquiries whether the child is reunited to his/her parents or not;
- Fabrication or induced illness, and the carer behaviour giving rise to it, need to form a specific part of the core curriculum for training all paediatricians;
- Failure to scrutinise the records of all members of the family, including siblings, can lead to a lack of awareness of very significant histories;
- All children admitted to hospital under a surgeon should also be under the care of a paediatrician. This is in line with the guidance that paediatricians should have overall care of children's wards and that no child should be admitted to an adult ward;
- There should be social-work support based in every Paediatric Unit and Child Health Department. Paediatricians and General Practitioners should always attend Child Protection Conferences and time must be made available for this to happen;
- Paediatricians must recognise the potential for causing severe distress to some families, particularly when the suspicion of FII (Fictitious or Induced Illness) turns out to be incorrect. Better use of the guidelines should give families the knowledge that they have been evaluated fully, fairly, and appropriately;
- There should be regular liaison meetings in every borough between police, social services, and medical and nursing health staff from primary care and from specialist services; and
- A review of the operation of complaints procedures when there are issues which relate to child protection should be undertaken urgently.

## TREATMENT AND PROGNOSIS

Unfortunately there is no specific effective treatment for fictitious disorders. The parents seldom fully engage in psychiatric treatment. Available evidence suggests that mistreatment of children is likely to reoccur unless the child is removed from the perpetrator. Prognosis for these children seems to be poor (Bools *et al.*, 1993). In many follow-up studies there is evidence of a low survival rate for these children. Rosenberg (1987) found short-term morbidity in all patients and long-term morbidity in 8% of survivors. Skau and Mouridsen (1995) found that in 23 cases located of Münchausen Syndrome by Proxy and non-accidental poisoning at least five of the children were known to have died. Anderson and McKane (1996) found mortality was 9%, with the recorded methods of death being suffocation, salt poisoning, other poisoning and uncertain substances. Children who do survive may suffer destructive joint changes, mental retardation, cerebral palsy, and cortical blindness. There are usually serious disturbances in psychological development ranging from conduct to emotional disorders to school-related problems, including school-avoidance and difficulties in attention and concentration (Bools *et al.*, 1993). These children may eventually develop Münchausen Syndrome themselves and take part in the fabrication of the illness (Meadow, 1984).

## SUMMARY

This chapter dealt with fabrication or inducement of illness, which can cause severe failure to thrive and sometimes can lead to death. The issues of labelling the disorder and controversy regarding definition, as well as the origin of the Münchausen Syndrome and the Münchausen Syndrome by Proxy, were briefly discussed. Findings from a few research studies were presented and major lessons deriving from the projected were elaborated on. The characteristics of the victim, perpetrator, siblings, interaction between abuser and the victim, and the histories of eating disorders by the perpetrator were brought to the reader's attention. Three cases dealt with by the author were presented to illustrate both the problem and its effects on children. The chapter ends with a few remarks made regarding difficulties in providing effective treatment and concludes that the only reliable solution to protect the child is to remove the child from the perpetrator's care.

# Section II

# THE FRAMEWORK OF ASSESSMENT

# A FRAMEWORK OF ASSESSMENT
# OF FAILURE-TO-THRIVE CASES:
# ECOLOGICAL APPROACH

*The first duty of a State is to see that every child born therein shall be well housed, clothed, fed, and educated, till it attains years of discretion.*

John Ruskin, 1867

## INTRODUCTION

As was shown in the previous chapters, the most significant feature of children who fail to thrive is disturbance in their physical growth, in particular inadequate weight gain for the child's chronological age. The question, 'How do we know that a child's growth is a cause for concern?' needs to be asked, and the factors contributing to the child's poor growth and development need to be explored through comprehensive assessment.

Each country provides different universal services for children and their families. In the United Kingdom, as well as in many other Western countries, during the first two years after birth an infant's weight, height, head circumference, and general psychosocial development are routinely checked and recorded by a health visitor. Each child is issued with a *red book* where progress is systematically recorded and discussed with the parents. It is expected that not all children will grow and develop at the same rate, and there will be some variation. In order to see how well a child is growing and developing, the measurements are compared with charts showing the expected range of measurements from that particular population. If a child is persistently showing a growth rate lower than most of the population, then this is taken to be cause for concern, and the child is diagnosed as failing to thrive. As failure-to-thrive syndrome can have a detrimental effect on a growing child, investigations are then carried out to find out the cause of the growth failure and to work out appropriate intervention and treatment strategies based on assessment findings.

To have a good understanding of what leads to failure to thrive, a multi-factorial, holistic framework of assessment needs to be adopted. Additionally, a multi-disciplinary approach is necessary to include medical, nutritional, and psychosocial factors in the assessment content. Existing literature shows a tendency to focus on factors associated with the assessor's professional remit and expertise. The assessment and formulations of the problems unfortunately tend to be somewhat fragmented, because of different theoretical stances and beliefs that are associated with failure to thrive.

## A NEW FRAMEWORK FOR ASSESSMENT

In the United Kingdom a new framework for assessing children in need was issued by the Department of Health in 2000, with the intention of providing holistic, child-centred, and much more targeted help for children, based on needs assessment. The assessment framework is multidimensional, exploring parental capacity, children's developmental needs, and family and environmental factors. Ecological theory is adopted, postulating that children's development is influenced by the quality and capacity of parenting which, in turn, are influenced by the characteristics of their families, social network, neighbourhoods, communities, and the interrelations among them (Bronfenbrenner, 1979).

A good understanding of all-round child development is required, with knowledge about developmental hazards and crises in order to make appropriate judgements about whether the quality of child care is good enough to meet a range of different and complex developmental needs which have to be addressed during each stage of the child's life. The philosophy of the new framework aims to redirect assessment focus from the risk-and-blame culture to the developmental needs of children, and ways of meeting these needs in the families and communities in which they live, by the provision of services for those who require help. Additionally, it is rightly argued that the 'wait-and-see' approach needs to be avoided when dealing with cases where evidence suggests a poor prognosis for change in parenting, thus promoting quicker decision-making to avoid further deterioration and increase of difficulties which may lead to significant harm for the child's growth and development. There is emphasis on providing better distribution of resources for all children in need of help, and to narrow the gap between protection and family support.

This chapter will discuss assessment of failure-to-thrive children and their families using an ecological approach. A range of relevant factors, as indicated in the assessment framework triangle (*see* Figure 9.1), will be linked to failure-to-thrive problems and relevant research findings. Various assessment instruments will be provided, many developed by the author and tested for suitability over many years. Issues such as measurements of physical

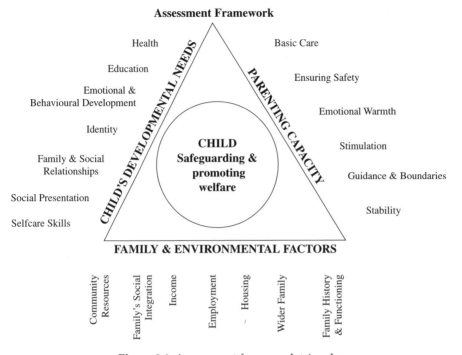

**Figure 9.1** Assessment framework triangle
*Source:* Department of Health (2000) *A Framework for Assessment of Children in Need and Their Families*. London: The Stationery Office. Crown Copyright material is reproduced with the permission of the Controller of HMSO and the Queen's Printer for Scotland.

growth; provision of nutrition; feeding styles and feeding problems; parent–child interaction and relationships; attachment-behaviour; and individual characteristics and developmental attainments will be discussed. Additionally, parenting style and competence; provision of physical and emotional care; socialisation of children by parents; environmental factors; and family functioning will be taken into account.

## Dimensions of a Child's Developmental Needs

### Health—Physical Growth

There is still a lot of disagreement amongst professionals as to when exactly a child's poor growth should give cause for concern and also about specific measures that should be adopted. With regard to physical measurements, weight-for-age, height-for-age, and weight-for-height have all been used, alone or in combination. Growth charts appropriate to gender are used which give the range of growth expected at various ages, although there is controversy as to which are most appropriate and accurate. As Bithoney (1984) notes, many researchers and practitioners use the *Stuart charts*, which are based on measurements of middle-class white children in Boston, MA, and the growth curves of the National Centre on Health Statistics (NCHS) have also been suggested as the best norm data, not only in the United States but also in other countries.

The *Tanner–Whitehouse charts*, which were used in Britain for 30 years to assess height, weight, and head-circumference, are now out of date. New growth charts, called *The 1990 nine-percentile United Kingdom charts*, have been used for over a decade now. It is claimed that the new charts describe the growth pattern more precisely. They consist of nine percentiles, whereas the former charts had only seven percentile lines, the lowest being the 3rd percentile. The lowest percentile on the new chart is the 0.4 line—only one child in 250 will fall below this line—which is a much better indicator for both the causes of concern and the reasons for the referral. The gap between each pair of percentile lines is the same (two thirds of a standard deviation), which it is said will simplify interpretation of unusual growth patterns.

Regardless of what chart is used, these measures are commonly divided into percentiles or hundredths. The simplest common criterion for growth failure in the United Kingdom is a drop below the 0.4 percentile for weight for children of that age. It means that only 250 children in the population will fall into this category. The cut-off point in the United States is the 5th percentile. Furthermore, to state that a child is failing to thrive, a child's weight needs to remain below either the 2nd percentile or 5th percentile for a period, e.g. one month (Wilensky *et al.*, 1996).

The World Health Organisation, on the other hand, does not use percentiles at all: instead, it uses standard deviation scores (SDS), also known as 'Z' scores, which can be converted to percentiles if the measurement is normally distributed. Since SDS are more suitable for the extremes of growth status seen in the developing world, the WHO curves are set at $-3$, $-2$ and $-1$ SD score below the median and 1, 2, and 3 SD above, corresponding to the 0.14th, 2.3rd, 16th, 84th, 97.7th, and 99.6th percentiles respectively. *See* Figure 9.2 (sample of weight chart).

Apart from being below the lowest percentile, a child can fall down across percentiles, e.g. from 50th to 25th or 9th percentile. Falling between percentiles might mean several things and the reasons need to be assessed. It can simply mean natural slimming due to increased activity at the toddler stage; it can be due to some kind of illness, e.g. infection, tummy-bug etc., when as a rule a child's intake of food is poor and loss of weight follows. Once the child recovers and appetite improves the weight will increase quite quickly. Falling down across the percentiles can also indicate some traumatic events in the child's life, e.g. abuse, abandonment, disruption of attachment-relationship, separation, anxiety, emotional stress, or development of serious disease. In such

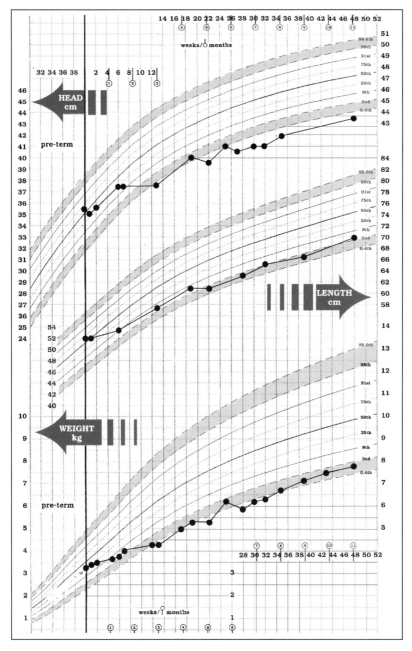

**Figure 9.2** Boys' growth chart: 0–2 years
Copyright © Child Growth Foundation

cases special attention needs to be given to the child's change of behaviour, emotional expression, and general physical appearance and functioning. *See* Figure 9.3 (falling down across percentiles).

The following cases demonstrate loss of weight for two different reasons:

> Jane was just over four years of age when she was referred to the paediatrician because of loss of weight, lack of appetite, irritable and defiant behaviour, and general change of mood. A preliminary medical investigation did not show any organic reason for failure to thrive. However, further assessments and direct observations of Jane's behaviour identified several features, indicating that sexual abuse might have taken place. Jane's change of behaviour coincided with her grandfather's coming to live with them after his wife's death. Further investigation confirmed the abuse;

and

> Tony, an 18-month-old toddler, developed a severe chest-infection, which lasted for a few weeks. He lost a considerable amount of weight as his appetite deteriorated, and he found it difficult to eat due to a persistent cough. Tony's weight dropped from the 25th percentile to below the 2nd percentile. His mood also deteriorated. He became irritable if pressed to eat, and withdrawn due to his lack of energy and his not feeling well.

Another factor which needs to be remembered is not only whether a child has lost weight or maintained its previous weight, but also whether a child is failing to gain weight at an appropriate speed for its chronological age in comparison to other children's speed of growth at the same age. Wright and Talbot (1996) advocate the use of a definition based on a fall from the 50th to below the 10th percentile, rather than one based on percentile position alone, since the reason for concern could be slow weight gain rather than simply that a child is small. Edwards *et al.* (1990) described the use of a downward percentile shift as a diagnostic criterion to provide a direct measure of growth velocity. This author suggested that the predicted growth trajectory should be calculated from weight attained at 4–8 weeks, a time when catch-up after birth will have already occurred. Corbett *et al.* (1996) postulated that this will reduce the likelihood of small children, who show stable growth-trajectories, being diagnosed as having FTT. MacMillan (1984) noted that the rule-of-thumb is that if a child crosses two major percentiles this should be seen as abnormal. The new major percentiles are considered to be the 99.6th, 98th, 91st, 75th, 50th, 25th, 9th, 2nd, and 0.4th, so that if a child, for example, drops from the 75th percentile to the 9th, it should be considered unequivocally significant.

It needs to be remembered that genetic factors play an important role and tend to determine the size of a child and the speed of growth. Small parents tend to have small children. However, it is also possible that one or both parents had failed to thrive as children, so their height and size might not represent their genetic potentials. Equally, there is a genetic endowment on

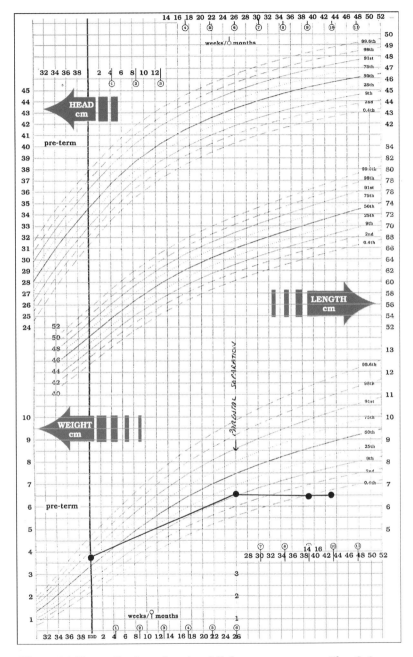

**Figure 9.3** Percentile chart showing fall-down across percentiles: 0–1 year
Copyright © Child Growth Foundation

growth which means that people from South East Asia or India should probably not be plotted on the standard Western charts. In addition, a child whose weight (US measure) for age is at the 25th percentile, but with the genetic endowment to be at the 80th percentile, is missed by the 5th percentile threshold. Care also needs to be taken when comparing the growth of children who are born prematurely or who are small for gestational age.

As we can see, weight-for-age is commonly used in tracking children's growth. However, weight and height are compounded in this measure. When a child's weight-for-age is low it is not clear whether the primary problem is low weight, short stature, or a combination of the two. Low weight-for-height is a measure of wasting and is often an early sign of malnutrition. Low height-for-age is a measure of stunting and is an indicator of chronic undernutrition. Taken together, height-for-age and weight-for-height provide a nonredundant, comprehensive picture of a child's growth status.

How to measure growth failure in children has attracted lively debate, and stimulated various research projects, which proved as varied and inconclusive as ever. Nevertheless, new anthropometric measures were developed in an attempt to predict the problem—'Z' scores are one of them. Weight loss can be measured in terms of SD or Z scores. Failure to thrive will be assumed if a child crosses the percentile curves of weight by two standard divisions (Goldson, 1989), or whose weight-for-age is more than 2SD below the population median (Mathison *et al.*, 1989).

Zamora and Parsons (2000) believe 'Z' scores to be the most accurate technique for classifying growth deficiency. A 'Z' score of 0.00 is equivalent to the 50th percentile. A 'Z' score of 2.00 SD corresponds to a percentile of 2.3, and is currently recommended by the WHO as a cut-off point for growth deficiencies. Using 'Z' scores in everyday practice is more complicated as it requires computer software for the calculation of faltering in growth. Hobbs and Hanks (1996) used 'Z' scores and converted these (approximately) to percentiles as follows:

50th percentile—Z score $= 0$
3rd percentile—Z score $= -2$
97th percentile—Z score $= +2$

According to Hobbs and Hanks, the changes in 'Z' score represent real gains in growth in relation to the population as a whole and can be mathematically compared, in contrast to weight gain, which can only be interpreted in terms of *expected* weight gain. It means that a child may gain weight but fall further behind its peers. They believe that weight is the most sensitive measure to assess when a child has not achieved its full potential for growth.

Raynor and Rudolf (2002), on the basis of their study of a randomised control trial of 83 children, concluded that weight alone is a good measure of FTT since no other marker is more predictive than another. They go further, and say that such measures can be ascertained using the Gomez calculation, weight SD scores, or simply the position on the weight chart. There is no simple anthropometric measure which highlights the degree of risk for a child. Clinical skills and experience are most important to determine which child is failing to thrive (and how severely), and which child is simply showing growth-faltering or is just small. They concluded that taking into account growth over time, development of dietary status (as well as psychosocial factors) is essential to determine the severity of FTT in children.

## ORGANIC FACTORS INFLUENCING GROWTH

Bithoney (1984) noted that organic factors may influence growth. He observed that some of these appear to play a causal role, while others have been shown to be associated with deficient growth. He highlighted organic factors which may cause failure to thrive, and which, if not taken into account, may lead to an erroneous diagnosis of non-organic FTT. These include heredity, constitutional short stature, gestational factors, minor congenital anomalies, and under-nutrition. For example, illnesses such as central nervous-system malformations can interfere with the complex regulations of appetite, sucking, swallowing, and digestion. Infection may make the child too lethargic or too weak to eat. On the other hand, disorders such as cleft lip may have little impact on the primary aspects of feeding, but may interfere with the parent–infant feeding interaction style, and this may secondarily disturb the feeding process. As Woolston (1984) observes, some physical illnesses, such as diarrhoea, may primarily be a result of the malnutrition. However, the diarrhoea may also exacerbate feeding disorders by making the infant less efficient at calorie and fluid absorption. Some children would require medical examination and necessary laboratory testing to exclude possible organic reasons for their failure to thrive and to receive appropriate treatment. Although the majority of children who fail to thrive have nothing wrong with them physically, some need to undergo investigation if there is no improvement in spite of intensive and skilful intervention, as was demonstrated by Isabella's case (*see* page 33).

## FEEDING/EATING

The most common factor in FTT is the feeding/eating behaviour of children and parental interaction/management of the feeding process. As we have seen in the previous chapters, feeding difficulties lasting over a prolonged period can lead to serious under-nutrition and distorted parent–child interaction during the process of feeding. Additionally, and more worryingly, early feeding difficulties can disrupt, in some cases, the formation of secure attachment of babies to parents and bonding of parents to children. Feeding/eating times tend to be stressful events for both children and parents. Mothers tend to be anxious, impatient, forceful, worried and angry when trying to feed a

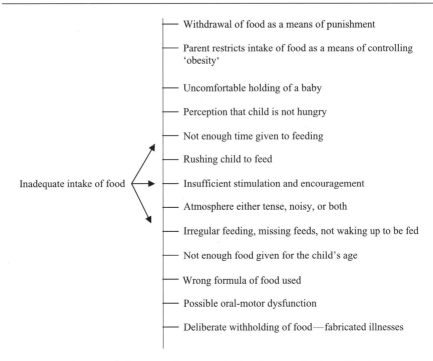

**Figure 9.4** A range of reasons for inadequate intake of food

child. Children, on the other hand, are fearful, uneasy, tense and apprehensive when being fed. Feeding, instead of being a time of mutual pleasure and enjoyment, becomes a battle of wills and aversive interactions. A consequence is that the child does not get sufficient food to promote appropriate growth.

Parental reactions to feeding difficulties differ, as does the interpretation of food refusal. Some simply feel that the child is not hungry and will eat better next time so feeds/meals are missed on a regular basis. Some lead a chaotic life, and children are neglected. In those circumstances children are fed irregularly when parents happen to remember to feed a child. The bottle is propped up in the pram for the child to feed, or another small sibling is asked to feed the child, or even to prepare a bottle. The food taken (more often than not) is not even half of the required amount for the child's age. Such children are permanently half-starved. This is not often picked up, as parental attitudes towards a child may be positive, but family life is so dysfunctional that the child's poor growth and starved appearance get lost in the midst of other concerns. In such cases there are no feeding difficulties—the child simply does not get sufficient nutrition.

It needs to be remembered that children may be starved, either deliberately by withholding food on the basis of fabricated illnesses (*see* Chapter 8), or being given inadequate food in quantity and quality because of parental attitudes to food and preoccupation with weight control. (*See* Previn's case, page 48.)

However, the evidence arising from a majority of studies has constantly shown more feeding difficulties among families with children who fail to thrive than controls (Iwaniec, 1991; Dawson, 1992; Hanks & Hobbs, 1993). Mothers are reported to be less sensitive, infants more negative while being fed, and vocal interaction infrequent in comparison with controls. Most children in the samples of Drotar (1991), Drotar *et al.* (1990), Hampton (1996), Hanks and Hobbs (1993), and Iwaniec (1983) experienced significant feeding problems, such as spitting up, poor sucking, storing food in their mouths, refusal to take solids, rumination, and taking excessive time to feed. Feeding difficulties emerged soon after birth. For example, Raynor and Rudolf (1996) reported that a concerning number of mothers described difficulties in feeding their infants starting in the first three months of life.

Skuse *et al.* (1994) found that a substantial number of infants studied were reported as having slept through feeds during the first year of life, and their parents were less likely to wake them for feeds. The authors pointed out that many mothers did not wake them up for feeding, and found that the children who slept through feeds had lower weights for their age. Iwaniec (1995) reported many mothers' lack of awareness or recognition that their children were extremely thin and that the amount of food they consumed was inadequate for their age. Additionally, a child's slow feeding was often interpreted as meaning it was not hungry.

During the assessment attention should be given to the following:

1. *Recording of daily food intake*: if possible, samples through a whole week should be obtained to see whether there are any differences and what pattern of eating behaviour and intake of food is evident over several days;
2. *Observing 2–3 feeding sessions (at different times)*: if possible, video should be used to record one or two sessions. Observation of parent–child interaction is essential to see reactive and pro-active behaviour of parent and child, the feeding style of the parent, the amount of food, and the type of food taken; and
3. *Particular attention should be paid to non-specific symptoms* such as intermittent vomiting, spitting up, diarrhoea, and respiratory tract infection which are very common in malnourished children. Dental problems might contribute to refusal to eat as they might cause pain, and there may be other neurological problems leading to difficulties in swallowing and sucking.

Infants and young children who fail to thrive may have some organic features that contribute to, but do not explain, their growth failure. It has been found that a significant degree of oral-motor dysfunction is common, such as problems with sucking, chewing, and swallowing (Lewis, 1982; Skuse, 1993). Consequently, parents may be faced with a significant, yet subtle and

| Date | Time | Food Amount | Method of Feeding | Time Taken | Mother's Feelings |
|------|------|-------------|-------------------|------------|-------------------|
| Wednesday 20 October | 8.30 am | ½ Weetabix, a little milk | being fed | 45 minutes | exhausted, depressed, bad start to the day |
| | 10.00 am | 100 mls milk | | 10 minutes | |
| | 11.45 am | ½ potato, 2 pieces of carrot, few pieces of lamb, gravy | began herself, but then refused to swallow meat. Mother ended up liquidising the child's lunch and feeding it to her, almost by force | 1 hour 20 minutes | angry and depressed |
| | 3.00 pm | 3 spoons of yoghurt, 1 biscuit | fed herself | 20 minutes | very tired |
| | 5.30 pm | 1 chip, 2 spoons of baked beans | being fed, refused to eat fish | | gave up, asked her father to feed her |
| | 7.00 pm | cup of drinking chocolate | | 10 minutes | |

**Figure 9.5** Daily eating record (a sample)
*Source:* Iwaniec, D. (1995) *The Emotionally Abused and Neglected Child*. Chichester: John Wiley & Sons Ltd

often unappreciated, obstacle to ensuring the child ingests adequate nutrition for growth. Contextual features, such as inappropriate positioning during feeding, may also compound these problems, such as being fed in a noisy, distracting room; or being fed in the pram with a bottle propped in the mouth.

Lewis (1982) identified the following oral-motor indicators, which should be considered for assessment purposes:

- difficulty in positioning and handling the child during feeding;
- excessive feeding time (greater than 45 minutes);
- absent, weak, uncoordinated, or delayed sucking;
- chewing and swallowing problems;
- tongue-thrusting resulting in food loss;
- persistent, involuntary tongue-biting, spoon-biting, or nipple-biting;
- intolerance of developmentally appropriate food texture; and
- excessive drooling.

## DEVELOPMENTAL DELAYS

It is widely recognised that a child's early experiences can have long-lasting effects on its later development (Rutter, 1995b). Cases of non-organic FTT are particularly worrying since many of these children show poor developmental outcomes in language, motor, cognitive, social, and affective areas. Their mental abilities tend to suffer, as found by Dowdney *et al.* (1987), Illingworth (1983), Reif *et al.* (1995), Skuse *et al.* (1994), and effects can be long-lasting (Iwaniec, 2000, and Iwaniec & Sneddon, 2002). The detrimental effects of early malnutrition may be extensive given a rapid period of growth, particularly brain growth. Since brain growth and synoptic connections occur within the first two years, if there is inadequate intake of food to support that growth, then brain growth will be affected. Grantham-McGregor *et al.* (2000) concluded that children younger than two years are particularly vulnerable to the effects of malnutrition, since head circumference and height in the first 24 months are more significant predictors of IQ at 11 years of age than more recent or concurrent measures. Woolston (1984) defines developmental delay as either a deceleration of the acquisition of the new developmental milestone or actual regression in certain areas. The measurement of developmental delays may be particularly useful for prognosis and provision of necessary intervention to rectify the problem. For example, Corbett *et al.* (1996) found that even in relatively mild failure-to-thrive cases there are long-term adverse cognitive deficits and that a velocity-based measure could be a useful predictor of cognitive outcomes. It was found that IQ can be reduced by 10–20 points, which is potentially reversible if positive changes occur in a child's life or if appropriate intervention and treatment take place (Kristiansson & Fällström, 1987; Hutcheson *et al.*, 1997; Iwaniec, 2000). Reif *et al.* (1995) found that five years after assessment children who failed to thrive had more learning difficulties and evidenced developmental delays also in language, social, and emotional areas in contrast to the studied control group. Developmental delays are also associated with poor stimulation, a low level of interaction at home, disorders of attachment, separation, and rejection. Some of these children are neglected both physically and emotionally, so there is limited verbal, social, and emotional contact between the parent and the child which, in turn, leads to poor developmental attainments. The use of the *Bayley Scale of Infant Development* provides comprehensive measures on all-round child development.

### Emotional and Behavioural Development

The interactions between parents and children (particularly the early ones involving communication between mother and baby) are of crucial significance in a child's development. What a baby needs is close, confident, and caring physical and emotional contact with the parent (be it mother, father, or other carer) in order to be healthy, vigorously develop, and thrive. The absence of such continuing nurturance and physical intimacy can bring about anxiety in a child, fretting, and disruption of biological function. One of the indices of basic trust and security in an infant (in Erik Erikson's sense) is stable feeding behaviour. In order for eating to be nutritionally beneficial and enjoyable it requires conditions that denote a relatively benign and calm state of psychosomatic harmony.

Good emotional development, establishing in a child a sense of security and safety, is determined by parental responsiveness. This last is a complex and many-sided phenomenon, but there are at least three different elements that make up what one might assess to be sensitive responsiveness: these are tendencies to react promptly, consistently, and appropriately in response to a child's crying and other signals of distress.

Parents who are sensitive and attentive tend to have children who are securely attached to them as they feel they can always rely on their parents when they need them. Parents who are consistently responsive to children's efforts to seek closeness or comforting engender secure attachment, while parents who are inconsistent, rejective, and insensitive can produce insecure attachment styles in children. In a well-functioning attachment system the care-giver is sensitive and psychologically available to give comfort, support, and contact as well as opportunities for environmental exploration.

*Secure attachments (infant-to-parent) may be indexed by the baby's:*

1. interest and attentiveness when with the parent (looking, gazing, listening);
2. relaxation and/or calmness in the company of the parent;
3. dependence behaviours—e.g. holding, proximity-seeking (later when more mobile going for comfort and help)—directed at the parent;
4. evident preference for the parent to others;
5. curiosity and exploration using the parent as a 'base';
6. pleasure, enthusiasm, joy (e.g. smiling, vocalizing) in the presence of the parent; and
7. protest, displeasure, concern when separated from the parent: comforted when he/she returns.

However, research on attachment of failure-to-thrive children to their mothers suggests that a considerable number of children are insecurely attached (Kotelchuck *et al.*, 1981; Iwaniec, 1983; Crittenden, 1987; Ward *et al.*, 2000), as fully discussed in Chapter 6. Research has repeatedly demonstrated that an insecure-attachment history is a risk factor for mal-adaptation in a few areas of development. One of the mechanisms through which insecure attachment affects mal-adaptation is the inner working model, which portrays early parent–child interaction, and shapes future behaviour and ability to form positive relationships with peers and adults. Without help, or better experiences, children's abilities to form meaningful and warm relationships may

Table 9.1 Types of attachments, parental behaviour and child's reactions (outcomes)

| Types of attachments | Carer's behaviour | Effect on child's developmental outcomes |
|---|---|---|
| Securely attached children | Sensitive; responsive to signals of distress; warm, reassuring; supportive; encouraging; patient; comforting; available; concerned; engaging; protective | Self-confident; high self-esteem; social leaders; empathic; popular; show good developmental attainments; open; trustful; sociable; skilful in interacting with others; adaptable; mature emotionally; stable; friendly |
| Avoidant/anxious | Hostile; rejective; critical; persistent rebuffing; unsupportive; unresponsive to signals of distress; uncommunicative; avoiding physical contact with a child | Unselective attachment; treats parents and strangers alike; over-friendly with strangers; poor self-confidence; poor concentration span; disruptive; destructive; developmentally delayed; difficulty in building relationships with peers; attention-seeking |
| Anxious/ambivalent | Neglectful; unsupportive; disorganised; insensitive; dismissing; chaotic | Apprehensive; confused; passive; detached; withdrawn; developmentally retarded; poor self-confidence; chronic doubts; poor socialisations |
| Disorganised/ disoriented | Unpredictable; frightening; frightened; changeable; secretive | Confusion; anxiety; undirected expression of fear and distress; dazed or disoriented facial expression; emotional and thought conflicts; disorganised behaviour; apprehension |

be affected. They may carry such negative representations into adulthood and parenthood. It is important, therefore, to assess the quality of attachment and to apply corrective measures to prevent long-term negative consequences. Table 9.1 gives a description of each type of attachment, parental behaviour, and children's reactions.

## BEHAVIOURAL DEVELOPMENT

Children's development is viewed in terms of the accomplishment of crucial socialisation tasks. Those tasks will be learned and skills acquired if the socialising agents, such as parents, provide models of behaviour as well as guidance from which to learn. Children need to be educated and helped to achieve social competence and to behave in a pro-social age-appropriate way. Parents need to recognise that each child comes to this world with different temperament characteristics, and individual behavioural styles which might pose different child-rearing problems or challenges. Some children are very easy to bring up. They eat and sleep well, they are happy, and easy to satisfy. Others are far more challenging to rear and will require more time and energy to look after. They might be very sensitive, difficult to feed, and to satisfy. Some will learn new skills and ways of behaving quickly and enthusiastically, while others will find mastering developmental tasks frustrating and difficult. Because human infants are so totally dependent for so long on their primary care-givers, their developmental outcomes will reflect the quality of care and attention given to the specific needs of a child. If their basic needs are met they are thought to develop a basic trust in parents, and thus to evolve a nucleus of self-trust, which is indispensable for later development. When children's needs are not met, their physical, emotional, cognitive, and behavioural development is quite likely to be arrested. In infancy, curtailed development will tend to show itself in insecure attachment and delayed psycho-motor development; in pre-school children it will be manifested in disturbance in social and emotional behaviour; and in school-aged children it will show itself in serious learning deficit and behavioural problems.

If practitioners are familiar with a child's individual attributes and rearing difficulties which may stem from it, they can advise parents how to manage certain types of behaviours and reactions. For example, a difficult child requires fair but firm and consistent rules and routines and behavioural boundaries to help them through the socialisation process. Slow-to-warm-up children, on the other hand, require parental patience in teaching them different skills. These children are more timid and less confident in trying new things. Once they learn a skill, however, they do it well. Parents are advised to wait and encourage instead of rushing and criticising.

Some failure-to-thrive children present deficit behaviour—conduct problems—and emotional disturbances. Table 9.2 shows distribution of various behavioural individual characteristics.

## Identity

As children grow they begin to identify themselves, firstly as part of the family, then as part of neighbourhood and community. If a child is of a different race or origin (geographically and/or socially) than the people in their family, or the majority of people in the neighbourhood or community, they may need to develop awareness of the differences in their origin, culture or way of life. They need to grow up knowing, for example, that although they might look a bit different to other children in the neighbourhood, they are equal to them in every respect. If a black child happens to be placed in a white

**Table 9.2** Individual behavioural characteristics (temperament attributes)

| | Easy child | Difficult child | Slow-to-warm-up child |
|---|---|---|---|
| **Rhythmicity** | Rhythmic in biological functioning, e.g. eating, sleeping, naps. The carer can organise daily activities as the child is predictable | Unpredictable in biological functioning. Difficult to establish routine in sleeping, feeding, toileting, etc., if changes from day to day | |
| **Activity** | | | Unlike easy and difficult children, slow-to-warm-up children are very low in activity. They sit a lot, move slowly, and walk rather than run. They do everything slowly |
| **Adaptability** | Adapts relatively easily to new circumstances and changes: e.g. from liquids to solids; from baby-bath to big bath; from cot to big bed; from home to school, etc. | Takes a long time to adapt to new food, textures, smell, and different types of food. Adaptation to new things (such as big bath, bed, different room, nursery, school, people) is long | Takes a long time to adapt to new foods, new textures, smells, etc. Adaptation to new things is long, e.g. from liquids to solids; from baby-bath to big bath; from cot to bed; from home to school, nursery etc. |
| **Approach/ withdrawal** | Gets used to people easily and interacts with them without too much apprehension or distress | Gets withdrawn, upset, uncooperative, and stubborn when exposed to less well-known people. Difficult to engage | Withdrawn when approached by people, do not get involved, avoid new people, uncooperative, stubborn |
| **Intensity** | Reactions, e.g. crying or laughing, are moderate. Can be distracted or pacified easily | Very high in intensity, loud crying, loud laughing and talking, very involved whatever it is doing | Low in intensity, quiet. Does everything and reacts to things in a calm, low-key way |
| **Mood** | Positive in mood, happy, jolly and easy to satisfy | Frequent negative moods lasting a long time, difficult to jolly out of a bad mood. Often looks miserable and unsatisfied | Frequent, negative moods lasting a long time but expressed in a quiet manner. Tends to be miserable for prolonged periods of time |

**Table 9.3** Types of behavioural and emotional problems of FTT children

| Behaviour | Often | Occasionally | Seldom |
|---|---|---|---|
| Withdrawn | | | |
| Unresponsive | | | |
| Lethargic | | | |
| Uncommunicative | | | |
| Reluctance to play or to engage in activities | | | |
| Inability to stand up for him/herself | | | |
| *Acting-out behaviour:* | | | |
| Demanding | | | |
| Defiance | | | |
| Irritability | | | |
| Whining | | | |
| *Emotional problems:* | | | |
| Head banging | | | |
| Rocking | | | |
| Destructiveness (destroying personal belongings) | | | |
| Self-biting | | | |
| Scratching | | | |
| Cutting | | | |
| Attention-seeking | | | |
| Poor concentration | | | |
| Fire-setting | | | |
| Sad, miserable expression | | | |
| Aimless wandering and inactivity | | | |
| Not speaking to other children or people, particularly parents | | | |
| Not being interested in play of other children | | | |

*(Cont.)*

Table 9.3 (*Cont.*)

| Behaviour | Often | Occasionally | Seldom |
|---|---|---|---|
| Excessive dependence on the presence of familiar figures, e.g. nursery nurse, teacher, social worker, etc. | | | |
| Lack of emotional reactions to people or events | | | |
| Comfort habits: sucking thumb, masturbation, keeping special objects | | | |
| Vomiting | | | |
| Diarrhoea | | | |
| Soiling and smearing | | | |
| Wetting | | | |
| Over-eating | | | |
| Under-eating | | | |
| Disturbed sleeping | | | |
| Regressed behaviour such as reverting to baby-like language | | | |

foster-carer's home the child has to be brought up being aware of his/her origin and, furthermore, helped to identify with other children or people of the same race and culture. Children who are emotionally ill treated are at particular risk of suffering from low self-esteem, which affects development of appropriate self-identity. Being often denigrated by the care-givers brings about self-depreciation and/or lack of self-confidence.

## Social Presentation

Children like to be dressed and look the same as other children, especially when they are at school or in other public places. They need to be clean, washed, and wear well-laundered clean clothing of the right size. They need to be properly turned out so they do not stand out as dirty, smelly, infested with lice, for example, and looking shabby. As children need to build up social relationships with peers it is essential that they are helped to integrate into their peer groups. In order to be accepted and thought of as worthwhile and fun to be with by other children they need to look more or less the same as the rest. Neglected children who also fail to thrive tend to have social-presentation problems, especially those whose parents are alcoholics or live in impoverished, dysfunctional families. FTT in these children is the result of chronic neglect and omission of meeting basic needs. Social presentation of these children can be quite striking as they look thin, small, dirty, and shabby. They lack self-confidence and their self-esteem is poor. They tend to be socially isolated because of their appearance and, at times, disturbed behaviour. Additionally, these children are often not liked by teachers as they are not appealing or pleasant to be with.

Social presentation of the majority of failure-to-thrive children is good or very good. They come from all backgrounds and social classes, and their physical appearance and presentation give an impression that they are well cared for, which, of course, can be very misleading, as shown in the cases of Jimmy and Mark (page 91).

## FAMILY AND SOCIAL RELATIONSHIPS

Families of FTT children are not a homogeneous group, and they do not differ substantially from any other family that has problems with child-rearing. As a rule there is only one child that fails to thrive in the family. It is often observed that the relationships, level of mutual attachments, and physical growths of other children are good and not causing any concern. An FTT child, due to difficulties in feeding and poor growth, tends to elicit stress, worries, low self-efficacy, and feelings of child-rearing incompetence. If the problem persists, there is observable tension between the child and the mother, and often between the parents themselves as well. Additionally, siblings, and the FTT child in some cases, show alienation and lack of interest in their poor-growing brother or sister. They tend to pick up parental behaviour and attitudes towards such a child very quickly and behave in a similar way. Thus, the failure-to-thrive child can become socially isolated and lonely within the family.

Psychosocial short-stature children are singled out, rejected, and discriminated against. The cause is often associated with attachment-bonding problems, bereavement in the family, loss of a previous child, or some form of tragedy at the time of the child's birth, or the child representing a shameful part of the family history, e.g. illegitimacy.

Relationships between parents and extended family members are fraught, as various family members blame the parents, but, more specifically, the mother, for the poor quality of care afforded to the FTT child. There are noticeable poor relationships between the parents, and many were found to separate or divorce some years later (Iwaniec, 2000). Equally, social contacts and relationships with neighbours, friends, and professions fluctuate between claiming to be very good and very bad, depending on whether a person agrees with the parents or not.

It needs to be remembered that there may be a very damaged person living in the family who may inflict a lot of pain and generate fear, or abuse a child secretly. Violent fathers, drug-abusing or alcoholic parents, mentally ill family members, or persons with a learning disability can cause many difficulties. Such persons may sexually abuse a child, or may emotionally torment a child and other members of the family. An abuse of power over a vulnerable child who is singled out or scape-goated is evident in some FTT cases. When assessing family relationships we have to be open-minded, and rigid classification of bad and good needs to be avoided, as there are various shades of social relationships which are not necessarily damaging, even if they are qualitatively different.

## SELF-CARE SKILLS

Socialisation is the major developmental task of all children as they acquire step-by-step new skills and become more independent and able to do things without the help of others. These skills will be learned if a child is shown how to do things and is given the opportunity to try and experiment to do things alone or with a little help from carers.

Neglected children and children who fail to thrive tend to be delayed in self-care areas, partly because of low mother–child interaction, indifferent relationships, and poor stimulation (Hanks & Hobbs, 1993). The level of attention given to the child needs to be taken into consideration as well as parental awareness of when and how they should encourage self-skills learning. When assessing the family careful attention should be paid to identifying realistic and unrealistic expectations of the parents, as to what a child can or cannot do at a certain age. There are simple milestone measurements available, and health visitors can assist in developmental assessment. Child observation is a good way to put knowledge of developmental theory into practice.

## DIMENSION OF PARENTING CAPACITY

### General Overview

It is often amazing how well the majority of people, especially the young, adapt to their parenting role and become wholly successful and caring parents. They do this job effectively and willingly in spite of many other demands on their time and energy. Let us look at what this requires, and what stands in the way of good parenting.

Adequate parenting requires a number of skills that are far from being simple—part common sense, part intuition, part empathy, and part of what we have learned from being parented as children. Most parents successfully carry out the complex tasks involved in child-rearing, using a variety of methods in very diverse family, cultural, and social circumstances. Some, however, find bringing up children difficult, frustrating, and unrewarding. There are many reasons why some parents are inadequate in their parenting role. Contemporary parents are often inexperienced in the care of children. They may be unaccustomed to babies because they were brought up in small families and were not given responsibilities for caring for their younger siblings, unlike the case in past years. They may themselves have been brought up in neglectful and uncaring homes, or been abused or ill treated, and had no opportunities to acquire a better parenting style and understanding of children's developmental needs. They might be living in adverse social and economic circumstances that could affect the quality of everyday child care. Some might be ill, have learning disabilities, or suffer from depression, so they cannot tune into a child's emotional needs. Additionally, lack of support and guidance, as well as social isolation brought about by diminished extended-family and community resources (from where, traditionally, help was provided) contribute to poor and often ill-informed parenting. Growing numbers of single, young, and immature mothers (who may be socially isolated and unsupported), often living in poverty, are unprepared for the demands of child-rearing, and therefore unable to provide basic physical and emotional care and nurturing for their off-spring.

Failure-to-thrive children come from all families: well-to-do and poor; with young, and more mature parents; middle-class and well-educated; and working-class and poorly educated. As FTT studies usually cover deprived areas to select research samples (even community projects), we do not have a true or representative picture of social backgrounds and parental social characteristics. The parenting capacity is multi-dimensional, and child-rearing practices may differ over time as they are influenced by different personal structural and child circumstances. Belsky (1984) convincingly argued that competent parenting is multiply determined and proposes that influences fall into three categories:

1. The parents' characteristics;
2. The contextual sources of support (e.g. marital/partner relationship, family unity and support, help and support from extended family, friends, neighbours, and wider community); and
3. the child's characteristics (e.g. temperament, physical appearance, health, child's behavioural responses to the parents).

Belsky further suggested that the above factors exert a different level of influence (with *the parents' characteristics* being the most significant factor), then *the context of support*, and lastly *the child's characteristics*. It is clear that the level of interaction between various components influences the quality of care a child receives. Parental characteristics such as sensitivity, patience, commitment, flexibility, affection, health, intellectual capacity, and sense of duty and responsibility will be positively activated if there is family support, especially coming from the partner who will take equal responsibility for parenting the child. Additionally, if there are easily accessible community resources to assist parents with a failure-to-thrive child it will help the parents further to cope with difficulties. At the same time a child's characteristics will powerfully influence the way parents interact, care, and feel about them. A child who presents constant feeding problems, cries a lot, appears to be miserable, and gives little positive feedback to the parents might strain the development of a good relationship. Assessment of parenting capacity has to take into consideration the nature of the relationship between parent and child. The 'goodness of fit' between the characteristics of the child and parent needs to be assessed within the context of their relationship. What is important when assessing parenting of FTT children is not so much how well informed, skilful, and competent they are but, more importantly, how those skills and the information are translated and expressed when dealing with the child within the context of parent–child relationship and the strength of bond within the family. The following questions during interview provide general information about child-rearing attitudes:

1. What kind of problems do you have with Susan? Can you describe each of them?
2. How do you handle these behaviours? Can you give me an example of how, for instance, you deal with Susan's defiance?
3. How do you discipline Susan?
4. Can you describe the rules and routines in your family?
5. How do you correct and teach her to behave well?
6. How do you teach her to learn different life-tasks and skills, such as eating, dressing, toilet-training, playing, and so on?
7. Do you praise Susan and show pleasure in her achievements?
8. How much time do you spend with her and what do you do when you are together?
9. Do you cuddle, hug, kiss, and smile at Susan?
10. Do you play with her and do you enjoy doing it?
11. How often do you speak with Susan and do things with her?
12. Do you enjoy Susan's company?
13. What do you like about Susan? Please describe these likeable qualities to me.
14. What are your expectations of Susan?
15. What do other members of the family think about her?
16. Can you describe how you get on together?
17. How does she get on with her brothers and other children?
18. How does she get on with other adults when she is in their company?

19. Did you want to have Susan? Was she a planned child?
20. What was your life like when you were expecting her and when she was a baby?
21. What kind of pregnancy, labour, and birth did you have with Susan?
22. What was she like as a baby in terms of feeding, sleeping, contentment, responsiveness, and health?
23. What were the major difficulties experienced when she was a baby?
24. Did you feel close to her when she was a baby and how do you feel now?
25. Can you tell me when she sat, crawled, walked, and said her first words and sentences?
26. How would you like to change the present situation so you and Susan are happier together?
27. What assistance and help do you need to make things work for Susan and the family?
28. Would you be prepared to work with us so that we can improve the present situation?

## Basic Care

Failure-to-thrive children require basic provision of physical care common to all children, such as food, shelter, clothing, appropriate hygiene, and adequate medical and social care. Failure to thrive may be the result of poor physical care, inadequate provision of nutrition, and the inability to respond to the child's emotional needs, but equally (and more frequently) it is a combination of feeding/eating problems, parent–child interaction during the process of feeding, and parental worries and anxieties associated with the child's poor weight gain, physical appearance, associated developmental delays and behavioural problems. However, basic care of children who fail to thrive also requires careful observation and identification of subtle clues which are demonstrated by parental attitudes towards food and weight or parental emotional relationships with the child. Some children appear to be extremely well provided for physically, and material standards are high, but emotional care is mechanical, showing absence of pleasure in being with the child and limited mutuality and physical and emotional togetherness. Occasionally, crippling over-protection is identified, which requires attention and detailed assessment.

The nutritional aspect of basic physical care requires careful and comprehensive attention, such as provision of the appropriate quantity and quality of food for the child's age, regularity of feeding/eating, and the manner in which the child is handled during eating/feeding time (Hanks & Hobbs, 1993; Iwaniec, 1991). The questions in Table 9.4 need to be asked when assessing physical and nutritional care of the FTT children.

Table 9.4 rates the quality of nutritional care provided for the child based on direct observation, food-intake recording, and interview data. The higher the scores, the greater the cause for concern over the child's welfare.

**Table 9.4** The quality of nutritional and physical care of a child

Rate the quality of nutritional and physical care provided for the child, based on observation and interview data. The higher the score, the greater the cause for concern over the child's welfare.

Name: —————————————— Date: ——————————————

Overall Rating: ——————————————

| Section A<br><br>Nutrition | Most of the time<br>1 | Sometimes<br>2 | Not very often<br>3 |
|---|---|---|---|
| Is the child regularly fed? | | | |
| Is the child given enough food for their age? | | | |
| Is the child being picked up when fed? | | | |
| Is the child encouraged to eat by being prompted and praised? | | | |
| Is food presented in an appetising way? | | | |
| Is the food suitable for the child's age? | | | |
| Are the signals of hunger or satiation properly interpreted? | | | |
| Is the manner of feeding comfortable and anxiety free? | | | |
| Is there availability of food? | | | |
| Is the child handled patiently during feeding/eating? | | | |
| Is the child encouraged to eat? | | | |
| Is there reasonable flexibility in feeding/eating routine? | | | |
| **Physical care** | | | |
| Is there awareness of the child being too thin, small, or unwell? | | | |
| Is the child's medical care being seen to, such as: medical examinations, vaccinations, eye and hearing tests etc? | | | |
| Is medical advice sought when the child is unwell? | | | |
| Is there recognition and concern about the child's well-being? | | | |
| Is the child appropriately dressed for the weather? | | | |

*(Cont.)*

**Table 9.4**  (*Cont.*)

| | | | |
|---|---|---|---|
| Is the child changed and clean? | | | |
| Are medical or other health or welfare agency appointments being kept? | | | |
| Do the parents administer required medication for the child? | | | |
| Is the safety for the child observed? | | | |
| Is the child supervised and guided? | | | |
| Is the child protected from a smoking environment and other unhealthy substances? | | | |
| **Total for Section A** | | | |

**Section B** rates parental attitudes and behaviour regarding feeding and food.

| **Section B** | **Most of the time 3** | **Sometimes 2** | **Not very often 1** |
|---|---|---|---|
| Does the care-giver appear angry during the feeding/eating period? | | | |
| Is there evidence of frustration during the feeding/eating period? | | | |
| Is the child punished for not eating? | | | |
| Is food withheld as a means of punishment? | | | |
| Does the care-giver restrict the child's intake of food to prevent possible obesity? | | | |
| Does the care-giver restrict the child's intake of food and variety of food due to fabricated illnesses, allergies, etc.? | | | |
| Are the care-giver's attitudes to food and eating negative (e.g. dislike of food, preoccupied with healthy food, strictly vegetarian, or vegan?) | | | |
| Has the care-giver a history of being anorexic, bulimic or experienced other eating problems? | | | |
| **Total for Section B** | | | |

## PARENTAL CHARACTERISTICS

Adequate parenting may depend on many factors. Cognitive, socio-economic, and historical characteristics of the care-givers may influence the way they look after and care for their failure-to-thrive children. Low maternal education is considered to be a risk factor (Drotar & Sturm, 1988). Skuse *et al.* (1994) found that mothers of children who began growth-faltering before six months of age were found to have significantly higher IQs than mothers whose children began growth-faltering after 6 months of age. In some instances the pattern of caring and paying attention to the children's nutritional and nurturing needs is very similar to that of their parents when they were children. It is either very rigid and demanding, with little space for flexibility and patience, or neglectful (quite often unintentionally), stemming from lack of understanding and knowledge about child-rearing and children's developmental needs. For example, a care-giver may not understand the importance of feeding-formula preparation, and (trying to save money) may over-dilute the more expensive formula so that it lasts longer, while not realising that this means the child will be inadequately nourished. Equally, some care-givers were found to deliberately dilute the formula to prevent the child gaining more weight because of fear of obesity and dislike of plump babies. Furthermore, some will wilfully withhold food as a result of an imagined/fabricated illness to attract sympathy and attention to themselves. Fortunately, these are isolated cases but are deadly serious and dangerous. The assessor has to pay particular attention when food allergies are reported, frequent visits to the doctor or out-patients' clinic are documented, and nothing is ever found to indicate eating or digestion problems. The child, as a rule, is put on a strict diet by the care-giver, resulting in starvation and failure to thrive.

Most care-givers, however, are just ordinary mothers who find feeding their children difficult. Such difficulties accumulate parental anxieties leading to forceful feeding, resulting in the child's fear and apprehension of feeding/eating and distortion of the relationships, particularly in terms of trust and a sense of security.

## CARE-GIVER CHARACTERISTICS

The following care-giver characteristics require attention:

- frequent depressive moods;
- post-natal depression;
- experiencing feelings of loss, and abandonment, or bereavement;
- low self-esteem and self-confidence;
- feeling helpless and inadequate;

- distorted perceptions and attitudes towards a failure-to-thrive child;
- lack of affection and bonding to the child;
- difficulties in enjoying the child's company and getting pleasure out of being together;
- worries and anxieties about the child's poor weight gain and development;
- limited interaction with the child;
- finding the child difficult to manage generally, but specifically during feeding time;
- physical and emotional distancing from the child;
- a poor marital/supportive relationship;
- being socially isolated and unsupported;
- belief that they will be accused of deliberate physical and emotional neglect (cognitive distortion);
- feelings of guilt and failure as a parent; and
- being rigid or chaotic in child-rearing.

## Ensuring Safety

Ensuring that the child is adequately protected from harm or danger is an extremely important factor to consider when doing assessment. It is particularly important when failure to thrive is persistent, and of long duration, and when universal and targeted interventions have not been effective. This applies to psychosocial short-stature children and more serious cases of chronic neglect, rejection, or other forms of ill-informed parenting and distorted perceptions (Blizzard & Bulatovic, 1993; Skuse et al., 1996). Some children are simply starved, as withdrawal of food is used frequently as a means of discipline to control behavioural problems. Some children are locked in the bedroom for long periods, and occasionally climb through the windows to escape punishment. Physical abuse like smacking, pushing, or pulling is not uncommon when care-givers meet a child's resistant behaviour to their requests or commands. Skuse et al. (1996) found that substantial numbers of children in their sample were sexually abused as well. In severe cases of long-term duration children may harm themselves, e.g. cutting themselves with a knife or sharp object, setting fires, head-banging, etc. They tend to eat non-food items, which can upset or even harm their digestive system. We need to be alerted to the possibility of deliberate starvation, fabrication of illness, or active inducement of illness (such as deliberate poisoning, giving a child laxatives to induce diarrhoea, or insisting that a child is allergic to many brands of food), thus starving the child. The disorder of Münchausen Syndrome by Proxy by care-givers is associated with growth failure in children.

Practitioners should be alerted to possible mistreatment or mismanagement if a child improves rapidly when living away from home, e.g. short-term foster-care, hospitalisation, or being placed with an extended family. In cases like that the assessor should examine what is done differently to produce the desired outcome for the child. It might be anxiety-free interaction that encourages the child to take more food and to feel at ease when in adult company. It can also mean that a child is given an adequate amount of food at the right frequency, or that abuse or neglect which occurred at home has been terminated. Since FTT is multidimensional, and controlling mechanisms are various and varied, great care must be taken to avoid assumptions that it is parental, deliberately maltreating behaviour which is responsible for triggering and maintaining the problem.

## EMOTIONAL WARMTH

### Ensuring the Child's Emotional Needs are Met

It is now widely accepted that a child needs a close, confident, and caring physical and emotional contact with the care-giver in order to grow well, be healthy, and develop vigorously. The absence of such continuing nurturance and physical intimacy can bring about anxiety in the child, fretting, and disruption of biological functions. It has been recognised that infants and small children deprived of warmth, parental care, and lack of responsiveness to their emotional needs may develop profound depression or acute withdrawal with consequent lack of appetite, loss of weight, and serious developmental delays (Bowlby, 1988a). One of the indices of basic trust and security in an infant is stable feeding behaviour. In order for eating to be nutritionally beneficial and enjoyable it requires conditions that denote a relatively benign and calm state of psychosomatic harmony.

Most parents of FTT infants are attentive to their children's emotional needs and do their best to provide emotional warmth when interacting with them, but tend to lose confidence when refusal to eat and poor physical growth take place. The parents feel rejected by the child as they reject their basic provision of care (which is food). Researchers such as Iwaniec (1995), Drotar (1991), and Raynor and Rudolf (1996) argue that failure to thrive can be a result, in some cases, of emotional neglect demonstrated by lack of pleasure at being with the child, or limited physical contact (such as holding, cuddling, smiling at, playing, initiating communication, responding to the child's signals of boredom, and being less responsive to the child's nurturing needs). Additionally, parental attitudes towards these children, if problems persist, are reported to be troubled and confused (Iwaniec & Sneddon, 2002). The emotional bond between child and parent tends to be weaker, as demonstrated by lower frequency of mutual interaction and reported lack of pleasure at being together and enjoying the child's company. Consequently, such behaviours and attitudes do not facilitate development of secure attachment as a source of safety and reassurance when in distress.

**Table 9.5** Qualities of emotionally caring parenting

| Emotional needs | Some defining criteria |
|---|---|
| 1. Affection | Affection includes physical contact, admiration, touching, holding, comforting, making allowances, being tender, showing concern, communicating |
| 2. Security | Security means continuity of care, a predictable environment, consistent controls, settled patterns of care and daily routines, fair and understandable rules, harmonious family relationships, the feeling that one's home and family are always there |
| 3. Responsibility | Responsibility involves discipline appropriate to the child's stage of development, providing a model to emulate/imitate, indicating limits, insisting on concern for others |
| 4. Independence | Independence implies making opportunities for the child to do more unaided and make decisions, first about small things but gradually about larger matters |
| 5. Responsiveness | Responsiveness means prompt, consistent, appropriate actions to meet the child's needs |
| 6. Stimulation | Stimulation means encouraging curiosity and exploratory behaviour, by praising, by responding to questions and play, by promoting training/educational opportunities and new experiences |

*Source:* Iwaniec, D., Herbert, M. & Sluckin, A. (2002) Helping emotionally abused and neglected children and abusive carers. In K. Browne, H. Hanks, P. Stratton, and C. Hamilton (Eds) *Early Prediction and Prevention of Child Abuse: A Handbook*, pp. 249–265. Chichester: John Wiley.

Apart from basic physical and nutritional care it is necessary to assess the emotional care of the child within the family. Direct observation and interviews with the care-givers will provide information about the way the child is nurtured and emotionally supported in mastering developmental tasks and being socialised according to the child's age.

The assessment should examine the care-givers' responsiveness to the child's signals of distress and pro-social communications. These are aimed at identifying caring parenting as discussed in Table 9.5.

## PARENT–CHILD INTERACTION

Parent–child interaction is a two-way process, which powerfully affects the way parents and children relate to each other, perceive each other, and influence each other's behaviour. The quality and quantity of mutual interaction is not only determined by the parental behaviour towards the child, but also by the child's input (whether positive or negative) that affects this two-way process. If parents receive positive feedback from the child, like smiling, taking food, responding to attention, then they will try to engage with the child more often. On the other hand, if a child gives back little in terms of showing pleasure in seeing the parent, then the care-giver will interact less. There are many reasons why failure-to-thrive children are passive and their responsiveness is more flat. Being undernourished brings about lethargy and withdrawal, which, in turn, creates an impression that the child prefers to be left alone. Consequently, parent–child interaction is poor in quality, infrequent, and of short duration. Children who fail to thrive tend to be nervous and apprehensive when in their parents' company, which indicates a painful and anxiety-provoking interaction and relationship with the care-givers (Iwaniec, 1999). When observing parent–child interaction and exploring the quality of the emotional bond during the early stages of a child's life, it is often apparent that disappointment, or unfulfilled dreams of a perfect child, are turned against the offspring. A downwards spiral of destructive interactions rolls on, preventing development of secure bonding of parent to child.

Parent–child interaction is at the core of indicating the quality of relationship and general well-being of FTT children. The following checklists (Tables 9.6–9.8) provide useful information about the frequency and quality of interaction between the failure-to-thrive child and its parents, the child's responsiveness and reaction when in the parents' company, and interaction between siblings and the FTT child.

### Rating Criteria

| | |
|---|---|
| Often | Indicates good quality of parenting and positive relationship with the child; |
| Seldom | Indicates emotional neglect and necessity to provide family support to stop escalation of negative feelings and poor provision of nurturing; |
| Almost never | Indicates severe risk of emotional abuse and prevention of developing secure attachment to parents. |

### Stimulation

Stimulation means promotion of the child's learning and intellectual development through various activities, interactive methods, play, and socialisation.

In order to help children to understand the world around them and to make sense of things they observe and hear, a great amount of parental attention is required to inform the child's learning on a daily basis. Most parents do that automatically. They point out different things to the child, saying what it is, and they attract the child's attention to new objects or experiences,

**Table 9.6** Child's reactive and proactive behaviour

| Child's reactive and proactive behaviour | Often | Seldom | Almost never |
|---|---|---|---|
| Is the child: | | | |
| 1. playing freely | | | |
| 2. laughing/smiling | | | |
| 3. running | | | |
| 4. talking freely | | | |
| 5. coming for help | | | |
| 6. coming for comfort | | | |
| 7. cuddling up to mother/father | | | |
| 8. responding to affection | | | |
| 9. responding to attention | | | |
| 10. at ease when the mother/father is near them | | | |
| 11. joining in activities with other children | | | |
| 12. not frightened when approached by parents, or corrected | | | |
| 13. eating/feeding satisfactorily | | | |
| 14. asking for food—indicates hunger | | | |
| 15. seeming to be at ease during feeding/eating time? | | | |

*Source:* Iwaniec, D. (1983) *Social and psychological factors in the aetiology and management of children who fail-to-thrive.* PhD thesis. University of Leicester.

showing them pictures or demonstrating how a toy works. Parents also do things deliberately with children to stimulate their learning and to enhance the child's curiosity about things around them. Parents will read or play with them, using age-appropriate material to get them involved. For example, they will take a child to a farm to show them animals, so the child can link real things with pictures in the book. Later on, they will guide their social learning, instruct them in what is right or wrong, and reason with them to promote better understanding and problem-solving through play.

Infants need attention and stimulation to help them develop basic skills like sitting, crawling, walking, talking, and the social behaviour of participation and sharing. Many parents of failure-to-thrive children engage with their children's curiosity and provide necessary materials like toys, books, etc. to occupy and entertain them. Some, however, spend little time with their children as they find him/her unrewarding and seldom involve such a child in family activities. Interaction with the child tends to take place when it is absolutely necessary, such as feeding, bathing, changing, and even then it tends to be silent, with little communication and stimulation taking place. Some failure-to-thrive children are reared in social isolation, spending a lot of time in the cot in the bedroom or in the pram in the garden or a different room. They are perceived as preferring to be alone as such children seem to be happier and more at ease when left to their own devices. It is not surprising

**Table 9.7** Mother/father reactive and proactive behaviour

| Mother/father reactive and proactive behaviour | Often | Seldom | Almost never |
|---|---|---|---|
| Are the parents: | | | |
| 1. talking to the child | | | |
| 2. looking at the child | | | |
| 3. smiling at the child | | | |
| 4. making eye contact (loving) | | | |
| 5. touching (gently) | | | |
| 6. holding (closely, lovingly) | | | |
| 7. playing | | | |
| 8. cuddling | | | |
| 9. kissing | | | |
| 10. sitting the child on the lap | | | |
| 11. handling the child in a gentle way | | | |
| 12. giving requests (as opposed to commands) | | | |
| 13. helping the child if it is in difficulties | | | |
| 14. encouraging the child to participate in play and other activities | | | |
| 15. concerned about the child | | | |
| 16. picking the child up when it cries or when it is hurt | | | |
| 17. answering the child's questions | | | |
| 18. not ignoring the child's presence | | | |
| 19. emotionally treating the child the same as other children | | | |
| 20. handling children consistently? | | | |

*Source:* Iwaniec, D. (1983) *Social and psychological factors in the aetiology and management of children who fail-to-thrive.* PhD thesis. University of Leicester.

that some of these children suffer from developmental delays because of severe lack of stimulation and social isolation.

Some care-givers are so obsessed with tidiness and cleanliness that toys and free play are not allowed, or the child can only play with one thing at a time. There are, of course, families that cannot afford toys, or toys they get are totally inappropriate for the children's age. Some do not attach much value to playing and doing things with the child. Cultural differences are quite high and often misunderstood. When assessing these children the level of parental involvement (both physical and verbal) must be taken into consideration. It is necessary to establish how much time is spent with the child on an average day and what is the content of mutual involvement. Direct observation is a good method to assess parental involvement and availability.

**Table 9.8** Siblings' reactive and proactive behaviour

| Siblings' reactive and proactive behaviour | Often | Seldom | Almost never |
|---|---|---|---|
| Are the siblings: | | | |
| 1. playing with the child | | | |
| 2. talking to the child | | | |
| 3. participating in activities | | | |
| 4. accepting the child | | | |
| 5. treating the child well | | | |
| 6. pushing the child away and rejecting it | | | |
| 7. blaming the child for everything that happens | | | |
| 8. protecting the child | | | |
| 9. helping the child when in difficulties or in trouble | | | |
| 10. scapegoating the child | | | |

*Source:* Iwaniec, D. (1983) *Social and psychological factors in the aetiology and management of children who fail-to-thrive.* PhD thesis. University of Leicester.

A 'typical day' history is a very useful tool to establish how much time parents or other people spend with the child and what they do when they are together.

## GUIDANCE AND BOUNDARIES

Guidance enables the child to regulate its own emotional state and to develop an internal model of conscience and appropriate behaviour, while also promoting pro-social interpersonal behaviour and social relationships.

In order for children to be well prepared for life and to become well adjusted, they must acquire a vast amount of information about the environment in which they live, the culture to which they belong, and the prevailing moral code that guides their behaviour. Thus, a child's socialisation process will depend upon parental ability, awareness, willingness, and motivation to give the necessary information to provide an appropriate model of behaviour. This depends on reasoning, instruction, supervision, and guidance to ensure social learning as a basis for future life and well-being. By observing appropriate parental behaviour and being provided with discrimination learning as to why certain things are painful to others and should not be done, and what is pleasurable and appropriate and should be done, helps a child to develop a good sense of empathy and fairness. Teaching socially appropriate behaviours in relation to self and others needs to start in infancy and expand during the toddler stage. Assessment needs to cover awareness of the existence of fair rules and routines; boundaries of what they can and cannot do; understanding of rules; provision of sensitive instructions; and availability of guidance and supervision. Additionally, children have to learn to consider the needs of others, learn to share and wait, and to control frustration.

One reason why some children are unable to develop and regulate their own emotional state in a positive way and build social relationships is because they are not provided with an appropriate model of behaviour and are not guided through their learning. Tension, anxiety, uneasiness, fear and apprehension when in the care-giver's company (which often originates from difficult feeding interaction) do not lend themselves to building predictable expectations of what is required and why. From early on the child needs to learn that there are rules which need to be followed. These rules must be simple and easy to understand, and, above all, they have to be fair. Setting up boundaries is important as the child is then able to develop internal models of moral values, conscience, and social behaviour which are appropriate and expected. Children who have a difficult relationship with the care-givers will find it difficult, if not impossible, to develop an internal moral code which derives from positive experiences and examples. Some failure-to-thrive children who are rejected or who are living in a neglectful home lack positive experiences to build their own moral behaviour. They feel worthless, have low self-esteem, and find it difficult to deal with social problem-solving.

## STABILITY

Stability involves the provision of a stable and nurturing family environment which is considered to be persistent and predictable for all family members. Stability in a child's life will create a strong sense of belonging and will help it to go through various social adjustments during the developmental journey. A sense of permanency in a child's life and familiarity with its surroundings are the first basis for building secure attachment. Stability applies to people and places, and creates feelings that people who matter will always be there when the child needs them. It means continuity of care, a predictable environment, a settled pattern of care and daily routines, harmonious family relationships, the feelings that one's home and family are constantly present, 'always there for you'. Frequent changes of home, partners, care-givers, daily-minders, nursery or schools destabilise a child's life and create a sense of insecurity, emotional upset, or disturbance. Removal of children from home should be considered as a last option in the care plan but, equally, they should not be moved from one foster-home to another.

**Table 9.9** Assessment of parenting

The following questions need to be asked when assessing parenting.
Is there evidence which would indicate:

- acceptable/unacceptable physical care, e.g. feeding, dressing, changing nappies, bathing, keeping clean and warm, acceptable sleeping arrangements, safety,
  *as evidenced by*
- positive/negative attitudes towards parental duties and responsibilities
  *as evidenced by*
- positive/negative attitudes towards the child
  *as evidenced by*
- parental lifestyle which might be contributing to the child's poor care and attention
  *as evidenced by*
- harmful habits (alcohol, drug abuse, criminal behaviour, prostitution)
  *as evidenced by*
- personal circumstances affecting positive parenting (single parents, poor housing, poverty, social isolation, poor health, unemployment, mental illness, immature personality)
  *as evidenced by*
- level of partner and family support
  *as evidenced by*
- parents' intellectual capabilities—level of education, cognitive abilities
  *as evidenced by*
- passivity, withdrawal, inertia—learned helplessness
  *as evidenced by*
- parental childhood experiences of parenting
  *as evidenced by*
- awareness of children's developmental needs
  *as evidenced by*
- concern about the child's physical and psychosocial well-being
  *as evidenced by*
- ability to interpret child's behaviour and respond to it in a sensitive and helpful way
  *as evidenced by*
- availability of clear and fair rules and routines and boundaries
  *as evidenced by*
- showing affection and demonstrating a positive bond with the child
  *as evidenced by*
- the level and quality of parent–child interaction
  *as evidenced by*
- the level and depths of parent–child relationship
  *as evidenced by*
- the help and assistance that were provided for parents to overcome parenting difficulties
  *as evidenced by*
- what use they made of the help available to them
  (a) level of co-operation with workers
  (b) working constructively towards set goals
  *as evidenced by*
- whether they are able to understand what is going wrong in their parenting and whether they are able and willing to work at it.

## FAMILY AND ENVIRONMENTAL FACTORS

### General Overview

Parents have responsibility to provide the quality of care that will meet the basic developmental needs of children, but in order to fulfil these obligations their needs as parents and family have to be met too. Parents, as people, have certain requirements, such as basic material needs for shelter and subsistence, and psychosocial requirements for support, security, recognition, approval, guidance, advice, assistance, education, and resources. The essential needs of reasonable shelter and financial provision are seen as foundation elements of life and, if unattended to, can create such an overpowering set of needs themselves as to make it pointless to consider others.

Over and above these, more specific parents' needs arise at different times in the family cycle and with change of situation or lifestyle. It is not enough to assume that intellectual understanding and competence at skills of parent-craft are sufficient to make for a satisfactory family environment. Emotional responses also require understanding—their proper interpretation, sensitivity, and willingness to accommodate other people's feelings within the family.

Nevertheless, parents are adults and are, quite rightly, expected to take the child through his/her early life journey in a responsible manner. There is no doubt that parenting entails sacrifices of time, money, interest, and energy, and that parenting creates, as well as interferes with, life opportunities.

### Family History and Functioning

Family unity and mutual support help parents to cope with many difficulties and stresses associated with the bringing up of children. A family with a failure-to-thrive child needs to pull together to resolve early feeding and caring problems, to avoid failure to grow and possible failure of bonding and attachment. Parental background history often indicates the poor quality of parenting they received but, in particular, lack of emotional nurturing and support as they grew up. Forty-seven per cent of Iwaniec's (1983) sample stated lack of warmth, empathy, consideration, and physical closeness when they were children. They were seldom helped and assisted when they became parents. They felt that they were better parents, although their behaviour did not always show better nurturing of their FTT children. Additionally, the marital relationship was problematic in 50% of the cases, and at the 20-year follow-up 55% of parents were not living together (Iwaniec, 2000). In cases of parental support and family harmony, coping with a failure-to-thrive child was mutually shared and relatively quickly resolved.

One of the most difficult aspects concerning parental background history is the assumption that current difficulties are the result of parental abuse as children or some form of ill-treatment. This is clearly not the case with all FTT children and their families. Many parents have survived childhood adversity and consciously become very caring parents. There is, however, a correlation between a lack of parental warmth, sensitivity, and support, and failure to thrive in children (Iwaniec & Sneddon, 2001). However, some parents have a history of emotional and physical abuse and neglect: attention, therefore, should be paid to these areas of parents' lives.

The effectiveness of different kinds of support as a factor influencing parenting is reported in Van Bakel and Riksen-Walraven's study (2002). They found that a high level of marital support and satisfaction was associated with skilful parenting. The quality of marital or partner support was also consistently found in FTT studies as a stronger predictor of good problem-solving (at the early stages of the child's growth-faltering) than network support. The wider community-based network support did not fully compensate for lack of spousal support and relationship satisfaction as couple and parents (Iwaniec et al., in press).

There is a clear indication that, when assessing family functioning in failure-to-thrive cases, we need to pay careful attention to the relationship of parents and their mutual support in parenting, as the quality of the relationship seems to influence parental responses to the child. Family cohesion, therefore, requires assessment in FTT cases. The following questions need to be explored:

- Do members of the family spend a fair amount of time in shared activity?
- Are segregated activities, withdrawal, or avoidance rare?
- Are warm interactions common and hostile ones infrequent among family members?
- Is there full and accurate communication between members of the family?
- Are valuations of family members generally favourable and critical judgements rare?
- Do individuals tend to perceive other members as having favourable views of them?
- Are members visibly affectionate?; and
- Do the members show satisfaction and good morale, and are they optimistic about the future stability of the family?

## Family Stress

Family stress has been observed as more common in families with children who fail to thrive (Iwaniec et al., 1985a). These include: chronic illnesses in the parents, siblings, or extended family; prior divorce, current separation, and emotional tension between parents; single mothers with young children; depression; social isolation; and lack of available support (Drotar et al., 1981). In

**Table 9.10** Family functioning

| Is the family able to: | Most of the time | Occasionally | Almost never |
|---|---|---|---|
| 1. Resolve conflicts? | | | |
| 2. Make decisions? | | | |
| 3. Solve problems? | | | |
| 4. Encourage development of a sense of individuality in each member of the family? | | | |
| 5. Respond effectively to change/stress? | | | |
| 6. Respond appropriately to feelings? | | | |
| 7. Promote open communication, so that members are heard, not interrupted, not spoken for, shut up? | | | |
| 8. Avoid collusion across the generations leading to conflict? | | | |
| 9. Produce closeness between family members to promote meeting their physical and emotional needs? | | | |
| 10. Work together as parents to promote children's welfare and good development? | | | |
| 11. Support each other when faced with problems? | | | |
| 12. Have good organisation in running daily life? | | | |
| 13. Put children's needs before their own? | | | |
| 14. Avoid open conflict between parents affecting other members of the family? | | | |

addition to the above-mentioned factors, family life is often seen to be filled with conflict and tension, rather than being a source of emotional support (Hathaway, 1989). It is of enormous advantage to have a good network of social support to help cope with these demands. However, several studies have found that the mothers of non-organic failure-to-thrive children are socially isolated, depressed, and lack energy and initiative to organise their lives in a more enjoyable way (Bithoney & Newberger, 1987). Mothers are thought to be less available to bond with a baby when their emotional resources are depleted (Drotar & Malone, 1982). Good assessment of family functioning may help in devising appropriate interventions, such as couple therapy. In order to understand the current situation, a good family history should be taken, which might shed light on our understanding of presenting problems and to address these when planning intervention.

Questions in Table 9.10 deal with various aspects of family functioning and need to be examined when carrying out family assessment.

## Income

Failure to thrive is also associated with poverty. Children from low-income families are lighter and shorter than those living in materially more affluent homes with better incomes (Dawson, 1992). As almost all studies of failure to thrive have been done in low-income populations little is known about it in affluent ones. However, classifying into social class can sometimes be misleading. For example, Skuse *et al.* (1994) examined two groups of children who failed to thrive: one with early onset (within six months of birth), and one with later onset (after six months of birth). Although both groups had similar amounts of money coming into the house, there were different patterns of managing money. Iwaniec's (1983) sample consisted of 40% of middle-class families, where there was no financial hardship but a high level of emotional indifference and marital instability.

## Housing

Assessment of accommodation is considered to be fundamental when looking at children's and parents' needs. Failure-to-thrive children are often brought up in impoverished, badly heated, and poorly maintained housing. It has been found (Iwaniec, 1983) that some of the children have frequent colds and infections, often due to poor heating and inadequate clothing. Additionally, frequent changes of housing because of rent arrears or conflict with neighbours prevents establishing meaningful contact and mutual support with neighbours and the wider community. It has been reported (Hanks & Hobbs, 1993) that basic living amenities are poor, which has a negative impact on the child's health and safety. Studies of failure-to-thrive problems are done in mostly disadvantaged inner-city areas. There is poor understanding of how widespread it is.

## Employment

Failure to thrive is associated with low-income families and general economic hardship. Most parents tend to be unemployed and live on various benefits. Poor growth is often embedded in a context of family economic disadvantage (Drotar *et al.*, 1990). Children living in families who have been unemployed for considerable time or have never been at work are lighter and shorter than children who live in better-off homes (Dawson, 1992). However, those parents who are employed tend to be happier, better organised, more mature and, as a rule, engage in providing family support to resolve the child's poor growth. Better self-esteem leads to better functioning, self-satisfaction, generating and influencing positive and self-fulfilling parenting.

## Family's Social Integration

Families of failure-to-thrive children tend to be socially isolated. They have little contact with neighbours and are inclined to avoid people in order to escape criticism and perceived disapproval of their parenting style. As their self-esteem is low, they anticipate rejection from the people living in the same community. It is not surprising that parents are apprehensive about inter-acting with neighbours or other people in the community for fear of being blamed for the child's poor weight gain and miserable appearance. For a child to fail to thrive in our weight-obsessed culture, to appear neglected in our child-abuse sensitive society, is a mortal blow to a mother's self-esteem; it is a highly public, deeply humiliating condemnation of the caring mother, who is experiencing child-rearing difficulties. Many mothers of FTT children do care about their children, as indicated in various research projects (Batchelor, 1999). Parents seldom interact, and there are some whose lifestyle alienates them from community integration and support: this is often due to alcohol abuse, drug-use, the children's unkempt appearance, or poor social behaviour. Such parents seldom get support from people living near them. As a result, they become isolated, unsupported, and are consequently de-pressed. These, in turn, have serious effects on children, especially infants and toddlers, as their mothers become physically and emotionally unavail-able and unable to meet their basic needs. When such problems are identi-fied, an effort should be made to connect them with local groups, such as a mother-and-toddler group, or mothers' groups, and efforts should be made to provide day-care services so that the child can meet other children and get some much-needed social stimulation.

## Community Resources

It is now widely recognised that availability of necessary facilities and suitable services in the community where the parents live serves as a buffer to prevent abuse and neglect, and ensure better developmental outcomes for children. Easy access to health services, schools, and day services, such as family centres, nurseries and playgroups, enables parents to use these services when they are needed more independently. This is particularly important for parents whose children require frequent medical and social-care attention. Failure-to-thrive children need to be seen by the GP and health visitor to mon-itor their growth, development, and health (quite frequently, to start with). Parents also need advice and help with prevailing feeding/eating problems. As some failure-to-thrive children are developmentally delayed they might need day-care services to help them make good the developmental deficit. Hobbs and Hanks (1996) found that families living near, or having easy access to, health centres or multi-disciplinary failure-to-thrive clinic frequently took

**Table 9.11** Process and stages of involvement in failure-to-thrive cases

| | |
|---|---|
| *Stage 1* | Identifying that child's weight is below expected norms and its general well-being is questionable |
| *Stage 2* | Advice and help provided by the health visitor or GP re. feeding, caring and management |
| *Stage 3* | If there is not improvement, and parents are doing their best, referral to the paediatrician to investigate any possible organic reason for the child's poor growth and development |
| *Stage 4* | Medical investigation if felt to be necessary |
| *Stage 5* | If there is non-organic reason for failure to thrive, and child welfare continues to cause concern, referral to social services for psychosocial assessment and care plan in the community |
| *Stage 6* | More serious cases (if there is evidence of rejection, emotional indifference or more serious neglect) to be conferenced |
| *Stage 7* | Treatment/intervention programme to be worked out and negotiated with the care-givers |
| *Stage 8* | Monitoring child's growth and development—either in outpatients' clinic, by GP, or health visitor, until child's growth is appropriate for the chronological age |
| *Stage 9* | Monitoring child/care-givers' interaction and relationship and general well-being of the child by the social worker and/or health visitor |
| *Stage 10* | Case closed when there is evidence of systematic improvement in child's growth and development, and care-givers'/child relationship for at least three months |

their FTT children there and received the necessary advice and reassurance which proved to be beneficial to the child. More important, however, was the manner in which those parents were dealt with: those who were given a sympathetic ear and opportunity to discuss worries regarding a child's poor growth and development also managed to resolve some of the interactional problems much more quickly. Good awareness of what and who is available in the neighbourhood may help to facilitate child and family needs at the onset of failure to thrive, thus preventing further deterioration.

## CONCLUDING COMMENTS ON ASSESSMENT FRAMEWORK

The new assessment framework is a good guide for practitioners to do their work. There is, however, nothing new or revolutionary about it, apart from avoiding words such as risk, abuse, and dangerous parenting. The philosophy underpinning the new framework of assessment means to be universal, applicable to all children in need, and based on the child's developmental requirements. If those developmental needs are to be met, at appropriate stages, then the 'wait-and-see' approach has to be avoided, in order to eliminate escalation of problems leading to significant harm. There is no doubt that better assessment is needed, of children and of parenting capacity, and that this is carried out on a multi-disciplinary basis, followed by appropriate and targeted intervention, to resolve presenting problems. Failure-to-thrive children have to be assessed and helped on a multi-disciplinary basis, as are other children at risk or in need of services.

It is well known that intervention is likely to be most effective in providing better results for children when it is done early in a child's life or the problem development. Stepping in early, as a preventive measure, will secure better outcomes for the child, will be cheaper in the long run, and less hurtful for everybody. However, there need to be time limits within which improvement has to take place. Children cannot wait indefinitely as they grow quickly, and problems grow with them at a remarkable speed. If parental capacity cannot accommodate the child's needs, and services provided are not used or refused, then alternative arrangements need to be made promptly and decisively. It is suggested (Adcock, 2001) that adoption or placement with a suitable relative should be considered after a time-limited intervention. This new thinking as to how to deal with children with poor parenting prognosis for change, and whose needs are unlikely to be met while living with parents, is based on numerous findings from committees of enquiry and research commissioned by the Department of Health. One questions, however, the availability of family-support services, which, if provided promptly and for long enough, might do the job effectively under Section 17 of the *Children Act* without reverting to more drastic measures. Most parents care about their children and, providing that help is given at the right time and in the right volume, change might occur.

Nevertheless, there are parents who cannot provide adequate parenting for various reasons and whose children are permanently neglected, and therefore deprived of opportunities to meet their potentials. A prompt decision, following comprehensive assessment, is essential to avoid negative snowball effects and to facilitate meeting developmental needs.

Adcock (2001) described the compounding effects of a negative process in failure to thrive in the following way:

> Deficits or dysfunctional behaviours at one developmental period will lay the groundwork for subsequent dysfunctional behaviours. Deficits, manifest at one stage, continue to exert an influence at the next stage unless an intervention occurs. For example, malnutrition in infancy may lead to impaired intellectual or cognitive functioning in toddlers which, in turn, lead to impaired performance as an adult.

## SUMMARY

Assessment of failure to thrive was widely discussed using a holistic, child-centred approach based on ecological theory, addressing child development, parental capacity, and environmental factors. A new framework of assessment introduced by the Department of Health in the UK was used to capture current thinking and research evidence of failure to thrive in children. The framework of assessment aims to promote family support in the community and to refocus its attention from protection to prevention. This extensive chapter has covered each aspect of the assessment triangle and provided various instruments to assist in the assessment process. The extent of discussion, covering individual factors, is dependent on its relevance to FTT and, more specifically, on the age of a child at a referral point.

# INTERVENTION AND TREATMENT OF FAILURE-TO-THRIVE CHILDREN AND THEIR FAMILIES

## CONSIDERATIONS ARISING FROM FAILURE-TO-THRIVE INTERVENTION RESEARCH, AND A WAY FORWARD

# 10

# LEVELS OF INTERVENTION

*Can a woman forget her sucking child, that she should not have compassion on the son of her womb? yea, they may forget . . .*

The Holy Bible, *Isaiah*, **xliv**, v.15

## INTRODUCTION

The best and most appropriate ways to help failure-to-thrive children and their carers, and when to intervene, vary considerably amongst cases and should be determined by comprehensive assessment. As we have seen, failure to thrive in children seldom arises as a result of a single factor, but rather as a combination of amalgamated difficulties adversely affecting a child's physical growth. Since failure to thrive appears to be multi-dimensional in nature, it is important to examine each of these dimensions in order to work out an appropriate care-plan.

Intervention programmes can take many forms, follow different routes, and may require the use of various methods and approaches to deal effectively and suitably with the problems presented by the child and the carers. It is now generally accepted that a combination of interventions, and use of different therapeutic methods and services produces better results in the long term than a single approach (Wolfe & Wekerle, 1993; Iwaniec, 1995, 1997; Black, 1995; Batchelor, 1999). Equally, full participation of care-givers in recognising the problem, planning and decision-making regarding choices, and the nature of helping strategies have proved to enhance more positive outcomes (Hobbs & Hanks, 1996; Iwaniec, 1997). For example, resolving feeding and stimulation problems at home may be enhanced and speeded up if a child attends a day-nursery and is fed and cared for by people who do not show anxiety or put pressure on a child to eat, and who behave in a relaxed way. Equally, the use of the family centre can help both the child and the parent at the same time. By attending parent-training sessions and learning from other parents' experiences, the mother may become better informed about the child's nutritional and nurturing needs, and the child may be helped by reducing developmental deficit and improving social competence by being with other children. Additionally, mothers can be helped by having opportunities to socialise with other parents, thus reducing social isolation and feelings of helplessness.

Increasingly, it has been recognised that failure to thrive more often than not is the result of child-rearing deficits combined with various personal and structural problems, rather than deliberate parental action (although abuse and neglect feature in some cases). Helping parents in more effective child-rearing practices and providing appropriate services should, therefore, dominate methods of intervention. The available evidence suggests that monitoring alone of more serious cases is insufficient to produce long-lasting changes in children's lives and the lives of their parents (Wolfe, 1990; Iwaniec, 2000). However, according to Wright (2000), one fifth of failure-to-thrive children have immediately improved following advice given by a health visitor. Those problems were obviously not too serious and of relatively short duration, where advice and reassurance were sufficient to produce the desired change. Those results also indicate that early identification of FTT can be resolved relatively quickly at a universal level of intervention. More proactive skill-teaching approaches are advocated, where parents can be involved and take responsibility for problem recognition and problem-solving, which would, in turn, generate a sense of achievement.

There is not a single or simple way to deal with more complex cases; neither is there an identified single approach or method that could claim exclusive success. Intervention strategies need to be tailored to the specific requirements of the individual families in their special circumstances. For example, if FTT is due to child-rearing deficit, then parent-training, including developmental counselling, may be the most suitable approach to adopt. If, on the other hand, it is due to acute feeding problems, oral-motor dysfunction, and anxiety associated with feeding, then modelling a more relaxed approach on what to feed, how to feed, hold, communicate, and generally interact during the process of feeding is advocated. If it is, however, due to a poor relationship and weak bonding, then a step-by-step approach of reducing ambivalent feelings towards the child will be required using various techniques of attachment-work to improve the emotional bond and quality of relationship between parents and child. Parents who present obsessive behaviour and attitudes towards weight and diet may need cognitive restructuring or other types of psychotherapy to change or modify their beliefs, feelings, and behaviour. Parents who chronically neglect their children might need continuous practical help and supervision on a long-term basis to secure reasonable nutritional and physical care of a child.

In order to know what to do when a child fails to thrive we need, first of all, to find out why this is so. Once the triggering factors and maintaining mechanisms are identified, then we can work out what to do using theoretical bases to guide intervention, and decide who should be involved to help resolve these difficulties in a way which would feel comfortable for the parents and beneficial to the child.

## LEVELS OF PREVENTION AND INTERVENTIONS IN FAILURE-TO-THRIVE CASES

Before discussing various types of therapeutic interventions in cases of FTT, it would be worthwhile looking at the policy, legal framework, and service availability to all children and families. Most countries, especially the more developed ones and welfare states, have legislation and policies to promote children's health, development, education, leisure activities, and protection from harm and abuse. This simply means that there are services available to safeguard child welfare, set up and financed by either central or local governments, and delivered by statutory or voluntary organisations. The governments also use the private sector to provide necessary services for families and children in need on their behalf. In cases of failure to thrive this involves carrying out assessments, monitoring, and treatment if necessary in order to obtain the required outcomes for these children. In child-welfare work such actions as assessment and monitoring of the case may lead to positive conclusions, but also to state intervention if required changes are not achieved and the child is suffering or may suffer significant harm. If there is evidence that a child is in danger of harm, and possibilities to produce the required change are unlikely, then reception into care may be advocated.

In child welfare and protection most countries have three levels of intervention: universal; selective; or court-sanctioned targeted services or interventions. In the United Kingdom there is an additional level which comes before court intervention. It is often called the *registration level*.

### Universal Prevention/Intervention

*Universal* prevention and intervention are available to all people in the United Kingdom. These include: community and hospital medical services; education; social services; and other local services which are open to all citizens. In respect of advice given regarding children who fail to thrive, assistance and monitoring are provided as a matter of routine statutory work by health visitors, earlier on by a midwife, and by the community or hospital paediatricians, if needed. Families have free access to the GP, health centres, and welfare agencies so that the child's progress can be supervised at a low-key level. The health visitors monitor the child's physical growth in terms of weight, height, and psychosocial developmental attainments. During home visits health visitors provide advice on how to feed and what to feed, how often and what

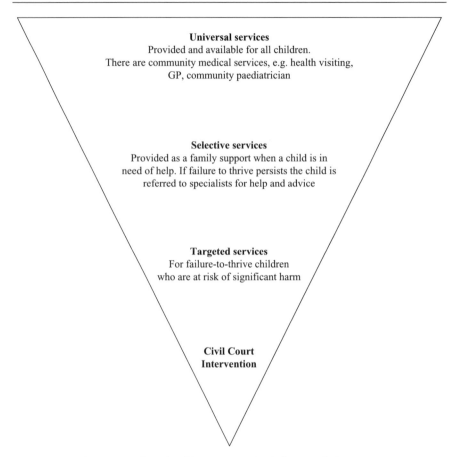

**Figure 10.1** Levels of intervention in failure-to-thrive cases

formula to use, when to introduce solids, and how to manage feeding and eat-ing difficulties. They also advise on how to manage some difficult behaviours, how to discipline and stimulate the child, and how to provide appropriate physical and emotional care. But as their caseload is large their help is usually limited to statutory assessment, advice, support, and monitoring. As a rule, however, more serious cases are referred to child care specialists for further assessment and treatment.

The child's early growth and development, as we can see, is regularly mon-itored and measured by the health visitors as part of their statutory duties. It is difficult to estimate how many children who show weight problems or feeding difficulties are helped early on as a result of routine work.

Babies who present more persistent growth-faltering are seen by health visitors at home or at the health centre on a more regular basis in order to be weighed and to enable the appropriate advice and help to be provided. The majority of infants who fail to thrive in the first few months of their lives usually steadily improve once their mothers become more relaxed, confident, and skilful in their parenting role, and when the children adapt to daily routines. First-time parents, single mothers, and those without extended family support seek help, advice, and guidance more often because of lack of experience in child-rearing.

Some of these children might need to be referred by the GP to the paediatrician if progress is slow. Some fail to thrive because of illness, and therefore need to be investigated medically to find out if there is an organic reason for their poor growth and development. Such children will be seen in out-patient clinics or as in-patients if observation and testing are required. It is immensely important to eliminate or to confirm any medical reason for FTT as a matter of good practice in order to prevent distortion of parental perceptions as to why children behave in difficult ways which may lead to interactional problems if not decisively dealt with. In many countries such services are available, so problems of early feeding difficulties and poor growth are seldom considered a result of parenting problems. However, if, after repeated visits to the GP, several admissions to hospital, and general lack of progress, nothing appears to be organically wrong with the child, the next level of intervention will be necessary.

## Effective Selective Prevention/Intervention

*Selective intervention* refers to specific, more intensive family support when a problem or problems cannot be resolved at a universal level. Selective intervention is voluntary, and aims to prevent further escalation of difficulties and to provide suitable services and/or treatments for parents and children who are in need of help.

The concept of *family support* (as a preventive measure) was introduced in the United Kingdom following the implementation of the *Children Act 1989* in England and Wales (*c*.41) and the equivalent in Scotland (*c*.36) and Northern Ireland in 1995. It replaced and widened the *Children and Young Persons Act 1969* (*c*.54), which was passed in order to provide services to prevent children coming into care. The philosophy behind and the aims of the *Children Act 1989* were to redirect child-welfare work from focusing almost exclusively on child abuse and protection to more child-oriented care-work within the family and community. Family support means allocation of services for children 'in need', or 'at risk' of not meeting developmental potentials because of the economic, personal, or other difficulties experienced by parents. Furthermore, *family support* emphasises interventions with agreement from, and in partnership with, parents. The concept of 'need' was left deliberately wide in order to reinforce the emphasis on preventive support and services to families. Of

---

course this lack of precision as to what is meant by 'in need' and how to put it into practice in everyday work has created a lot of confusion and led to misinterpretation of the concept. Most importantly, however, the ruling has not been backed up with adequate resources to make the philosophy of family support work.

In assessing individual needs, attention has to be given to the existing strengths and skills of the families concerned, in order to enhance their awareness, skills, and strengths to overcome difficulties. The emphasis is to keep children with their families and to avoid state interference. It is also stressed that families who are experiencing difficulties have the right to receive sympathetic support and intervention in their lives, regardless of whether the 'need' results from family difficulties or the child's circumstances. In this spirit, the assessment of need has to be undertaken in an open way, and should involve those caring for the child, the child him/herself and other significant persons. A holistic approach to looking at a problem and solutions is a key principle in the *selective intervention* of failure-to-thrive children.

The majority of children whose FTT is more persistent, and where there are concerns expressed by professionals or parents, will come into a category of *selective intervention* using various family-support services as well as drawing on a range of therapeutic methods.

## Indira's Case

Indira, a third child in the family, was born at full term, weighing 3 kg (6 lb. 9³/₄ oz.). Both parents and two brothers, 6 and 4 years old respectively, were delighted with the newcomer to their family.

Indira was difficult to feed while on liquids but things got worse when solids were introduced. She would spit food out, heave, store food in her mouth, vomit, and have diarrhoea. Each feeding-time was long, and very stressful to all members of the family as everyone was trying to feed her and to occupy her during mealtimes.

In spite of extensive efforts to feed and look after her, Indira did not grow satisfactorily. From the age of 2 months until 1 year and 5 months she remained either just above or just under the 2nd percentile. Additionally, Indira tended to catch colds and infections more frequently than average child, and there were periods when she was either irritable and oppositional or withdrawn and uncooperative.

The mother's approach to her feeding difficulties was quite rational and appropriate at first, but as time went on she became anxious and preoccupied to the point of obsession with feeding her child at all costs so that she would gain some weight. As a rule Indira would win each battle, leaving the mother in tears and totally defeated. Both boys became attention-seeking and resentful of Indira as the mother did not have time to spend with them and paid little attention to their emotional needs. The father became so concerned about the rapid changes in the family life and functioning, and lack of appropriate assistance regarding Indira's poor growth and emerging behavioural problems, that he brought Indira to the health centre insisting that they must get help otherwise there would not be a family to take care of any of them as his wife had reached breaking-point.

Indira was referred for more intensive intervention to deal with the family crises triggered off by Indira's refusal to eat and her poor physical growth. Three major problems were identified:

1. Feeding difficulties due to mild oral-motor dysfunction;
2. Indira's difficult temperamental attributes exacerbating feeding problems and general compliance; and
3. The mother's feeding style and interaction were anxious and riddled with worries about Indira's life and safety.

Because of the problems stated above, daily attendance at a day-nursery was organised, so that Indira could be looked after by people who were calm, consistent, and persistent, and who were instructed to feed Indira in a matter-of-fact way and make a fuss only when she ate well and at a reasonable speed (*see* discussion on treatment, Chapter 12). While Indira was in the nursery (which she loved), the mother was seen by the therapist to address her fears, anxiety, perceived sense of inadequacy as a mother, low self-esteem, and depressive moods. Relaxation training, cognitive counselling, and restructuring brought about good results in the way she felt about herself as a woman, mother, and wife. Indira's weight gain and increased food intake, in terms of quantity and variety of food consumed, improved family interactions and reduced tension which had been a part of daily life for a long time.

## Effective Targeted Prevention/Intervention

The third level of intervention applies to cases where intensive selective intervention does not produce the desired outcome and where parental participation and commitment to resolve the problem are poor. It usually applies when attempts to work in partnership with parents to protect a child's welfare and to improve the quality of care fail to materialise or if there are serious concerns about neglect or abuse.

Failures to produce a minimum standard of care, and concerns expressed by professionals involved, lead to a multi-disciplinary case-conference meeting, where the problems and solutions are discussed. The case-conference is called by social services, and all the professionals who know the child and the family are invited to attend, as are the parents. The case-conference is reserved to situations where there is evidence to substantiate the suspicion or allegation of 'serious' abuse or neglect. Different societies will have different views of the borderline between 'serious' and 'not-so-serious' abuse—and what is considered abusive in one country might not be in another. The threshold criteria and level of tolerance may differ substantially.

The case-conference in the United Kingdom is the key forum for deciding the way forward in more serious cases. A central consideration should be the degree of risk of further harm to the child's growth, development, and safety in the current situation. However, in the mix of professionals and parents and the varying levels of knowledge of the family, this central issue can often be overlooked. The case-conference decides if the child's name should be placed on the *Child Protection Register*. If the child is registered, this should be followed by a full and comprehensive assessment to determine whether concerns expressed are justified, what action should be taken, or what further help is needed to resolve presenting concerns. The outcomes of the comprehensive assessment are presented to the *Assessment Review Case-Conference*, where it forms the basis of the *Child Protection Plan*. Further *case-review meetings* are convened at six-monthly intervals where the *Child Protection Plan* is reviewed and, where a child is assessed as being at low risk of further abuse, consideration is given to removing the child's name from the *Child Protection Register*—so-called deregistration.

## What is the Difference between Family Support Services and those Offered for Child Protection?

The initial difficulty in assessing the relationship between family-support services/selected interventions and those deemed as child-protection *targeted intervention* is the problem of defining either with any great clarity. Gibbons (1995), in discussing family support and child protection within England and Wales, points out that the concepts are used by different people in different ways. In some circumstances a service may be deemed a child-protection service and in another a family-support service. A very wide range of services offered to very different families in varied situations is described as family support. These services may include children who are failing to thrive and their families. At one extreme are routine health and welfare services provided in varying degrees to all. At the other extreme are family-support services—intensive crisis-related services where the main outcome measure is whether protective removal of children into care can be avoided. The dilemmas, disadvantages, and potentially damaging effects of the concentration on child protection are exemplified by the growing consensus from research that children on the *Child Protection Register* may be *less in need* than many of the children who are not as their health and development are less severely impaired.

---

### Jonathan's Case

Jonathan was referred by the community paediatrician at 11 months of age as she felt that he had made little progress regarding weight gain and psychomotor development, in spite of attempts made by the health visitor to help the parents and to monitor progress. Jonathan had only gained just over 3 kg (6 lb. 9¾ oz.) since birth, and presented as a very wasted, withdrawn, and neglected child. Both parents were young and inexperienced in child care and had little understanding of nutritional and nurturing needs of children. Jonathan was not fed regularly, was not given the required quantity and formulæ advised by the health visitor, and was seldom picked up when being fed. Jonathan was not brought to the clinic to have immunisation, and appointments to do developmental assessments were not kept. Additionally, both parents abused alcohol, and were often found intoxicated, leaving Jonathan unattended. The father, when under the influence of alcohol, refused the health visitor access to the house and insisted that there was no need for her to be consistently interfering with their lives. As the situation became seriously dangerous to Jonathan's health, a case-conference was called to discuss the case and to work out strategies for intervention: this case-conference was also attended by the parents. The professionals attending the case-conference decided to put Jonathan's name on the *Child Protection Register*, and referral was made to the multi-disciplinary Child Treatment Research Unit to provide intensive treatment and support for the family. This treatment consisted of:

1. Setting up a feeding schedule, with provision of age-appropriate food and quantity;
2. Modelling and rehearsing of an appropriate style of feeding;
3. Increasing positive interaction to enhance stimulation and developmental attainments;
4. Allocation of Family Aid by social services (15 hours a week) to supervise basic child care—bathing, dressing, changing, putting to sleep, feeding, and responding to signals of distress and interpreting them appropriately;
5. Developmental counselling for both parents; and
6. Monitoring alcohol consumption and providing education regarding the negative effect of excessive drinking in terms of health and child care.

Intensive intervention produced positive outcomes for Jonathan. Within six months he gained 5 kg (11 lb. $^1/_4$ oz.) and grew almost $3^1/_2$ cm ($1^1/_2$ in.) in height. He became more alert, more responsive, and his physical appearance substantially improved. The parents' skills and, above all, their awareness of Jonathan's physical and emotional needs increased to levels where they could function more independently as care-givers. At a second case-review Jonathan's name was taken off the *Child Protection Register*, but the case was monitored by the health visitor on a regular basis to keep the momentum of positive change going in the right direction.

## Civil Court Intervention

The fourth level of intervention applies to children who are *at risk* of significant harm or who *have suffered* significant harm and where action urgently needs to be taken. Such children require, as a rule, removal from an abusive or dangerous environment as a matter of safety through the Court system. The criteria for significant harm vary between countries and over time. In countries where child welfare and protection are legislated for and observed, substantial services at all levels are available, while in less developed countries there are very few and they are difficult to access (Gough, 2002).

Some children who present persistent growth failure (due to seriously inadequate or dangerous parenting) come into this category of intervention. This might include persistent and severe physical and emotional neglect, rejection, deliberate withholding of food, or fictitious fabricated illnesses, resulting in child starvation and, in more serious cases, psychosocial short-stature children. In the majority of these cases the parent–child relationship is extremely poor and there are obvious attachment disorders. There is an observable lack of a parental emotional bond with the child and a lack of commitment to welfare and well-being. The reasons for this sad and dangerous state of parenting vary from immature, ill-informed parenting style associated with inter-generational deficit, to psychological disturbances in cognitive functioning, mental illness, learning disabilities, or persistent alcohol or drug abuse. In such cases application for a Care Order to the Court is necessary to protect the child from harm (or even death) and to determine a care-plan for the future. The decision to take the case to Court is usually based on the multi-disciplinary case-conference agreement informed by the comprehensive assessment.

Most children, when removed from home, are placed in foster-homes on a short- or long-term basis, and some will be considered for freeing for adoption if the possibility of rehabilitation back home is remote or impossible. Sometimes the child is placed with its extended family if this is considered safe and the family is willing. Such kinship care can be arranged voluntarily without taking a case to Court. Not all such placements are satisfactory and some are highly inappropriate (Lernihan, 2003). In the majority of cases parents of children in care have a right to reasonable access to their children. They can see them quite frequently, and access is either supervised or unsupervised. If the child was removed from home because of Münchausen Syndrome by Proxy, or because of sexual abuse, the access visits would be supervised, as they would also be in cases where the parents are addicted to alcohol and/or drugs. The frequency and nature of access visits in the United Kingdom is advocated by social services and determined by the Court.

Recent years have seen some changes and less rigid arrangements for adopted children. So-called 'open adoption' is considered for each child, which gives a range of possibilities for contact with birth-parents such as: two or more face-to-face contacts a year and contact in exceptional life-events, as well as exchange of photographs, birthday cards, or letters. The nature of contact is determined by the best interests of the child in terms of security, stability, and social adjustment. It is well known that children who grow up away from home but who are aware of their origin, and, better still, have occasional contact with their biological parents, have a better-developed sense of identity and less unrealistic and disturbing fantasies about their parents. The 20-year follow-up study of children who failed to thrive as children (Iwaniec, 2000; Iwaniec & Sneddon, 2001 and 2002) found that children who were adopted satisfactorily overcame acute adversity of childhood experiences and became well-adjusted individuals and parents in later life. Children in long-term, undisrupted and well-selected foster-homes have done equally well. Those, however, who had frequent admissions into care on a voluntary basis, but remain at home, have done less well in terms of stability, attachment to peers and romantic partners, educational attainments, employment, and self-esteem.

It is very important to emphasise that children in this category require intensive intervention when placed in substitute care in their own right to eliminate or minimise emotional disturbances and to make good developmental deficit. Provision of day-care services, play therapy, and systematic, positive monitoring of behaviour by various forms of reinforcement is essential to avoid break-up of the placements. Substitute carers require support and active help to guide them to understand and deal with children's difficult behaviour and disturbed emotions. Some of the intervention methods which are suitable will be discussed in Chapters 12, 13, and 14.

---

### Gary's Case

Gary (aged 3 years) was referred to the NSPCC by an anonymous caller who stated that a family that had recently moved into the area was causing serious concern for various reasons, but the way in which a little boy (estimated by the caller to be about 18 months old) was being treated by his mother was a particular source of alarm. The mother would 'throw him' out of the house and he stood, crying, in the cold weather, and was not allowed into the house in spite of the child knocking at the door and asking to be let in. He was left on the street a long way behind the mother as he could not walk as fast as she wanted him to. He often begged for food from strangers and picked up scraps of food from waste baskets. The caller reported that the boy looked ill, thin, and very anxious.

The home visit revealed that Gary was rejected by his mother. She stated that he was nothing but a problem to her, that she did not like him, and found it excessively difficult to cope with his bizarre eating behaviour, disturbed toileting, destructiveness, and complete defiance. The visiting official was shocked when he learned that Gary was 3 years old, as he did not look bigger than 18 months old, and his development was seriously retarded in all areas. It was observed at the time that he avoided his mother, was frightened when she came near him, and would not respond to her requests or commands.

A case-conference was convened and Gary was put on the *Child Protection Register* under the category of emotional abuse and physical abuse. The parents refused to attend the case-conference and the mother stated that she was not bothered about the case-conference decision one way or the other. The comprehensive assessment that followed confirmed that Gary had suffered significant harm and was frequently abused physically by his mother and occasionally by his father. He spent a lot of time locked up in his bedroom and was deprived of food as a means of punishment on a regular basis. He was seldom spoken to, apart from being told off, never cuddled or played with, and never attended to when he hurt himself or needed help and assistance. He presented typical and acute behaviour of a psychosocial short-stature child such as: bizarre eating pattern; sleeping problems; serious destructiveness; aggressive defiance; and toileting disturbances, such as smearing of faeces and urinating in inappropriate places.

Both parents insisted that Gary needed medical investigation as there was something wrong with him, and that it was he who needed treatment, not them. Gary was admitted to hospital and stayed for three weeks, more as a safety measure and break for the child than in order to investigate him for a disease. Nothing was found to indicate his poor growth. The mother visited him only twice, each time for only half an hour. During that time Gary put on weight (4 kg [8 lb. 13 oz.]), and his preoccupation with food decreased somewhat. He became less destructive and began to play more with other children. On returning home Gary rapidly lost weight and his behaviour worsened. He started attending day-nursery as a safety measure and to provide a source of stimulation, but presented as a very disturbed and damaged child.

Attempts to involve the parents in treatment were met with refusal, and they requested that Gary should be fostered out for his and their sake. The multi-disciplinary case-conference decided unanimously that application for a *Care Order* should be made in view of adoption.

## SUMMARY

This chapter introduced the concepts of multi-factorial interventions in failure-to-thrive cases. It discussed the necessity to approach intervention comprehensively, addressing both the child's and parents' problems. Four levels—*universal, selected, targeted* and *Court intervention*—have been elaborated on and three case studies have been included to illustrate *selected, targeted*, and *Court* levels of involvements.

# SOME THEORETICAL APPROACHES TO FAILURE-TO-THRIVE INTERVENTION

*It is a reproach to religion and government to suffer so much poverty and excess.*
William Penn, 1693

## INTRODUCTION

Failure to thrive has been grounded in a number of theoretical perspectives which will be outlined briefly here. Ecological, behavioural, cognitive, and attachment theory have all formed the theoretical frameworks on which to base the design and implementation of failure-to-thrive research and intervention strategies. These perspectives will each be addressed here from the viewpoint of theory, explaining why failure occurs, and methods of intervention used by different researchers and practitioners to solve the problem. As there is no space to present other theories and their link to failure-to-thrive interventions, the above four are used to illustrate practice-theory-driven working methods.

## APPLICATION OF ECOLOGICAL THEORY TO FAILURE-TO-THRIVE TREATMENT STRATEGIES

Ecological theory such as Bronfenbrenner's ecological model of child development (1979; 1993) has been applied to failure-to-thrive research, assessment, and intervention strategies. Bronfenbrenner's (1979) model uses systems theory to place development within a multi-level interactive social context with reference to the influences of the child's proximal microsystems and mesosystem. Expansion of Bronfenbrenner's model includes three processes through which contextual factors influence development as being of relevance to failure-to-thrive interventions. These processes include: first, a person-context model, by which children's characteristics (for example gender or age) mediate between contextual factors and development; second, a process-context model, by which processes operate differently in different environments. However, of most relevance to failure to thrive, according to Black (1995), is the person–process-context model (which is a combination of both the person-context model and the process-context model), and which posits that processes vary by environmental context and the characteristics of the child. By basing interventions on ecological theory, growth and development can be affected positively by first addressing critical relationships to promote improved nurturance. The view is that application of ecological theory to failure-to-thrive intervention strategies can help ensure that potentially critical variables and processes are not overlooked.

## Theory as Applied to Failure-to-Thrive Intervention

In a review of strategies for evaluation of and intervention in cases of infants diagnosed as failing to thrive, Black (1995) recommended the application of Bronfenbrenner's ecological model of child development (1979) as a theoretical framework for such intervention, which would take into account multi-factorial components to encompass family, ecological, and cultural factors. However, it was found that there was a tendency to focus on FTT as a nutritional deficiency rather than a multi-factorial problem. Ecological theory recommends that while planning an intervention it may be useful to gather information on proximal and distal variables that may contribute to the child's growth failure, together with information regarding potential mediating variables such as poverty and associated family problems.

Failure-to-thrive interventions undertaken from an ecological perspective have focused on children's characteristics postulated to mediate contextual factors and development (*person context*); for example, the child's cognitive, motor, and language development, including child temperament, gender, and individual differences (such as the age of the onset of FTT). Parental characteristics (*person context*) include parental history, health beliefs, psychological functioning, previous attachments, personality, coping style and strategies, cognitions, attitudes, and behaviours towards the child. An ecological approach to failure-to-thrive intervention also incorporates environmental influences on behaviour (*process context*). Finally, the aspect in which FTT researchers are perhaps most interested is the manner in which the child, parent, and environment act to influence interaction styles and behaviours (*person–process context*). This is demonstrated through focusing on how individual and environmental factors act together to influence interaction styles and behaviours, a process often conducted in the client's home.

As failure to thrive is conceptualised as a psychosocial problem, family-focused intervention may be the optimal strategy to promote improvements in health and development (Drotar & Crawford, 1985; Drotar, 1991).

## Methods

Methods used in failure-to-thrive interventions based on an ecological perspective include taking a detailed history at the assessment stage to elicit information regarding proximal and distal, individual, and environmental factors that constitute the person–process context (as demonstrated in Chapter 9). The information gathered at the assessment stage then informs the intervention methods. Such interventions often include formation of a therapeutic alliance with the parent, provision of support, modelling and practising developmentally appropriate parenting behaviour (Olds *et al.* 1994). Problem-solving is taught to parents and often centres on improving feeding and interaction patterns. Nutritional advice also forms part of the treatment process.

## Ecological Interventions

Black *et al.* (1995), who conducted a failure-to-thrive treatment programme and a follow-up study grounded in an ecological perspective, found evidence that home-based intervention initiated during infancy and toddlerhood among children who failed to thrive can influence development and family relationships when they reached the age of 4 years. However, the findings also illustrate that such early home intervention may only be effective among children of mothers who do not report high levels of negative feelings. Outcome was found to be mediated by the mothers' low or high levels of negative emotions, with decline in cognitive development particularly found in the children of mothers suffering from depression, hostility, and anxiety, effects which the intervention failed to reduce. The relationship between risk factors, maternal affectivity, and environmental factors appeared to have an effect upon the success (or otherwise) of the intervention; however, mothers with severe psychological problems could be so overwhelmed by any one problem that intervention had limited success. Given these findings, the authors concluded that such an intervention will be more successful for some and less so for others, with mothers benefiting most who had more positive attitudes and feelings. Parents with high levels of negative emotions may, according to Hutcheson *et al.* (1997), benefit from intervention directed towards changes in order to improve their function as parents.

According to Black (1995), many interventions are family-focused. However, not all such interventions meet the multiple needs of the children and families in question. In her account of 'Family-focused interventions', with emphasis placed on the importance of examining person-centred models as defined by Bronfenbrenner (1993), she points to the mixed outcomes of a number of such intervention programmes, including, in some cases, failure to promote positive changes in infant growth and development (e.g. Haynes *et al.*, 1984), and improvements in cognitive development (e.g. Drotar & Sturm, 1988) when compared to control and comparison groups. Black concludes that home-visiting, while effective in some respects, should be supplemented with additional services in FTT intervention programmes, and recommends that an intervention strategy combining home intervention together with multi-disciplinary services may be the most effective method to achieve positive long-lasting outcomes (*see* Chapter 12 for further discussion on the effectiveness of multi-model intervention).

## APPLICATION OF BEHAVIOURAL THEORY TO FAILURE-TO-THRIVE TREATMENT STRATEGY

In order to make sense of a complex world, people learn in the first weeks of life to develop strategies and techniques with which to guide behaviour. Behavioural theory concerns the processes through which people apply knowledge they have gained from interactions with their environment to guide their daily functioning, and works on the principle that behaviour is learned, maintained, and regulated as a cumulative result of a person's interactions with, and feedback from, his or her environment. Individuals, according to this theory, learn (through a process of positive and negative reinforcement) that particular behaviours and paths of action are associated with, and tend to result in, particular consequences, thus resulting in conditioning (the person strives to engage in positively reinforced target behaviour) and extinguishing (the person actively avoids negatively reinforced target behaviour).

Behavioural theory has been extensively applied to theories of child development where it has been shown that children use information learned from their experiences with care-givers and the environment to make judgments about the world around them on which they base their actions and essentially 'learn' how to behave. It has been demonstrated that care-givers and their children condition each other's behaviours and interactions through a process of responsiveness or unresponsiveness to cues and signals, synchronicity (or lack of it) in interactions, and sensitivity (or lack of it) to natural cycles and circadian rhythms, including cycles of attention and inattention, cycles of 'up' and 'down' time, sleep–wake cycles, feeding, hunger, and digestion cycles.

Behavioural theory has been usefully applied to the treatment of FTT. It allows researchers to conceptualise and address particular problem behaviours at a number of different levels and perspectives. Using behavioural theory, researchers and practitioners can look at each case from the viewpoint of the child, the parent, the family, and the social and natural environment. Distal and proximal factors shaping and maintaining problem behaviours may be identified and addressed in order to gain a better understanding of the origins of and solution to the problem. Thus the reasons why certain problematic behaviours or interactions have emerged may be better understood, including identification of which conditions or factors elicit or reinforce undesired or unrewarding behaviours, which conditions are missing (that, if in operation, would positively reinforce desired behaviours), and which outcome conditions either control or reinforce problem behaviour or extinguish/punish desirable behaviour. Herbert (1993) refers to the importance of establishing what is to be gained or the motives behind maladaptive behaviour, or, in other words, 'what is the pay-off for such behaviour?'

A behavioural-theory-led assessment of FTT takes into account both proximal and distal variables. Distal antecedents of failure to thrive could include child behaviours that are directly related to an organic disorder such as a hiatus hernia, pyloric stenosis, or any early illness that may have produced discomfort or pain while the infant was being fed. Through a process of negative reinforcement as described above, the child may associate the feeding situation with previous pain or discomfort, and thus develop a lasting aversion to feeding beyond the duration of the medical condition, with a possibility of initiating maladaptive feeding interactions that could lead to FTT.

Proximal antecedents of failure to thrive have been found to include emotionally inappropriate behaviours directed at the child, such as rejecting behaviours characterised by absence or withdrawal of affection from the child (who may for a variety of reasons be viewed in a negative manner by the parent). Parental hostility and rejecting behaviours may be presented in a variety of overt and covert forms during feeding interactions, and may lead to the development of an association between feeding and fearful, distressing experiences. Hostile maternal behaviours that may condition an aversion to feeding in children and reinforce food refusal include force-feeding, excessive feeding, shouting, obvious impatience, criticism, nagging, scolding, smacking, hurrying, and aggressive, violent, or rough handling during feeding interaction. Children may also learn that certain behaviours during feeding may influence parental behaviours, thus may be reinforced to carry out or maintain maladaptive feeding practices in order to exert control and to manipulate their parents or gain associated rewards such as increased levels of attention. Iwata *et al.* (1982) noted two types of contingencies that occur in the light of the above. First, parental attention to the child's misbehaviour during feeding, once established, is likely to continue. Second, when a child's disruptive behaviour is positively reinforced by parental attention, the child's disruptive behaviour is likely to continue, thus resulting in high rates of parental attention to misbehaviour and the occurrence of misbehaviour, leading to the establishment of a maladjusted feeding interaction.

Just as behaviour is learned, it may also be 'unlearned'. Some have suggested that abnormal behaviour does not differ from normal behaviour in its development, its persistence, and the way in which it can be changed (Herbert, 1974; 1987). Abnormal behaviour is the result of faulty learning, but essentially the behaviour can be learned and unlearned in the same way as any normal behaviour. Based on this reasoning, once the mechanisms through which problem behaviours (such as disruptive eating and dysfunctional parent–child interactions) have emerged, factors that may maintain the problematic behaviour may then be deconstructed and 'unlearned'.

## Methods

Behavioural techniques that may be usefully applied to the treatment of failure to thrive are substantial, including positive and negative reinforcement, differential reinforcement, extinction, skills training, modelling, stimulus change, role play, exposure training, and various cognitive methods.

Behavioural interventions are especially usefully applied to resolving problems in interaction between failure-to-thrive parents and their children, due to the belief that interactions play a major role in shaping and reinforcing both adaptive and maladaptive behaviours. At the assessment stage of a behavioural intervention much information will be gathered regarding proximal and distal antecedents (as described above), in an attempt to determine the mechanics of the care-giver–child relationship, with particular focus on interactions. In addition, parental views and experiences (i.e. the forces shaping attitudes, beliefs, and behaviour) are examined, including information on attachment, health, food beliefs, attitudes towards the child, relationships with significant others, and so on. This information is used to tailor the treatment phase of the intervention. Findings from such assessments are also shared with the parent so that they, too, may gain a deeper insight into possible mechanisms maintaining the failure to thrive. In this respect behavioural techniques are user-friendly as they provide a platform from which to make sense of the underlying problems. Further, the techniques used, such as shaping, reinforcing through a process of essentially 'rewarding' desired behaviours, and 'ignoring' undesired behaviours, are easily understood by parents who may already make use of such techniques, albeit in an inefficacious or misguided fashion. Such techniques may, once modelled, be used effectively as tools by parents to engage in more successful interactions with the child, together with more successful feeding behaviours and outcomes.

## Examples of Behavioural Intervention

Kahng *et al.* (2001) investigated the use of a multi-component behavioural treatment for food refusal. In order to explore an alternative intervention approach, these authors carried out a study examining the use of a multi-component treatment for food refusal involving a 'response-cost intervention' and differential reinforcement of alternative behaviour.

The intervention was carried out with a 5-year-old failure-to-thrive boy who, at the onset of the intervention, was dependent on a gastronomic feeding-tube (G-tube) for 100% of his daily calorific intake. During the assessment, problem behaviours were observed and data were collected on behaviour during feeding, with a focus on acceptance, expelling, gagging, and vomiting, and summarised as a number of responses per minute. Treatment involved several components, including the removal or returning of preferred items of food, dependent on the acceptance or refusal of bites of food taken without accompanying problematic behaviours. The boy received brief praise contingent on acceptance, and behaviours (such as expelling) were ignored. The mother and grandmother were trained to implement the intervention.

The multi-component intervention led to an increase in food acceptance and a decrease in problem behaviour during the treatment phases (occurring over a four-month period). In addition, expelling, gagging, and vomiting decreased to zero during the final phase of treatment. He continued with high levels of acceptance and low levels of problem behaviour with his mother and grandmother. Meal length was increased and additional food items were introduced, together with a gradual reduction in tube-feedings, resulting in a weight increase from 16.7 kg to 20.3 kg (2 st. 8 lb. 6 oz. to 3 st. 2 lb. 3 oz.).

Foy et al. (1997) described the effectiveness of a multi-disciplinary intervention using rapid introduction of oral feedings designed to treat severe feeding refusal. The primary operative principles of this programme are exposure and response prevention, specifically prevention avoidance or rejection of food. The method of this programme was to introduce food in a continuous fashion (despite protests by the child) with escape behaviour extinguished through lack of reinforcement, in the hope that oral intake would become a normally reinforcing experience.

Participants in this study were 19 children with feeding difficulties who were fed at least 95% by naso-gastric or gastronomy tubes. The evaluation process included psychological evaluation of family interaction and parental anxiety, a medical examination with nutritional assessment, an occupational therapy evaluation, and a radiographic study of swallow. An oral feeding phase was carried out on an inpatient basis for three weeks during which tube-feeding was phased out gradually through a process of ignoring negative behaviours (such as coughing, gagging, and fighting), while rewarding positive behaviours (such as opening mouth or accepting food) with praise. Gradually, parents became involved in treatment once the child started co-operatively accepting bites. Twelve of the 19 children were successful in the oral feeding programme, with success measured as taking all calories by mouth at follow-up. The length of time from non-oral feeding to oral feeding ranged from 1 to 23 months. Of those who failed to be classified as successful, three were taking at least 25% of their calorie intake by oral feeding and four were taking less than 25% by this means.

Hampton (1996) described the work of the Children's Society *Infant Support Project (ISP)*, Wiltshire, which undertakes treatment of non-organic failure-to-thrive children and their families. The *ISP* uses a problem-solving-based approach and behavioural methods of intervention, and has a multi-disciplinary team including nursery nurses, social workers, and health visitors.

At the assessment stage (which takes place during visits to families) the ISP makes use of a referral form based on the work of Iwaniec *et al.* (1985b) to provide an inventory of the signs and symptoms of FTT. A weighting system developed by the *ISP* is then applied to enable prioritisation of need and provision of a measure of the effectiveness of the work. Weight, height, and head-circumference charts were used as baseline measures.

Methods of the *ISP* are based on social-learning theory, and behavioural methods of intervention, and include multiple videotaping of meal-times to record significant aspects of meal-time behaviour, and to carry out a functional analysis of feeding. Food diaries are also completed by parents. Checklists derived from other researchers are used to observe and assess parent–child interaction at meal-times, and summaries of findings are then given to parents, with care taken to avoid providing parents with conflicting advice from the multi-disciplinary team. The most common intervention decided upon with the parents is to ignore any unacceptable behaviours while strongly reinforcing any behaviours that are acceptable. Families were also encouraged to use community resources available: for example, the use of local clinics for regular weighings and measurements of children's growth.

An independent assessment conducted by Carole Sutton (1994) (an expert in behavioural approaches) examined outcomes for children and parents and the level of satisfaction following participation in the *ISP*. Progress was measured by a baseline to follow up a comparison of each child's weight and recording of FTT indicators pre- and post-intervention. Of 108 children, a total of 73 (67%) made progress regarded as satisfactory or better, based on weight gain and reduction in FTT indicator scale-score. Together with producing good outcomes for feeding behaviours, and positive parental ratings, there were cost-effective benefits of short-term intensive support interventions.

## APPLICATION OF COGNITIVE THEORY TO FAILURE-TO-THRIVE TREATMENT STRATEGIES

While behavioural theory holds that behaviours can be learned and unlearned through a process of rewards, punishments, and other experiences, it has been argued that

> we can never fully understand the nature of ... any ... behaviours ... without learning something about the thoughts that accompany them.
> (Bernstein *et al.*, 1994)

A cognitive behavioural approach to the study of human behaviour encompasses both an emphasis on the processes underlying learning and the mechanisms or mental processes through which people organise that learning. Cognitive behavioural theory holds that learning affects the development of thoughts and beliefs and in turn influences behavioural patterns.

Cognitive shortcuts or schemas have an adaptive function much like learning (conditioning and aversion), whereby people develop strategies of processing information based on prior experiences and beliefs in order to guide behaviour. The development of knowledge occurs in stages. Piaget, in the 1920s, coined the term 'schema' to describe the basic units of knowledge that individuals use to make sense of the world from infancy. Schemas may be positive or negative (Beck & Weishaar, 1989), and may guide the interpretation of events (Kendall & Lockman, 1994). Cognitive-theory-led failure-to-thrive research focuses on gaining a better understanding of the mechanisms underlying how parents acquire, store, and retrieve information regarding their roles as parents and their perceptions regarding their children.

Cognitive theory has been applied to parenting behaviour, and has been used in the development and implementation of failure-to-thrive intervention programmes. Self-defeating thoughts and beliefs about parenting abilities may affect a failure-to-thrive parent's ability to cope effectively with the parenting task, due to the fact that dysfunctional thoughts lead to dysfunctional feelings and consequently negative outcomes (Iwaniec, Herbert and Sluckin, 2002). A parent may have a dysfunctional schema of her/his child that could be due to preconceptions and expectations regarding it. Parents' schema of their child may also be altered and/or reinforced by psychological functioning of the parent, and by the health, appearance, and temperament of the infant (Derivan, 1982). Further, parents may have a dysfunctional schema of their own roles as parents. This could be due to child-related alterations to a parent's life-choices, expectations, or role-satisfaction as a parent. Furthermore, some parents may have inadequate models with which to guide their parenting behaviour, due either to a lack of experience in dealing with children, or to having experienced inconsistent parenting in their own childhood. It has been shown that parents with inconsistent parenting models are less able to tolerate or adjust to demanding infant behaviour or temperament than parents who experienced sensitive nurturing as children (Drotar & Malone, 1982). Dysfunctional parenting schemas may result in parents misinterpreting their children's behaviour, a factor that may lead to unsatisfactory interactions.

Parents may also lack confidence in their parenting abilities because of low self-esteem and low parental self-efficacy. Low parental self-efficacy has been shown to impact negatively on parental functioning by reducing parental competence (Coleman & Karraker, 1997). Low parental self-efficacy has also been found to affect parents' ability to cope with stressors (debilitating factors, as multiple stressors are associated with failure to thrive, including difficult feeding behaviours and interactions).

Beck and Weishaar (1989) discussed systematic errors in reasoning (*cognitive distortions*) that may be triggered by stress, a factor that, according to these authors, reduces people's ability to avoid distorted thinking. Such cognitive distortions include over-generalisation, magnification and minimisation, personalisation, and dichotomous thinking. Parents' beliefs in their abilities as parents will also be affected by perceived external expectations and perceived external ratings of abilities as parents, and for this reason many failure-to-thrive intervention theorists have emphasised the importance of fostering a supportive relationship with the parent, with care taken to avoid feelings of criticism or blame.

## Methods

Cognitive therapy is used to identify and correct negative, dysfunctional, or maladaptive cognitions relating to the parenting of the failure-to-thrive child. Attitudes and perceptions of parental duties and attitudes and responsibilities are also examined (Iwaniec *et al.*, 2002). Through a process of reassessing an individual's cognitive perceptions, negative perceptions can be replaced with healthier ones with the hope that healthier interactions and behaviours will ensue. This is achieved through a process of examining beliefs, identifying and challenging dysfunctional thoughts, and providing skills and experiences that promote adaptive cognitive processing (together with developing schemas to better cope with distressing situations).

Cognitive therapy involves discussion between the therapist and the parent, centred around examining the underlying beliefs currently guiding feelings, expectations, and behaviour. Once these have been identified, the therapist attempts to help parents to modify dysfunctional beliefs and thought processes. An essential component of cognitive therapy is that the parent is actively involved. Thus, parents must participate in the exploration of the manner in which their behaviour is guided by their own beliefs and information-processing. They must see for themselves the underlying mechanisms at work in order to understand why alternative information-processing strategies may be more productive and rewarding. Modelling of alternative methods of interaction or alternative feeding strategies may help parents widen the scope of self-imposed and child-related expectations.

The change in cognition occurs when a person believes that it will happen and says 'I can do it', 'I will make an effort to do more things with my child', and 'I will practise patience'. Little can be achieved if cognitive change does not take place. Change can only occur if a person is engaged in the problematic situation and experiences emotional arousal. Thus, a mother who finds physical contact with her child difficult may begin by imagining what it is like to sit a child on her lap (with accompanying emotions), and practises (during the course of therapeutic intervention) sitting a child on her lap and having other physical contact with the child. Reasons why particular emotions are aroused at each stage (e.g. it does not want to be picked up and loved) are examined and tested. In the case of a child who refuses to take food, conversation with the mother may show that she feels the child refuses to eat in order to spite or hurt her. Discussion then takes place about how this makes her feel, and suggestions are made concerning how these feelings can be tested as realities. Education about the developmental stage of the child and the occurrence of particular behaviour characteristics of most children of the same age may help changes in attitudes and beliefs. For example, a child's resistance to novel foods with different textures or smells (upon initial presentation) is to be expected and not to be taken personally. By exploring, with parents, various possibilities and reasons why a child is failing to thrive, and teaching them to take into account all the factors in the situation, cognitive change may occur, followed by changes in behaviour and outcomes.

Cognitive work points to the successful aspects of parents' lives, so that they can take comfort from those aspects and redirect their thinking to constructive strategies to problem-solving and feel good about them. For example, a mother who has difficulties in feeding her child usually experiences an overwhelming feeling of inadequacy and failure as a carer. Furthermore, such mothers think and feel that they are the only ones having these difficulties, and therefore believe that they are useless as parents, or, worse, that they are not loved by that particular child.

According to Iwaniec et al. (2002), when choosing cognitive methods of working the first task is to identify damaging thoughts and demonstrate their link with the child's negative outcomes. Parents are asked to record negative or unhelpful thoughts and try to link these to accompanying feelings in order to gain a clearer understanding of how their thoughts act to influence their behaviour. Parents are then helped to develop alternative ways of thinking and understanding in order to achieve cognitive change. For example, by replacing feelings of anger and frustration upon a negative feeding interaction a parent may learn to substitute feelings of hope, commitment, and determination.

Table 11.1 illustrates distorted thoughts and attitudes in relation to a failure-to-thrive child, and presents cognitive change.

## Self-Instruction as Stress Management

Meal-times for many parents are battlefields, with stress and anger rising high. It is very helpful and necessary to prepare for them so that the mother does not get stressed and defeated before she even starts. She must tell herself,

**Table 11.1** Dysfunctional thoughts, beliefs, and alternative ways of thinking

| Event | Belief | Feeling | Behaviour | Outcome |
|---|---|---|---|---|
| **Self-defeating thoughts and feelings** | | | | |
| Child fails to thrive | He refuses food to hurt me. I cannot cope | Anger, frustration, helplessness | Force-feeding, screaming, shouting | Food-avoidance behaviour |
| **Cognitive change—alternative ways of thinking** | | | | |
| Child fails to thrive | He is a difficult child to feed. There are many children like him | I can try different ways of feeding, and I can manage | Being patient and encouraging when feeding a child | Child eats more, puts on weight |

*Source:* Iwaniec, D. (1995) *The Emotionally Abused and Neglected Child.* Chichester: John Wiley & Sons Ltd

quietly instruct herself, how she is going to deal with the situation. She may say:

- 'This is not going to upset me'
- 'I know what to do'
- 'I am going to stay calm'
- 'I am going to take Susan to the kitchen and tell her what I am going to prepare for a meal'
- 'I am going to ask her to help me'
- 'I am going to smile, touch, and hug her while preparing a meal'
- 'If I realise that I am getting upset or tense, I will take a deep breath and tell myself that I am going to do my best and in a calm way'
- 'I am going to talk to Susan warmly and gently and try to make her feel relaxed and at ease'
- 'I will not put pressure on her, but gently prompt her to eat'
- 'I will not get angry if she refuses to eat. I will just leave it and try again later'

## SELF-CONTROL TRAINING

Novaco (1975) developed stress-management training, including anger control, to offer people skills in managing provocation and in regulating anger arousal. Components of this programme include a *situational analysis* (identification of situations that provoke thoughts and feelings in anger-inducing encounters) and encouragement to use self-statements and feelings associated with anger as cues for *positive coping strategies*. Parents are encouraged to conceptualise anger as a state which is aggravated by self-presented thought, and to view arousal as a series of stages rather than as an all-or-nothing state. Attention should be paid to identifying and altering irrational beliefs: for example, 'she is doing it on purpose to hurt me'; or 'she knows what to do, it is just sheer laziness'. Coping strategies include self-instructions that may be used, including those that encourage a focus on the task to be accomplished, and those that encourage other behaviours, such as getting a cup of tea or relaxing (for example, doing relaxation exercises for a few minutes or simply taking a few deep breaths). In other words, parents are advised to interfere with anxiety-provoking thoughts as soon as they occur, instruct themselves to do something else, or to think of something pleasant. A list of useful techniques in self-control is given below as a series of self-instructions:

1. Go to another room for a few minutes to get away from the child;
2. Count to 10, or count leaves on a potted plant;
3. Go to the kitchen to make a cup of tea;
4. Take two or three deep breaths;
5. Go to the bedroom and punch a few cushions;
6. Go to the garden, do some digging, walk around the garden to get rid of the tension and to calm down;
7. Go to the bathroom and read the newspaper for a few minutes;
8. Listen to some favourite music;
9. Do some heavy physical work, e.g. vacuuming, scrubbing floors, cleaning a messy shed, etc.;
10. Pinch yourself or put your hands under very cold water;
11. Sit quietly for a few minutes and reflect on pleasurable and soothing things instead of brooding about the child;
12. Try to recall positive aspects of the child's behaviour; and
13. Try to remember that children are small and immature and are bound to make mistakes or produce growing-up problems.

## APPLICATION OF ATTACHMENT THEORY TO FAILURE-TO-THRIVE TREATMENT STRATEGIES

Attachment theory (Bowlby, 1982) has been shown to be a useful theoretical framework for non-organic failure-to-thrive intervention strategies. Self-regulation of food intake is closely linked to affective engagement between parents and their children. As many parent–child interactions occur at feeding times, disorders in attachment (including associated inability to attend to infant cues and signals and to provide feelings of security) can lead to lack of appetite and the development of dysfunctional feeding patterns and behaviours. A number of FTT interventions have used attachment theory as a theoretical framework.

As has been discussed in Chapter 7, disrupted mother–infant communication plays a negative role in parent–child play and feeding interactions, and in the development of a child's attachment to his or her parents. This view is influenced by findings from attachment research indicating associations between failure to thrive and disorganised infant attachment, and unresolved mourning or trauma in parents, including unresolved attachment losses (Benoit *et al.*, 1989; Coolbear & Benoit, 1999; Crittenden, 1987; Valenzuela, 1990; Main & Hesse, 1990). The authors refer to prospective and retrospective evidence linking the quality of early parent–infant relationships (particularly in relation to the arena of responding to, sensitivity to, and ability to read cues and signals from children) with later serious socio-emotional and behavioural problems (Dozier *et al.*, 1999; Greenberg, 1999). Based on their own research findings Benoit *et al.* (2001) found that interventions aimed at increasing parent sensitivity may also have the effect of reducing the disruptive behaviours considered to contribute to disorganised infant attachment.

Chatoor *et al.* (1984) devised a multi-faceted conceptual framework for understanding feeding disturbances in order to facilitate diagnosis and treatment of FTT and growth disorders in infants and young children. Based on a developmental perspective, this classification system for feeding disturbances incorporates Mahler *et al.*'s (1975) concept of separation and individuation and Greenspan's (1981) developmental stages for the first year of life (which are homeostasis, attachment, and somato-psychological differentiation). Three distinct stages of feeding development were classified, together with an outline of deviation from 'normal' patterns of development purported to have a role in the aetiology of non-organic failure to thrive, including disorders of homeostasis, disorders of attachment, and disorders of separation and individuation.

According to this developmental framework, from birth to the age of 2 months, infants are preoccupied with achieving regulation of state, or homeostasis, in which the infant attempts to achieve a balance between internal state and involvement with the world with the assistance of care-givers (who attempt to provide an environment conducive to this). Failure of an infant to master self-regulation, including sucking, swallowing, and an ability to give signals to influence the timing of onset and termination of feedings, can lead to feeding difficulties together with impeded development of motor skills, language, and affective management. It is important, therefore, that the infant is able to deliver signals of hunger and satiation. Of equal importance, however, is the mother's ability to recognise and interpret these cues. If a mother is unable to interpret cues, she may under- or over-stimulate the infant. Between two and six months of age the infant engages in attachment with care-givers. At this stage regulation of food intake is closely linked to the infant's affective engagement with care-givers, as many interactions between the dyad occur around feedings. Disorders of attachment can result from a lack of engagement between the dyad, leading to lack of pleasure, lack of appetite and possibly severe dysfunctional feeding patterns (such as vomiting and rumination). Feeding characteristics associated with disorders of attachment include vomiting, diarrhoea, and poor weight gain.

Between 6 months and 3 years of age, the infant enters a development stage described by Mahler *et al.* (1975) as 'separation and individuation'. At this stage the infant learns means–end differentiation, and begins to understand that actions elicit consequences. Lack of somato-psychological differentiation, together with a struggle between autonomy and dependency, can get caught up in the feeding situation and result in an infant's emotional needs (including affection, dependency, anger, and frustration), rather than hunger needs, dictating behaviour. It is important that parents become aware of the importance of somato-psychological differentiation. Parents can be taught techniques, such as separating meal-times from play-times, in order to assist this development in their infants. This conceptual framework provides a developmental context in which to assist early identification of maladaptive feeding behaviour. Together with providing parents with the above knowledge, Chatoor *et al.* (1984) advise that professionals should teach parents to read infant cues, respond in a contingent manner, and encourage them to trust their infants' abilities in nutritional self-regulation.

Researchers have applied findings from attachment research to the management of FTT, including the knowledge that a parent's ability to recognise, interpret, and respond to a child's signals, together with synchronised and sensitive parent–child interaction, are crucial for the development of secure attachment relationships. While not all cases of failure to thrive are due to impaired care-giver–child interactions, dysfunctional emotional engagement between care-givers and their infants and disorganised attachment can lead to impaired ability to self-regulate feeding, dysfunctional feeding patterns, and difficulties in achieving somato-psychological differentiation (all of which can contribute to the infants' FTT). Failure-to-thrive intervention researchers, such as Benoit *et al.* (2001) and Chatoor *et al.* (1984), have used this knowledge to inform intervention strategies including working with care-givers to help them to become aware of such mechanisms and equipping them with strategies aimed at improving interaction and communication with their children.

Iwaniec *et al.* (2002) discuss ways in which children with attachment disorders can be helped, and in which parent–child bonding can be strengthened. According to Iwaniec (1999), in order to promote attachment security in infancy, proactive and sensitive maternal behaviour during feeding, bathing, and changing is required. Furthermore, it is essential that parents respond promptly, consistently, and appropriately to children's signals of distress. By holding children gently while engaging in activities with them, parents can help develop the attachment relationship with their child. Talking softly, making sure to establish eye-contact, and smiling will help the child to feel loved and relaxed, enhancing the quality of parent–child interaction, and ultimately promoting a secure attachment between the dyad. Further, such attachment-inducing behaviours also help to ensure that the care-giving atmosphere is calm and relaxed. The cognitive behavioural methods employed by Iwaniec (1997) in her failure-to-thrive intervention strategies include such methods where it is hoped that, by increasing the child's feelings of trust and security associated with the care-giver and the feeding scenario, an atmosphere more conducive to feeding and eating will be achieved.

## SUMMARY

Theoretical frameworks applied to failure-to-thrive intervention and treatment have been discussed. Four theories only (ecological, behavioural, cognitive, and attachment) were included in this chapter to illustrate the theoretical base for planning intervention. There are obviously other theories which could be taken into consideration, but there is insufficient space to do so here. Brief explanations as to why some children fail to thrive (based on different theoretical perspectives) have been outlined, as well as types of interventions proposed. Some examples of effective helping strategies linked to different perspectives and based on various research findings have been presented and discussed.

# MULTIDIMENSIONAL/INTEGRATED MODEL OF INTERVENTION IN FAILURE-TO-THRIVE CASES

*The burnt child dreads the fire.*

Ben Jonson, 1616

## INTRODUCTION

As has been discussed in previous chapters, failure to thrive is multi-factorial in aetiology; therefore intervention needs to be tailor-made, addressing different problems and using various methods and techniques (which may be based on a number of theories).

The package of intervention and treatment methods presented in this chapter has been developed by the author and her colleagues, and tested for effectiveness for more than 25 years in 298 cases. It is an integrated model, based on several theories emphasising multi-disciplinary, inter-agency approaches, and community-based interventions. It is also a child-centred model, where parents play a central role in problem identification and problem-solving, through working in partnership with professionals involved in the case.

## INTERVENTION

Intervention strategy with failure-to-thrive children in this model is typically carried out in a number of stages, with the main aim being to achieve a normal pattern of growth as quickly as possible. At the assessment stage the multi-factorial nature of failure to thrive is established through a process whereby diagnosis is confirmed and the potential elements causing and maintaining the FTT are explored. This process includes focusing on parent–child interactions; observing and recording of feeding behaviour and intake of food; preparing a feeding schedule and content; advising on general parenting style;

and enhancing parental capacity to meet a child's developmental needs. Environmental and economic factors, as well as parental history, are explored to provide a more holistic picture of the child and the parents.

Intervention with failure-to-thrive cases usually falls into two basic categories:

- addressing immediate and urgent needs or crises; and
- longer-term therapeutic work with more complex cases.

## Addressing Immediate Needs

The type of intervention at this stage varies substantially between cases. As a rule there are more problematic cases where provision of *universal services* has not had the desired effect. Quite often there are delays in referring a child, due to the belief that the toddler will grow out of poor eating and growing, and so the 'wait-and-see' approach is adopted (which in some cases leads to more and more problems as time goes by). Apart from growth-faltering, there are interactional and relationship difficulties as well as behavioural and emotional problems, which bring about crises in parenting and at times in family functioning. It is sometimes necessary at that stage to arrange a day-nursery for a child to break the cycle of aversive interaction and to provide a stimulating and anxiety-free environment; this may be particularly beneficial for children with developmental delays and unmet physical and emotional needs. At the same time it gives the therapist and parents more time and the opportunity to explore in depth problems associated with child care, family, and personal life.

Some families might need assistance with: welfare rights benefits; housing; health (in particular mental health, such as depression or other mental health problems); addictions (such as alcohol or drug misuse); financial problems; unemployment; marital frictions; or family violence. There might be concerns about other children's welfare and behaviour. These issues, once identified, need to be discussed with the parents, and appropriate referrals need to be made to activate help. It is important that parental problems are dealt with early on to reduce stress and to create an atmosphere where further therapeutic work can take place.

Many mothers of FTT children are isolated, feel depressed, and experience a profound sense of inadequacy as parents. They tend to think that people see them as poor mothers and that they deliberately neglect the child. This distorted thinking pattern leads to negative feelings and negative outcomes for mother and child. While there are some who neglect and reject their children, most do not.

It is important at this stage to organise support for the parents to break the social isolation and give some practical help—getting in touch with the extended family or neighbours (with parental agreement) to alert them to what is happening and ask them for assistance. Equally, exploring what is available within easy reach in the community (such as mother-and-toddler groups, play-groups, women's groups attached to community centres, churches, leisure centres, and local libraries) may be beneficial. Some parents, and in particular mothers, do take advantage of these facilities once they gain some self-confidence.

The author's model of step-by-step therapeutic intervention is presented below, and each component is then elaborated on in a more detailed way. The author's substantial clinical and research experience in this area indicates that giving advice to parents on how to deal with a failure-to-thrive child is not enough, especially when there are obvious tensions, worries, resentments, depressive moods, neglect, and growing interactional and relationship problems. They need more regular and intensive support and guidance and, at times, the direct involvement of a therapist in modelling the feeding of, playing with, reacting to, and relating to the child. Many parents (even those who have raised another child) tend to lose confidence as problems connected with a child's growth and general presentation intensify, and concerns are expressed regarding the child's appearance, indicating a possibility of poor quality of parenting. These parents need to be shown how to relax, how to feed the baby, and when and what to feed: they need to be supervised and reassured that what they are doing is right; they need developmental counselling to raise awareness about the children's physical and psychosocial needs; and they need help in their own right to become more effective parents and individuals.

## THERAPEUTIC HELP FOR PARENTS

Some mothers of failure-to-thrive children require personal counselling to explore what is going wrong in the parenting of that particular child and what effect it has on their behaviour and feelings. Many need cognitive work to deal with their dysfunctional thoughts and attitudes, and most need developmental counselling to explore the developmental needs of children and to learn how those needs can be facilitated. Even those who are well informed about child development welcome that opportunity to reassure themselves that they are doing things right, and that the child is progressing well. Some couples need assistance in resolving marital frictions, and in more serious cases (where intensive couple therapy is required) may need to be referred to a specialist in this area of work. Equally, help may need to be arranged for clinically depressed parents. It should be stressed that the chronology of intervention and treatment is important, particularly in the circumstances where therapeutic progress depends on parental engagement, full participation, and commitment to produce necessary change. For example, a seriously

**Table 12.1** Integrated model of intervention in failure-to-thrive cases

| PARENTS | CHILD | THERAPIST | COMMUNITY |
|---|---|---|---|
| Relaxation training to deal with anxiety and tension related to child's poor growth | Gentle interaction to bring child into relaxed state before meal-time | To provide modelling on:<br>• how to create an anxiety-free atmosphere for parent and child<br>• how to react during meal-time<br>• how to encourage a child to eat and make meal-time enjoyable<br>• how to play, communicate and engage in mutual activities | Asking extended family or neighbour to help |
| Putting into practice new feeding behaviour learnt through modelling | Asking child to participate, getting involved in preparing food and helping | | Asking health visitor to help |
| Getting into the habit of praising, hugging, smiling, kissing, being warm and affectionate, showing pride in child's achievements | Child getting reinforcement chart to be rewarded for good eating and other pro-social behaviour | | Arranging day-nursery or daily minder if necessary |
| Organising reinforcement chart and activity rewards for a child as a symbol of achievements | Play sessions with mother and then with other members of the family | To provide:<br>• developmental counselling to raise parental awareness of a child's developmental needs<br>• personal counselling for parents to get in touch with their own feelings and to enhance personality growth | If necessary, arrange investigation of physical illness by hospital |
| Getting involved in play and other activities with the child in a warm, reassuring way | Story reading as a means of increasing physical and emotional closeness with the mother | | Case-conference if there are worries of abuse or neglect or other form of maltreatment |
| Increasing physical contact: cognitive restructuring, dealing with unrealistic expectations, faulty perceptions, and emotional thoughts | | | |
| Stress management, anger control | | | |
| Group work as a means of learning new skills and getting social support | | | |

depressed mother needs help first, before being able to engage in resolving interactional and nurturing problems with her child. In other words, we cannot put 'the cart before the horse' in the therapeutic process. At the same time, the assumption that placing a child in the day-nursery (where care and attention are satisfactory) is enough to resolve parent–child relationships and interaction problems is unrealistic. Providing a day-nursery for a child may facilitate much-needed social stimulation, resulting in developmental catching up and accelerated physical growth due to better intake of food, but it seldom resolves the child's problems at home. Newly learned skills, emotional stability, and social stimulation have to be reinforced and nurtured at home by parents in order to provide continuity and sustainable positive change. So, helping strategies for a child have to go hand in hand with helping parents to be better equipped to care for a child in an informed and satisfactory way. No amount of intervention is going to produce long-lasting, meaningful changes to the child if an alcoholic mother is not going to stop drinking, a depressed one does not get treatment, a violent father does not stop terrorising his family, or if economic and housing conditions do not improve to at least a minimally acceptable level.

Most parents, but in particular mothers of FTT children (as case studies illustrate), are found to be very anxious, worried, helpless, and disillusioned about their abilities to parent a child: they tend to lack confidence in terms of self-efficacy, and their self-esteem is often at rock bottom. This learned helplessness is portrayed by depressive moods and apathy in some, and others show a high anxiety level expressed by an outburst of anger and frustration. These difficulties experienced by parents require attention and therapeutic help to prepare them and energise them emotionally to start helping their failure-to-thrive children. Relaxation, anger control, stress management, cognitive restructuring, and problem-solving may be used for some clients.

## CHILD-CENTRED INTERVENTION

The major therapeutic emphasis in every failure-to-thrive case is on the child, and whatever else is done with or for the parents and family is done to facilitate an effective resolution of problems facing the child. Parental co-operation, engagement, and commitment are essential to make adequate progress, so fully involving parents from the beginning as co-therapists, and establishing a working partnership with them, are beneficial for all concerned. Joint planning, involvement in assessment, active participation in intervention, and evaluation of each stage of the programme should be agreed and observed.

Child-focused intervention normally involves three stages, and each stage will be described and discussed below.

## Dealing with Insufficient Food Intake

The primary objectives of all failure-to-thrive cases are to increase food intake by children, and to improve the manner in which children are fed and dealt with, in order that they may gain weight and grow. As many children present feeding difficulties, and do not get sufficient nutrition into their systems, this problem is dealt with first in order to help the child to take more food, and to help the parents to better manage the process of feeding. Some children are simply not given a sufficient amount of food, because the signals of satiation and hunger are not properly interpreted: some parents may be unaware of how much milk or solid food a baby should take at a certain age and size; and sometimes a feeding formula is wrong, so the parents are advised and shown how to feed, what to feed, when to feed, and how much food is required for the child's age. Parent training and education play an important role here as well as frequent home visits to monitor the programme of feeding. Those parents who deliberately dilute the formula or restrict the child's food intake because they fear the child becoming obese need extra attention in terms of counselling and supervision of the case. Some of these parents have a history of *anorexia nervosa* and *bulimia*, so they need additional help to monitor the case. Occasionally, there is a need for greater surveillance if the child's weight remains problematic for a long time, in spite of intervention taking place. We also need to be alerted to the small number of cases where failure to thrive is the result of deliberate withholding of food or fictitious illness (such as alleged allergies to food, etc.). These children are suffering significant harm and require urgent case-conferencing and removal from the home for safety and protection.

## Stage 1: Resolving Eating Difficulties

When a child is given sufficient and appropriately prepared milk formula or food, but refuses to eat and presents difficult behaviour (e.g. crying, pushing food away, spitting, storing food in the mouth etc.), and the care-giver shows anxiety and tension while feeding a child, then gradual reduction of tension and anxiety is necessary to make the act of eating more enjoyable to the child. Much effort is put into making meal-times more relaxed for everybody in the family, and special and rewarding times for the child. The meal-time arrangements and feeding behaviour are discussed and modelled by the therapist, and then supported when a feeder (usually the mother) tries new ways of holding a child while being fed, encouraging by smiling, talking gently, and making a child as comfortable as possible. By direct modelling (demonstrating what to do, and the manner of interaction), the care-giver can learn by observation, and gain confidence in how to manage the process and to create a relaxed atmosphere prior to and during the meal-time. In order to create calmness and harmony between the feeder and the child, the feeder should speak quietly and warmly to the child, should smile, touch the child's cheek, and stroke its hair from time to time. An older child (e.g. toddler) can be taken to the kitchen to observe the mother preparing food and assist (figuratively speaking) in this task: for example, the child could be asked to pass something, or hold a carrot or tomato, etc. As food is prepared the mother tells the child what she is doing, thanking the child for helping her, describing (in an interesting and appetising way) the dish she is preparing in order to generate interest in food and eating. Food is arranged on a plate in small quantities in an imaginative and appetising way to stimulate interest and the desire to eat. A variety of shapes and figures can be created depending on what kind of food is being cooked: for example, the shape of a smiling face, fishfinger boy, a snowman, a tree, etc. A story may be invented about the shapes of food arranged on the plate to generate more interest and appetite, as this tends to speed up the process of eating.

## A fish finger champion story

Once upon a time there was a little boy (or girl) called (give the name of a child). He loved playing football and he wanted to be a footballer when he grew up, but he was very small and thin because he did not eat enough to grow strong and fast. One day a *fish finger champion* appeared on his plate and said: 'If you want to be a footballer you need to eat more and a lot of things to get strong and big. Show me how fast you can eat fishfingers, potatoes, carrots, and peas. You

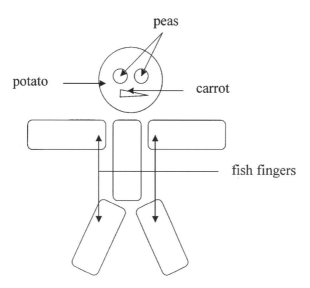

**Figure 12.1** Fish finger champion

must eat everything that is on the plate and I will be a very happy fish finger champion. If you eat well you will get a nice sticker to put on your special *Good Eating Chart* so everyone can see how good you are at eating. See you again sometime. Tomorrow, *smiling face* will be on a plate to talk to you or maybe a *snowman*. You will be able to choose from your food list.'

Most toddlers are fascinated by the characters or shapes on the plate, and by the story which accompanies it. The stories need to be devised to appeal

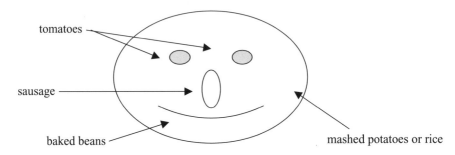

**Figure 12.2** A smiling face

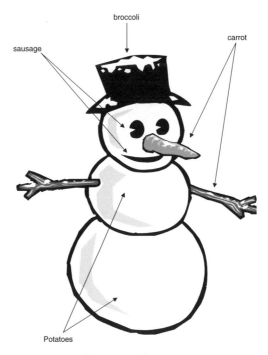

**Figure 12.3** Snowman

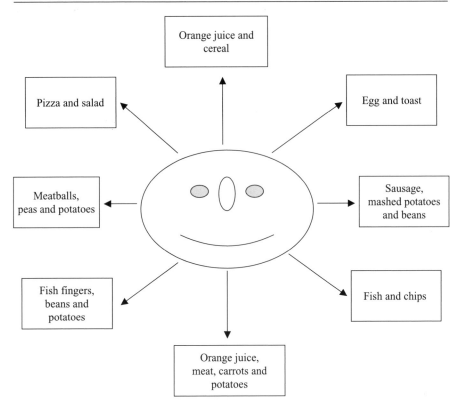

**Figure 12.4** Menu list: 'What am I going to eat this week?'

to individual children. It takes two minutes to arrange food in an interesting shape and most food is suitable for such displays. The benefits are quite extensive in terms of largely increased intake of food, the variety of food consumed, the speed of eating, and the pleasant atmosphere created during meal-times. In addition, there will be parental satisfaction in a job well done.

To keep the eating momentum going and to further reinforce good eating behaviour, a *Good Eating Chart* should be displayed for everyone to see how well a child is doing. The chart could be put on a fridge, kitchen door or other suitable place in the kitchen. Each reasonably well-eaten meal earns the child a sticker, which he or she puts on a chart with the help of a parent or older sibling. The child should be praised for being big and clever and it should be stressed that everyone is pleased with him or her and that he is going to grow fast and strong. The choice of sticker is important as it has to match the likes of the child and be wanted to be earned by the child. If a child likes a sport, e.g. football, then a variety of stickers of footballers are likely to appeal; other ideas might be pictures of cars, aeroplanes, animals, cartoons, TV-show or

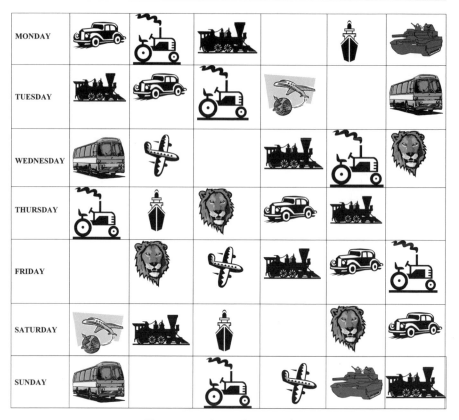

**Figure 12.5** A good eating chart

storybook characters, or toys—something depicting an interest or favourite particular to the child will motivate him/her to comply. The stickers can be purchased cheaply from a toyshop or bookshop, or made by cutting out pictures from various magazines and brochures.

Apart from symbolic rewards (a sticker chart) and social rewards (praise), activity rewards (in the form of parents and children doing things together) should be introduced. If a child earns two or three stickers for good eating, then this should be further rewarded by giving it a little toy, reading an extra story at night, taking the child to the park to play on the swings and slides, or presenting it with some other present. As parent–child interaction is problematic in many failure-to-thrive cases, mutual activities to increase positive contact together is of particular value and importance. Activity rewards, therefore, should be as frequent as possible. Increased mutual activities tend to improve relationships between parents and children, and reduce anxiety and apprehension when in each other's company. Additionally, by being

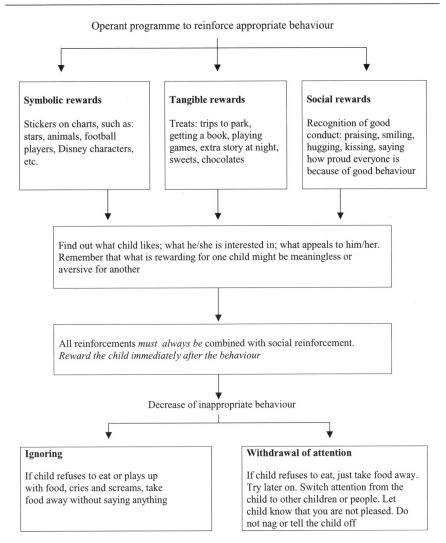

**Figure 12.6** Description and rules of symbolic, social and tangible rewards for good behaviour

appreciated, and when achievements are acknowledged in different ways, the child's self-esteem and sense of being liked is enhanced. What needs to be stressed here is that the therapist needs to be actively involved during the early stages of the feeding programme so as to model the style and tone of feeding interactions. Advice and instructions alone—a didactic approach— do not seem to work in more difficult, chronic cases (especially when parents have received a variety of advice and instruction earlier which did not work

**Table 12.2** Parental reaction to a child's eating behaviour

| We agree to perform the following behaviours: | | |
| --- | --- | --- |
| *If* Susan tries to take food, tries to swallow and opens her mouth | → | *Then* we will smile at her, tell her that she is a big girl, stroke her hair, touch her cheek, and will show pleasure in her behaviour |
| *If* Susan takes her food, does not spit or store food in her mouth | → | *Then* we will tell her how clever she is, that she is a champion and that we are very proud of her |
| *If* Susan eats what she is given within 20–25 minutes | → | *Then* we will tell her that she will grow fast and will be the strongest girl in the nursery/school or neighbourhood and that we love her for it |
| *If* Susan shows resistance and refuses to eat | → | *Then* we will leave her alone, will not pressurise her to eat, will not make any negative comments. We will try again in half an hour or so |
| *If* Susan plays with her food, throws the food on the floor and gets agitated etc. | → | *Then* we will remove the plate, say that we do not like her doing it and stop commenting on eating altogether and switch our attention from her for a few minutes |

for them), or when they did not get sufficient support and a helping hand, or where tactics and methods were not evaluated for suitability and modified according to needs. Once a care-giver becomes more confident and relaxed due to improvement in the child's intake of food and speed of eating, telephone calls to remind the parent what to do and to rehearse the process are sufficient in most cases.

Some parents, however, especially those with mild learning disabilities, and very young, single, and unsupported mothers, require longer input of therapeutic work, more involvement, and frequent reminders of what should be done and when. Apart from frequent telephone calls, a simple, written instruction as to how they should react and what to say when a child eats well or when there is resistance to eat should be provided.

### Treatment in the Nursery

Some parents' anxiety levels at the point of referral are so high, and their emotional energy so low, that it is in the child's best interests to be placed in the day-nursery, on either a full- or part-time basis. A resolution of feeding/eating problems in the nursery involves techniques similar to those used at home, but has the advantage of having other children at the table who are good eaters, and a nursery-nurse who is calm and emotionally uninvolved to supervise meal-times. It is assumed that, if the child watches other children eating well and enjoying food, the child's appetite will be stimulated, and the child prompted to start behaving in the same way. One nursery-nurse is trained to manage eating behaviours and other activities, and takes responsibility for effective implementation of the treatment programme.

The data collected (by using direct observation and videoing meal-times) produced interesting information. We have learned that when excessive fussy attention was given, some children responded less favourably. They tended to push the plate away, play with the food, store food in their mouths, walk away from the table, or disrupt other children's eating. When attention was redirected from a failure-to-thrive child to other children at the table eating well, the performance was much better. Comments directed to children who ate well, such as:

> What a great eater you are, Mark, you will be a football player soon and win all the matches!

or

> Fung Yee is a champion, she has eaten all her sausage already—it is nice, isn't it?

can help.

It would appear that being approached in a matter-of-fact way and only occasionally prompted in a low-key way increased the intake of food and speed of eating. Such children responded better to competition:

> Who will empty the plate first, second, or third?

or when attention was switched from them to other children at the table. It became clear that because of excessive pressure to eat at home, and parental anxiety, the child developed food-avoidance behaviour as a coping mechanism. By associating eating with excessive pressure and uncomfortable feelings, they perceived attention (even of a positive kind), at first, as leading to something they did not like. Once new experiences became internalised, new behaviour patterns emerged which were relaxed and normal. As we can see, direct observation and experimentation can help in the choice and further development of methods and techniques to deal with these problems. Intervention needs to be tailored to a particular child in his/her special circumstances with a specific set of needs and problems.

## Treatment in Hospital

Hospitalised, tube-fed children are particularly difficult to treat as they present diminished oral/instrumental abilities to eat. Additionally, they do not show any interest in food whatsoever, so various types of reinforcements do not have the same effect as they do with other children with eating disorders. The process is painfully slow, but satisfactory if the process of retraining is observed by everybody concerned.

The author has dealt with three cases of this kind, and each of them had achieved a satisfactory outcome within two to three months of treatment. Once the child reached an appropriate weight and felt physically well, the tube-feeding was gradually reduced and then withdrawn altogether. At first, the child was asked to sit at the table with children on the ward who had no problems with eating, and was asked not to eat, but just to observe and listen. The therapist was present for at least one meal a day, and a specially trained nurse supervised each meal-time. Then food (specially arranged and organised by the paediatric dietician) was put in front of the child. The child was praised by the therapeutic team if attempts were made to put food into the mouth, but it was done on a low-key level, and no pressure to eat was exerted. Comments were made about other children eating and enjoying the experience. Once the child had re-learned what to do with food once in the mouth (e.g. chewing and swallowing [which took three to four weeks]), the tube-feeding was completely disconnected in order to produce feelings of hunger and an urge to eat. Loss of weight is predicted at this stage, so it is important to stick to the programme and not to lose nerve because of slow progress and anxiety arising amongst professionals and parents. The dietician works out a menu (according to parental advice) containing food liked by the child and which the child found easy to swallow. At first the food is liquidised and taken one to two spoons at a time, then easy-to-chew-and-swallow food is introduced and presented in an interesting and exciting way (e.g. snowman—consisting of mashed potatoes, mashed peas, and mashed carrots—or a smiling face of mashed potatoes, gravy, minced chicken, and mashed carrots). At first little amounts of it are eaten, but as time goes on and as the hunger drive begins to emerge, the intake of food slowly increases. At this stage, symbolic and social rewards are put in place and massively reinforced by everybody. The child regulates the amount of food consumed, but is gently encouraged to take it in greater quantities. The likes and dislikes are monitored by the dietician. Emphasis is put on the child's learning to eat by mouth, and on what the child seems to like and is able to take, rather than on the nutritional value of the food. The range of food gradually increases once oral eating is mastered. These cases need to be followed up for a considerable time as the relapse rate is high, and booster treatment is often required once the children go home. To illustrate treatment of this kind Emma's case is given below.

## Emma's Case

Emma was 2 years old at the time of admission to hospital because of her complete refusal to take food. She was seriously undernourished, well under the 3rd percentile, and looked withdrawn and apathetic. Emma had a history of FTT almost from birth. Feeding difficulties emerged during the first few weeks of her life and became acute at the time of admission. The parents received some help over the two-year period from the health visitor, friends, and the GP—everyone, apparently, giving different advice as to what to do and how to handle the poor food intake. The parents were told that Emma's eating behaviour was difficult due to hiatus hernia , but that should mend itself: if not, it would be operated on when she got older. She had to sleep in a sitting position to reduce discomfort. The hernia was successfully operated upon when Emma was 2 years old. It was predicted that, by eliminating discomfort while eating, this would encourage a better intake of food once Emma fully recovered from the operation and hospitalisation. The parents were advised to exert their authority as there was no longer any reason for Emma to resist eating. This approach (as can be imagined) led to even more difficulties, as both parents began to believe firmly that Emma was simply playing up. The more pressure they exerted, the less she ate, and eventually she stopped eating altogether. She was hospitalised again and referred for more intensive therapeutic intervention as she lost even more weight and completely refused to take food. She was so wasted and lethargic that tube-feeding was introduced to keep her alive. She was tube-fed until she had reached an acceptable weight to start treatment in taking food by mouth.

## The treatment programme included:

1. The gradual introduction to taking food orally by observing other children eat, reinforcing eating in a matter-of-fact way, and not putting pressure on her;
2. Presenting food in an appetising and interesting way, and food that she knew and had eaten in the past;
3. Rewarding by praise (and ignoring refusal) each attempt to put food into her mouth, and to chew and swallow it;
4. Once Emma had learnt how to eat, and began to take larger amounts, she was discharged home with intensive follow-up and daily home visits for two months to monitor progress; and
5. To keep the momentum of progress going, and not to put too much pressure on still very anxious parents, a day-nursery was arranged (full-time for a month and then gradually reduced to three and then two days a week [*see* Treatment in the Nursery, page 226]).

## Treatment for the mother included:

1. Relaxation training;
2. Cognitive work—because of diminished self-efficacy and self-blame;

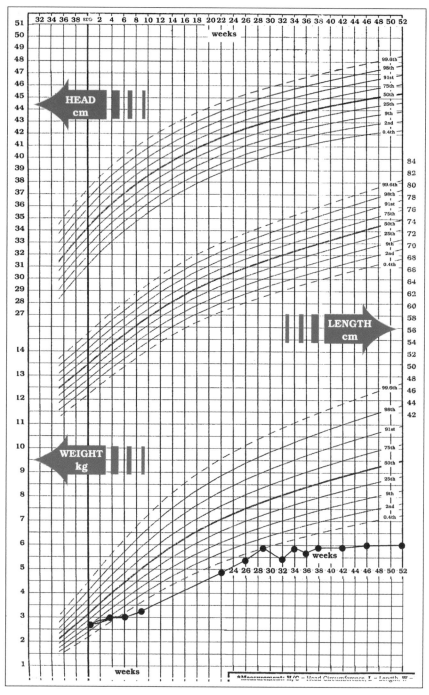

**Figure 12.7** Emma's growth chart: 0–4 years
Copyright © Child Growth Foundation

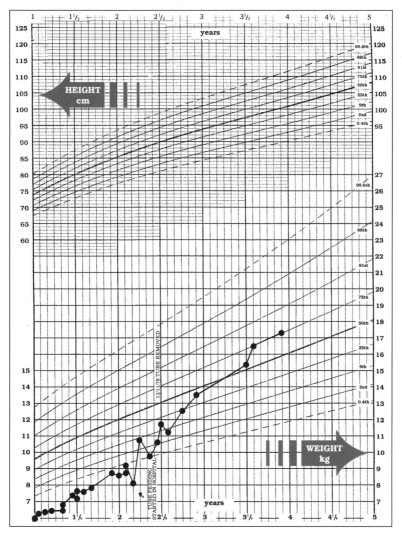

**Figure 12.7** (*cont.*)

3. Developmental counselling to provide information and to facilitate discussion about children's developmental needs and ways of managing children's behaviour;
4. Group work—to provide the opportunity to meet other parents with similar problems, exchange tips and ideas about mutual experiences, and provide social support; and
5. Both parents received substantial help in terms of setting up, negotiating, modelling, monitoring, and evaluating treatment at home. Task

distribution between parents, in relation to Emma, and other areas in their lives was negotiated, clarified and agreed.

The positive results of the multi-disciplinary effort to deal with acute growth failure and eating problems are demonstrated in Emma's growth chart (Figure 12.7). The following professionals were involved in organising, executing, and the follow-up treatment: paediatricians, a psychologist, a social worker, a dietician, hospital nurses, nursery-nurses, a health visitor, and the GP. The treatment (from admission to hospital to final close of the case) took eight months, two-and-a-half of them spent in the hospital.

The methods of treatment and approaches described in this chapter are applicable to many failure-to-thrive cases, and have proved to be successful in producing good outcomes.

### Stage 2: Increasing Positive Parent–Child Interaction and Building Secure Mutual Attachments

Some failure-to-thrive children are insecurely attached to their mothers, and the mothers, in some cases, are not strongly bonded to particular children. Interaction between the mother and the target child is based on duty rather than pleasure and desire to do things together or to be together. If they do interact, their behaviour is either passive or anxious. Fathers tend to have better relationships with the child, and the way they respond is qualitatively much more relaxing and encouraging to the child. They tend to come to fathers for comfort and reassurance far more often than they do to their mothers. They also talk to their fathers and ask for help and assistance more frequently in comparison to their mothers. Some of these children, about 40% in my sample, show fear and apprehension when in the mother's company, and look ill at ease when in the same room. In order to bring them closer together and to reduce ambivalent or negative feelings, structured interaction, increasing in time, is introduced as therapy.

This phase is discussed in detail with both parents and planned jointly to accommodate the date and time required to proceed with the programme. The rationale and methods are explained, negotiated, and written down so that each party knows what is expected—when, and who is going to do what. In most cases an agreement is drawn up specifying the mutual obligations for the family and therapist.

When parent–child interactions are highly (and sometimes mutually) aversive (a common finding), the mother is asked to play each day exclusively with the child, after her partner returns from work, for 10–15 minutes during the first two weeks, and for up to 25 minutes in the following four weeks. After the mother's session with the child the rest of the family (if applicable) might join in for family play or other activity session.

Play sessions are always modelled by the therapist so that the mother can see how they are done, how to encourage the child to participate, what toys to use, and how to speak to the child. During the first two to three sessions the therapist is present to assist the mother with play and to give advice when things do not go well. The best sessions are those which require cutting shapes and gluing pieces together: in other words making something together. Household junk can be used, e.g. egg or cereal boxes, cotton wool, pieces of paper, etc.

Mothers are encouraged—as a general principle—to look, smile, hold the hand, stroke the hair, and praise the child if there is good response and participation. This often requires careful programming if the child's behaviour is very timid. The mother's approaches are shaped by a series of successive approximations: they are encouraged to initiate as well as to react. After a few days, and in some serious cases even weeks, a mother is guided to seek proximity by sitting her child on her lap for 2–3 minutes, by hugging briefly, holding hands, kissing, and eventually holding it close (but gently), and speaking in a warm, soft, and quiet way.

Once the child feels more at ease, the mother is asked to sit the child on her lap for 5–6 minutes at a time, three to four times a day, holding it gently and lovingly, and reading a story or describing pictures in the book. The purpose of this exercise is to promote physical contact and experience pleasure in being close together, and to gradually enable the mother to discover qualities in the child which were not recognised before, and for the child to feel wanted, loved, and appreciated. As time goes on the child tends to sit more comfortably on its mother's lap, gets closer to her, puts its head on her shoulder, and responds spontaneously to what she reads or describes.

There were a few rejecting mothers in the sample who found this part of the treatment very difficult, and in three cases impossible to persevere with. Aversion in the other cases gradually lessened when the children began to smile back, seek their mothers' presence, and in other ways responded to their overtures. This period of therapy requires a lot of support for mothers and other members of the family. Fathers are particularly important here, to support the child and mother in a way which reduces maternal jealousy and resentment because the child relates better to the father than to her. In more persistent problems in this area (acute jealousy) extra in-depth psychotherapy is needed.

Frequent, brief home visits and telephone calls should be made to monitor the programme. In more serious cases it can take three months of hard work to bring a mother and child closer together and to the point of beginning to enjoy (or stop disliking/fearing) each other.

### *Video Recording and Feedback*

A variety of techniques can be used to increase parents' awareness and understanding of what is happening and how to correct inappropriate parental responses to their children. Very effective work has been done videoing the interaction of parents who persistently react with hostility to the target children and where attachment behaviour is riddled with insecurity. Examples of aversive parental behaviour are videoed and then played back to parents, so they can see and hear for themselves how they behaved and what they said. They are asked to pay particular attention to their tone of voice, eye-contact, facial expression, and general body language when they speak to and deal with the child. They are also asked to observe their child's anxious and fearful reactions to them, and the child's apprehensiveness when in their company. The impact of such behaviour on the child is discussed in terms of immediate pain and long-term consequences (such as prevention of developing strong self-esteem, a sense of belonging and security, and a general feeling of being loved and wanted).

Parents are asked to imagine how they would feel and how they would react if they were treated in the same way as they were treating their child. By asking them to reflect on their harsh and hostile behaviour, and asking them to put their feet into the child's shoes, see through the child's eyes, and feel through the child's heart, it is hoped that they will be able to get in touch with their own and the child's feelings which, in turn, will help them to empathise and recognise the pain and hurt felt by the child. Parents are asked to observe the role-play conducted by a therapist demonstrating warm, encouraging, and caring behaviour when doing things with the child. In turn they are asked to play with the child, which is videoed, played back, and discussed. If a video is difficult to get, an audio-tape can be used so that parents can hear what they say and the manner in which they say it.

### Stage 3: Intensifying Mother–Child Interaction

The third stage is planned to include two weeks of deliberately intensified mother–child interaction. The mother is to take the child with her almost everywhere she goes, and have it present when carrying out various tasks—within reason. She is asked to chat to him/her as much as possible, regardless of whether or not he/she fully understands what she is doing or saying. She is told to make a lot of eye-contact, and to smile, to cuddle, and to hug the infant as often as possible. This is done to generalise the already acquired positive interactions and feelings during feeding and play-time to other areas of the child's life and daily activities. It is hoped that the child will begin to feel at ease all the time and will use the mother as a safe haven whenever there is perceived danger or stress or he/she has need for help or comfort.

### Stage 4: Dealing with Behavioural Problems

Children still presenting behavioural problems at this stage of treatment can be helped by behavioural methods such as effective use of positive reinforcements: they are praised for good conduct or for even attempting to be-have in a pro-social manner. They are rewarded by favourable activities, e.g. story-reading, favourite foods, or special play. Parents are guided through the process in order to create a warm anxiety-free atmosphere, so children can begin to feel that they are liked and wanted (*see* Iwaniec, 1995; 1997, for further discussion).

## HELPING PARENTS

So far, therapeutic intervention mainly to help children has been discussed, but parents need help as well if they are asked to promote changes in the child's and family's life. The methods most frequently used by the author when working with parents of failure-to-thrive children which have been positively evaluated will be discussed below.

### Personal Counselling

The main task of counselling is to help parents reflect on the problems they are experiencing and to direct them to a better understanding of themselves and their behaviour. Counselling involves rigorous exploration of difficulties, clarifying conflicting issues, and searching for alternative ways to understand and to deal with the problems. The emphasis is put on self-help, calling on the inner resources of the person who is in difficulties, promoting personal growth and more mature ways of acting and reacting, thinking first and responding in a thought-through way. Personal counselling is necessary when a mother feels jealous of the child's affection for the father and the father's affection towards the child. It is also helpful to take a mother into her childhood and explore with her experiences as a child and how they might have affected the parenting of her children. These parents are often themselves emotionally deprived, and they have nobody to turn to for help; they also might be reluctant to approach child-welfare agencies for fear of losing their children. Counselling 'opens a door' to more sincere, anxiety-free sharing of true feelings and difficulties: however, it is not sufficient or even appropriate to use with very chaotic dysfunctional families riddled with violence, alcoholism, or drug abuse, who have little insight, and are unable to see or to accept their faults and the point of view of others.

### Developmental Counselling

One of the most important and necessary aspects of intervention is devel-opmental counselling, which is educational and informative in the sense of disseminating the knowledge we have of child development (for example, what is normal or appropriate to the child's age, sex, and level of ability, and suggesting to parents what are reasonable expectations for their child). Transmission of information about normal child development and basic child needs for 'optimal' development is often as important as suggestions about ways of dealing with worrying behaviours. Unrealistic expectations on the part of parents as to what the child should (or should not) do often leads to parent–child relationship problems and maltreatment. When pressure is put on a child to perform certain tasks which it is not developmentally ready to perform, then the child will get anxious, confused, and nervous, which, in turn, may bring about behavioural and emotional problems and a sense of helplessness. Parents often perceive a child as lazy and disobedient, and punish it for non-compliance with their requests: abuse can start here, when parents, dissatisfied with a child's performance, constantly criticise, rebuke, or deprive it of affection and treats, or call it stupid, thick, ignorant, or good-for-nothing.

Parents often compare their children, or a child, with those of friends and neighbours, so it is essential to counsel them about individual differences in speed of development and how to encourage a child to learn different skills. In the case of failure to thrive, where a child's development might be de-layed due to lack of stimulation, attention, and proper care, parents need to be guided and instructed on what to do and why. This is often the case with toddlers, when temper-tantrums and oppositional behaviour are interpreted as sheer naughtiness and wickedness, and not as inner frustration when striv-ing to master a skill. Bowel- and bladder-control is another example of often unrealistic expectations and faulty perceptions on the part of the parents.

Not infrequently those difficulties between parent and children have con-tributed to the child's behaviour problems in the first place and get in the way of the parent's practical efforts to implement a programme. We know that some children seem temperamentally resistant to socialisation and nur-turing, from birth (Herbert, 1993). Parents may have special sensitivities or anxieties with regard to this particular child which make it impossible or difficult for them to be firm or consistent when he behaves in a certain man-ner. High levels of arousal (anger, anxiety) on the part of the parents, plus a common non-compliance in the child, interact so as to disrupt its routines or even its socialisation. Parents often have fixed ideas about rearing children, which represent the standard of their parents or reactions against them. These matters may require discussion and a sympathetic hearing before the parents can sustain the modification of their own behaviour which (*inter alia*) is being required of them.

## Group-Work

Many mothers of children who fail to thrive are socially isolated and generally have little social support. As parenting takes a lot of time and emotional commitment, it is useful and beneficial to have a good network of social support to help to cope with these demands. In addition, family life is often seen to be filled with conflict and tension, rather than being a source of emotional support. Mothers appear to be less psychologically available to their children, because their emotional resources are depleted. Social isolation results in fewer or no opportunities to have child-free time or to talk to others about things other than child-related problems. These mothers also suffer from low self-esteem and lack of confidence as they feel that they are being blamed for their child's poor growth and unhealthy-looking appearance.

Parents' or mothers' groups may be particularly beneficial as they provide opportunities to meet other parents who are faced with similar problems regarding their children, and who may well experience similar stresses in other areas of their lives. There are many advantages for meeting in a group, such as a forum for peer support; the opportunity to exchange tips and ideas about parenting children; having time out of the house; the possibility of building a closer friendship with another mother; and opportunities to exchange telephone numbers so that contact can be maintained outside group meetings. Above all, it shows, to each individual member of the group, that they are not unique and there are other families coping with similar problems. In addition, members of such groups have chances to learn from formal and informal discussions, participate in role-plays, and get involved in group exercises.

Groups are organised in different ways according to what they aim to achieve and which problems they plan to address. Informal group-work for mothers of failure-to-thrive children can provide an excellent forum in which to tackle social isolation and feelings of helplessness and uniqueness. However, in order to be sustained and well attended, there must be a well-planned programme of activities, so that members feel that it is worthwhile to attend. Early sessions, in particular, have to be interesting and engaging, as they will determine the level of later success.

Informal groups should be run by the members themselves, with guidance and advice from a professional person they all know. This provides the best and quickest help to increase self-worth and a sense of competence. By planning, organising, contributing to the content of activities, by giving others advice or suggestions as to what works and what should be avoided in parenting, it provides feelings of importance and heightens the sense of self-efficacy. As time goes by, and they begin to experience satisfaction in activities which make them feel better as parents, they will become aware that their children and families are also deriving benefit, so will gain confidence that they are able to produce change in their own and their children's lives. Repetition of small achievements produced by the successful re-enactment of the performance of tasks in group-work will lead gradually to stronger self-esteem in other areas of these mothers' lives. The heightened self-efficacy leads to more vigorous, persistent, and probably more successful attempts to cope with problems, while problem-solving further increases perceived self-effectiveness.

Group-work for this client group can be run as well in a very structured way, similar to parent training, to teach parenting skills and practise them, as well as learning problem-solving techniques associated with other areas of parents' lives.

It needs to be remembered, however, that not all parents can 'learn in public', and not all will desire or need to belong to a group. Accommodating different needs and facilitating individual preferences is a key to successful outcomes. Group-work is one of them.

## SUMMARY

The multidimensional/integrated model of intervention developed by the author has been discussed above. Methods and techniques dealing with feeding/eating problems, interactional and relationship difficulties, and behaviour management, were fully elaborated upon, providing tips and ideas which were easy to follow by parents and carers. Various methods of helping parents (such as personal and developmental counselling and group-work) were briefly elaborated on, as was therapeutic work with children in hospitals and day-nurseries. This chapter also discussed how to respond to immediate needs of failure-to-thrive children and their parents, and fully described long-term intervention and treatment.

# 13

# APPROACHES TO FAILURE-TO-THRIVE INTERVENTION PROGRAMMES

*If we desire to change something in a child, we should first consider if that something could be changed with benefit in ourselves.*

Carl Gustav Jung, 1932

## INTRODUCTION

A number of different disciplines have been active in pursuing failure-to-thrive intervention research, and several approaches have been developed over the years to improve the effectiveness of such interventions. Indeed, the problem of failure to thrive has attracted a lot of interest, and has stimulated research on both sides of the Atlantic amongst different professional disciplines. It also has become very competitive, in terms of both research and ideology.

The fact that so many professions are interested and involved in researching and working with failure-to-thrive children and their families will make it worth while looking at multi-disciplinary co-operation and interagency work. Intervention led by health visitors will be discussed, as well as the role of social workers and their involvement in the intervention programmes. Additionally, co-operation between agencies and role-distributions amongst professionals involved with failure-to-thrive work will be examined.

## MULTI-DISCIPLINARY APPROACH

A multi-disciplinary approach has been strongly advocated and promoted as the optimum approach to intervention, reflecting the multi-factorial nature of the failure-to-thrive syndrome by many researchers (e.g. Hanks & Hobbs, 1993; Iwaniec, 1995; Batchelor, 1999; Wright, 2000, to mention a few). Dawson (1992), in a discussion of multi-disciplinary approaches to failure-to-thrive intervention, makes a reference to a number of ways in which intervention programmes can be and have been tailored to the individual needs of FTT families and children. He claims that it is necessary for assessment, treatment, and evaluation to be carried out by an inter-disciplinary team in order to meet the multiple needs that a child with FTT and its family may present, with different professions being better suited to deal with different aspects of the syndrome. For example, a nutritionist should evaluate the child's food intake and feeding behaviour, and a physician should look for medical aetiologies.

A good example of a multi-disciplinary FTT intervention programme is the work of St Elizabeth's Failure-to-Thrive Program developed in 1983 in Covington, Kentucky, as described by McMillen (1988). This programme is run by a team consisting of employees working in physical therapy, speech pathology, audiology, nutrition, social services, home health, and paediatrics. Interventions are informed by an assessment procedure, and include the education and support of parents of FTT children.

At the start of the intervention the children are assessed by each member of the team with an emphasis on team collaboration so as to inform the plan of intervention. Having identified the particular problem for each child, the intervention team monitors the child's progress through a series of visits in which they also educate the parents as to the child's special requirements. At this stage much emphasis is placed on the working relationship with the mothers whereby the members of the team endeavour to act as a positive educational role-model for the parents and also to establish rapport with the mothers and offer them moral support. The philosophy is to attempt to nurture the parents while also nurturing the child.

Further benefits associated with the application of a multi-disciplinary approach to FTT intervention are illustrated by Hobbs and Hanks (1996), who describe the first 18 months' work of a specialist clinic established in 1993 in Leeds (UK) to provide help for failure-to-thrive children and their families. The clinic was set up, within the National Health Service framework, for the treatment and management of these children, working on the premise that a multi-disciplinary team (in which professionals with knowledge and skills with children worked together) enhanced the chances of bringing the necessary changes. Work of the clinic was guided by the principle that management and treatment of FTT are rarely effective if dealt with by a single professional input, and that when medical and psychological aspects of FTT are combined into a single central focus on food and feeding, outcomes for those children are much better.

The clinic includes input from clinical psychologists, consultant community paediatricians, community dieticians, staff-grade community paediatricians, nursery-nurses, and health visitors, with the child and family being seen together. Time is also provided for home visits by a dietician, community paediatrician, and psychologist. Liaison with other professionals also occurs, whether inside or outside the clinic, with the health visitor having a lead role in the liaison. The authors also point out that working as a multi-disciplinary team has an added advantage of providing mutual support and mutual supervision for the professions involved in what can often be a challenging task.

This very progressive programme of intervention incorporates observations of some aspects of interactions, food preparation, and children's eating behaviour, which are then utilised to formulate a management programme. More specific and detailed analysis is undertaken using an interview schedule to chart certain aspects of the feeding process, yielding qualitative data which can then be compared with the eating behaviour of other groups of children.

Improvements are measured in terms of weight change from first to last attendance at the clinic. Based on data for 47 children (who attended the clinic on more than one occasion), there was an overall improvement from a mean Z score of –2.17 to one of –1.87, an improvement of + 0.30. For the four infants suffering from the most severe FTT (Z score below –4.0), all improved to –4.0 or better. Eight children deteriorated, although the deterioration was in general much lower than the overall improvements of the other children in treatment. The results clearly indicated the effectiveness of the approach, both in terms of the multi-disciplinary nature of the team, and the methods used to help these children and their families.

Hampton (1996) describes the multi-disciplinary *Infant Support Project (ISP)* in Wiltshire (UK) run by the Children's Society. The *ISP* used a problem-solving-based approach and behavioural methods of intervention. The team consisted of social workers, health visitors, and nursery-nurses. Assessment and treatment in this project were conducted in the child's home, and physical-growth measurements in the health centres. Close collaboration and written agreements on how to proceed with the cases, and what information to give to parents, was observed to avoid conflicting messages. The team's success in 68% of cases was linked to theoretically based assessment and treatment, and to rigorous evaluation of the progress by parents, team members, and an independent assessor. The team was led by the social worker with extensive experience in child care.

Failure-to-thrive syndrome presents as a complicated picture, rather like a jigsaw-puzzle, where pieces have to be put together thoughtfully to discover what is the subject, and what piece connects with which. A few people having varied expertise can assemble that picture much more quickly than one person alone. A multi-disciplinary approach is not only advisable, but essential, to assemble all pieces of the puzzle quickly and effectively. Of course, it is not always possible to have a special team dedicated to work with failure-to-thrive children, but working in that spirit with individual cases, and involving professionals from appropriate disciplines to look for solutions is always possible.

## NUTRITIONAL APPROACH TO MANAGEMENT OF
## NON-ORGANIC FAILURE TO THRIVE

Nutrition is a core element of non-organic failure-to-thrive aetiology. However, given that a focus on nutritional and dietary input alone has been shown to be of limited effectiveness in the treatment, and may even exacerbate problems (Batchelor, 1999), nutritional factors, it is believed, are best addressed together with psychosocial factors as part of a multi-factorial, multi-disciplinary approach to intervention and treatment.

While nutritional management has been shown to be ineffective in isolation, food consumption needs to be addressed to ensure calorific intake, and should include assessment of oral functioning, including an assessment of the mechanical act of feeding, assessment of family interactions around food, and an assessment of family beliefs and attitudes towards foods.

Maggioni and Lifshitz (1995) published a review outlining components of nutritional management of non-organic failure to thrive including assessment, management, and follow-up in which they provided a comprehensive set of guidelines and recommendations. They rightly argued that it is essential to rule out organic disease before firm diagnoses are made. Comprehensive examination is needed to ensure that food intake is appropriate for age, and that sufficient dietary intake, containing essential nutrients for growth, is attained. This nutritional examination should include making records of food consumption over 24 hours for a period of three to seven days: it should note the frequency of meals, feeding patterns, and intake of fluids. Maggioni and Lifshitz have stressed that mother–infant feeding, as well as non-feeding, interaction, should be taken into consideration. Maternal and infant behaviour and psychological expressions should be investigated to provide a more comprehensive picture of what is happening and why.

Particular attention needs to be paid to non-specific symptoms that may be present in these children's eating behaviour: for example, vomiting, spitting up, diarrhoea, storing food in the mouth, and heaving. These symptoms tend to reduce in frequency as more calories are ingested and retained, and may be linked to symptoms of under-nutrition: they can also be used as a baseline from which to measure progress. Factors that may contribute to FTT require checking: these might include swallowing or sucking problems due to (for example) mild brain injury. The authors advise that evaluation needs to become more intensive if initial advice given to parents about feeding does not lead to weight gain. They argue that nourishment involves much more than ingestion of food. Therefore, additional factors which affect nurturance should also be taken into account, including infants' individual differences, temperamental characteristics, adverse social or psychological environments, and parental beliefs and concepts of nutrition.

Nutritional management is described as the cornerstone of intervention as caloric intake is generally seen as the root of the problem. Nutritional therapy, according to the authors, has several goals including the achievement of ideal weight-for-height and correction of nutrient deficits, so enabling a catching up of growth; restoration of optimal body composition; and parental education in nutritional requirements and feeding of the child.

During recovery, catch-up growth requires the provision of up to 50% more protein and 30% more calories than normal. For this reason, Maggioni and Lifshitz argue that FTT children should be fed a high-calorie, high-protein diet, and that parents should be recommended to provide nutritious snacks. Benefits of high-calorie energy-dense nutritional intake include reduced recovery time, shorter stays in hospital, and a lowering of associated costs of both. The authors point out that by achieving rapid weight gain without inducing undesirable body-composition changes (especially fat accretion), hospitalisation for rehabilitation can be shortened and should therefore be a consideration in nutritional management.

Based on the premise that failure to thrive results from inadequate nutrition and energy intake, Moores (1996) published a review of dietetic practice in a community setting that set out to outline the effectiveness of intervention. In this review, methods of assessing nutritional intake are outlined, including weighed food intakes, taking a dietary history, 24-hour recall of food intake, and the keeping of food diaries: it concludes that the most appropriate method for assessing nutritional intake for FTT children is the use of a three-day diary, designed to prevent the possibility of making false records, and giving parents clear instructions as to how to use it. Food diaries form the basis of nutritional advice given during interventions with the non-organic failure-to-thrive child. Parental perceptions and attitudes to food and the child's eating can also be revealed and explored through the use of food diaries, in conjunction with food-composition tables provided by the manufacturers of foods, in order to calculate energy content, which, in turn, should be compared with the child's Estimated Average Requirements (EARs) as stated in 'Dietary Reference Values' (DOH, 1991).

Moores (1996) recommended that once the energy status of the child is informed by the food diary, nutritional intervention should be based primarily on increasing the calorific content of foods and encouraging parents to increase quantities and frequency of high-calorie foods in the children's diets. Many parents of non-organic failure-to-thrive children find this concept contradictory to their own beliefs concerning healthy eating: they therefore require guidance and explanations by the intervention team. Parents should also be encouraged to provide their non-organic FTT children with foods from each of the five food groups on a daily basis.

Batchelor (1999), in an overview of outcomes from nutritional intervention studies, notes a number of recommendations for interventions. She suggests that assessment and intervention should take account of the multi-factorial aetiology of failure to thrive, including the nutritional element, where intervention includes the child and the care-giver. She further points out that a

multi-disciplinary perspective on assessment and intervention will facilitate
the need to address both the nutritional and psychological dimensions of the
failure to thrive.

## HEALTH-VISITOR INTERVENTION

The use of health visitors as part of failure-to-thrive intervention programmes
requires future research to determine its effectiveness compared to the employment by other groups of professionals. However, it appears that whatever
the 'magic ingredient' associated with successful parenting outcomes, health
visitors are well placed and effective in parent-related interventions. Advantages associated with the use of health visitors in failure-to-thrive intervention
programmes have been identified in a number of research projects. Due to
their training, skills, and contacts with community services in working with
families (with an ideal logistic positioning through their daily visits with infants and toddlers for identifying failure-to-thrive children), health visitors
have the advantage of being perceived by parents to have a supportive and
educational role, and therefore are well placed to work with families in a
relaxed, sensitive, nurturing, and non-judgmental manner.

As has been discussed in Chapter 10, health visitors are usually the first
professionals to identify FTT as it is their duty to provide universal support
and surveillance for families with pre-school children. In order to further examine the belief that the skills of health visitors (such as knowledge of families
in their home environments) could be used to greater extent by hospitals in
failure-to-thrive intervention programmes, Wright *et al.* (1998) conducted a
randomised control trial that aimed to evaluate the effectiveness of health-
visitor intervention for failure to thrive in children under 2 years of age.

In the study developed by Wright *et al.* in the Parkin project in Newcastle
upon Tyne, England, 229 children (mean age 15.6 months), all identified as
FTT before they reached 2 years of age, received health-visitor advice and support. Children were randomly assigned to either the intervention (n = 120)
or control group (n = 109). The intervention group received structured intervention from a health visitor trained in the management of failure-to-thrive
programmes. The intervention involved extra participation by health visitors,
yet was incorporated within their normal routine work. Once a definitive diagnosis of failure to thrive was confirmed for each child, the health visitors
were encouraged to look for dietary problems, and to commence a programme
involving dietetic, paediatric, and social-work input. Seventy-eight families
(80%) accepted dietician input involving the keeping of a three-day food diary designed to inform specialist dietician advice. Medical examination by
the project paediatrician was taken up by 74% of the families. The health
visitor then monitored each family and obtained weight measurements until
the infant recovered. Health visitors joined team meetings to discuss future

management for persistent FTT cases (33%). Children were referred for social-work assessment as necessary. The control group received conventional health-visitor management with no additional failure-to-thrive training. An independent research assistant retrieved (and withheld) weights and medical information for these children annually throughout the study period.

Upon assessment, when each child was over three years of age, it was found that the health-visitor-led intervention was significantly more effective, with 91 (76%) of the intervention group recovering from their FTT compared to 60 (55%) of the control group. In terms of frequency of weighings, it was found that controls were weighed on many fewer occasions, with a number of these children (16%) having no weights taken after the initial screening, with five of these children having severe failure to thrive when last measured. Further, 31 (34%) controls had only one or two subsequent weighings, with 22 of these children still meeting the screening criteria for failure to thrive when last weighed. Ninety-two (97%) of the intervention group had more than three routine weighings after the programme began. At a follow-up home visit at a mean age of 45.2 months, children in the intervention group were found to be significantly nearer to an expected weight-for-age.

Based on results in weight gain, this study demonstrated that the employment of health visitors, when supported and trained in the recognition and management of children with FTT (under two years of age), can result in a better follow-up, and produce significantly better long-term weight-and-height gain in FTT children than conventional hospital-based management. Wright et al. (1998) also maintained that the results justified greater use of health visitors in failure-to-thrive cases, with the added advantages of this type of intervention, including cost-effectiveness, and the possibility of reduced hospitalisations, with fewer failure-to-thrive children going unnoticed by the medical system.

A much earlier study, carried out by Haynes et al. (1984), aimed to assess the effectiveness of lay-health-visitor intervention in cases of failure to thrive over a six-month period after diagnosis. Participants in the study included 50 hospitalised non-organic failure-to-thrive children, of which 25 mother–child pairs were offered lay-health-visitor intervention, plus community and medical resources, and another 25 mother–child pairs were instead offered community and medical resources, if thought necessary by the Child Protection Agency.

The intervention by lay health visitors was found to have had no effect on growth. While all of the children were found to have gained weight, weight percentiles were not significantly increased except in a few cases. It was found that of the children who did gain weight, diagnosis was made early in life. As anticipated, non-organic failure-to-thrive children grew along the expected growth curve. No measurable improvement in the infants' development was observed. Many of the failure-to-thrive children were found to have persistent delays in development: these were less severe when diagnosis occurred earlier in life. Positive outcomes (although not significant) included finding that where the mothers had more problems, children were not as negatively affected by their parent's behaviours as they might have been without diagnosis and intervention. Also, children may not have been as depressed as they could have been if they had not received additional stimulation and intervention. The members of the health-visitor intervention group were also found to maintain more contact with services than was the case with the other group, members of which were found to be much more likely to be lost to the system. Based on these findings, the authors recommended the use of more in-depth assessment and diagnosis procedures for both mother and child, with a focus on the quality of parent–child interaction, the identification of any psychological conflicts (or contextual stresses) which might interfere with effective care-giving, and with an emphasis on the identification of the type of intervention likely to be most effective for each case.

Given a perceived lack of evidence as to which forms of intervention are effective for failure-to-thrive children and their families, Raynor *et al.* (1999) carried out a study to determine the success of specialist health-visitor intervention. This study was the first to be carried out on children who were diagnosed on broader clinical grounds than weight alone as having nonorganic FTT. An attempt was also made to demonstrate broader results than previous studies, including growth and cognitive outcomes.

Failure-to-thrive children, recruited from referrals to an FTT clinic by general practitioners, health visitors, consultants, or clinical medical officers over a two-year period from April 1994 to February 1996, were selected at random to receive conventional care, or conventional care *and* additional specialist home-visiting for 12 months. Of the 83 children (aged 4 to 30 months) who participated in this study, 42 received specialist health-visitor intervention. The study included an assessment carried out by weekly home visits lasting 60–90 minutes, over a four-to-five-week period, in which parents were engaged in a semi-structured interview. Observations were carried out, including a video of a meal-time, and an assessment of parent–child interactions. The intervention was planned with the family in order to set achievable goals, and had a focus on eating behaviour. Work with mothers included meal-time management, and the alleviation of stress during meal-times. Further observations of parent and child together were carried out during several visits. Parents were given advice as to their children's nutritional needs (amount, frequency, and types of food), with emphasis on the need for a high-fat, high-carbohydrate diet, and were also offered counselling on personal problems, and referred to specialist agencies where required.

Outcome measures included growth, diet, use of health-care resources, child behaviour and development, maternal mental health, and maternal use of support services. No significant differences were found in primary outcome measures for the two groups. Both groups improved in developmental score and energy intake. Children in both groups showed good weight gain: however, it was found that children who were less than 12 months old in the intervention group showed a higher increase in weight SD score than the control group {0.82 (0.86) v. 0.42 (0.79)}.

The study failed to show that specialist intervention conferred additional health benefits on a failure-to-thrive child. However, positive feedback from the parents involved, together with a number of trends in the data, suggest that the intervention was successful in other ways. It was found that for the intervention group a more co-ordinated approach was provided, with significant savings in terms of health-service use, with controls having had significantly more dietary referrals, social-services involvement, and hospital admissions. Controls were also found to be less compliant with appointments.

Kendrick *et al.* (2000) conducted a systematic review and meta-analysis of the effectiveness of home visiting on improving parenting, and associated outcomes including the quality of the home environment as measured by the Home Observation for Measurement of the Environment (HOME) inventory. This review, while not specific to failure-to-thrive intervention research, includes two FTT studies, and may be used to inform health-visitor intervention programmes.

A meta-analysis of 12 studies identified as reporting HOME scores found that health visiting was highly effective in improving the quality of the home environment. Of the 27 studies involving health-visitor intervention which reported other outcome measures, 21 studies indicated the presence of significant treatment effects and associated improvements: only six showed no significant positive outcomes. Of the 17 studies within this group looking at mother–child interaction as an outcome measure, 12 studies reported significantly better mother–child interaction. These findings provided evidence that home-visiting programmes can be effective in improving outcomes and achieving significant improvements.

Important issues emerged. While home visiting has been shown to be successful in improving parenting, it is difficult to establish which particular part of home visiting is the crucial effective element, due to the multi-faceted, multi-disciplinary nature of most interventions. Also, there was not much evidence of a theoretical basis to explain the process through which the various interventions would achieve improvements in parenting outcomes.

Other sources also refer to the advantages associated with health-visitor-led intervention of failure to thrive. Based on practice evidence, Wright (2000) states that health-visitor home visits can achieve positive improvements, with an immediate success rate of 20%, as part of routine work.

Outcomes for children from health-visitor-led interventions include better long-term weight and height gain and less severe delays in development if the intervention is organised at an early age. Together with benefits identified for the child, parents have positively rated health-visitor intervention. Benefits for healthcare have been repeatedly pointed out, including fewer failure-to-thrive children falling through gaps in the system, or going unnoticed and undiagnosed. Further, health-visitor interventions have proven to be cost-effective, resulting in reduced hospitalisations, referrals to a variety of health-care services, and savings in terms of improved compliance and attendance at medical appointments. All in all, health-visiting interventions appear to provide wide-ranging outcomes, not the least of which is more effective management.

However, it has been recognised that health visitors require training in the recognition of FTT and the development of helping strategies which go beyond nutritional issues alone, and in addressing the quality and tone of interaction between failure-to-thrive children and their parents. Such training assists them to tackle more complex cases and recognise more serious problems at an early stage.

## SOCIAL-WORK INVOLVEMENT IN FAILURE-TO-THRIVE INTERVENTION

Social workers have been shown to make a valuable contribution to interdisciplinary teams treating children who fail to thrive. Working from a biopsychosocial perspective, the social-work approach integrates the biological, psychological, social, and legal components of FTT. In addition, social workers are well equipped to work in failure-to-thrive intervention teams due to their professional background (which includes working with families and understanding social and environmental issues). They also may have valuable links with community-support services, and an understanding of child care legislation, regulations, and procedures. Marino et al. (2001) have argued that social workers' skills enable them to work effectively in failure-to-thrive intervention teams.

Apart from their assessment skills, social workers are also well placed in post-assessment liaison. Additionally, they can provide appropriate emotional support and education on parenting. Furthermore, their knowledge of community resources which can be applied to initiate immediate community involvement will be of considerable help. They may be able to secure long-term follow-up, work with parents under very difficult circumstances, inform parents about progress throughout the treatment process, and provide models of positive parenting in a supportive environment to improve parent–infant interaction. If other agencies are involved, social workers can guide parents through these involvements and support them in what may often be anxiety-provoking situations.

Moore (1982) carried out a study in which supervised students of social work provided a supportive and nurturing intervention for non-organic FTT children's parents whose infants had been hospitalised at least once for the condition. This study was based on the premise that in order to avoid re-hospitalisation of non-organic failure-to-thrive infants, treatment should aim to develop parental understanding and knowledge of the issues involved, which was not usually achieved through traditional hospitalisation treatment alone.

Project Thrive was developed by the Family Protection Team, part of the Community Council on Child Abuse and Neglect, in co-operation with the University of South Florida Social Work Department, and was run by student social workers with non-organic FTT training. The aim of this study was to provide evidence that frequent intensive support and assistance with situational stresses can resolve non-organic failure to thrive in a cost-effective manner. Further aims were to prevent re-hospitalisation of the child and to stabilise weight gain at a rate appropriate to the child's age.

Work with the parents began in the hospital and was designed to encourage parents' efforts to care for and visit their children in hospital. The social workers ensured that such visits took place. Following the children's discharge from hospital, social workers, together with public-health nurses, co-ordinated home visits. Social-work visits occurred twice weekly (during feeding, where possible) for approximately two months. The purpose of these visits was to provide support, nurturing, role-modelling, education, and to monitor the baby's progress. Environmental needs were assessed, community support was located, and parents were referred to appropriate services when it was felt necessary.

The intervention proved very successful as none of the babies required re-hospitalisation, and all gained weight. Mean weight gain was 3 lb. 5 oz. (1.5 kg), and the mean period of time in the programme was seven weeks. A further success was listed as lack of necessity for foster-care referral during the study period. According to Moore (1982), this programme provided evidence for the efficacy of an intensive supportive social-work-driven approach to FTT intervention. Together with positive results achieved on outcome measures, the programme was economical (due to the involvement of students), and proved to be of benefit to parents, children, students, organisers, and state finances.

Iwaniec et al. (1985a; 1985b) conducted a multi-component behavioural social-work intervention with 17 FTT children and their families. This cognitive/behavioural social-work intervention successfully blended triadic behavioural social-work methods with community methods directed towards feeding performance and improving relationships between parents and children. A high level of success was reported, with improvements maintained for at least two years. Booster sessions were provided if there were relapses or if it was thought that extra help was needed to secure progress. All children were seen periodically in an out-patients' clinic to further reinforce progress, give parents encouragement, and acknowledge their hard work and success. Close collaboration of social worker, paediatrician, paediatric nurses, and, in some cases, dieticians (as well as carrying out regular reviews of cases

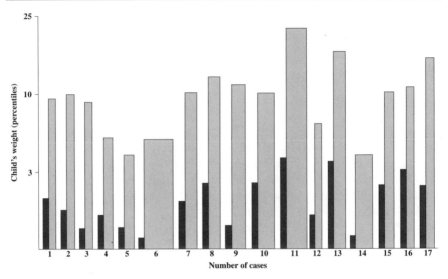

**Figure 13.1** Weight gain following intervention: black bars represent weight at
referral point and grey bars, weight gain after intervention
*Source:* Iwaniec, O., Herbert, M. and McNeish, A. S. (1985) Social work with failure to
thrive children and their families. *British Journal of Social Work* **15** (4). Reproduced by
permission of Oxford University Press

with parents in the out-patients' clinic), maintained good growth progress
for the child and established a good relationship between the team and the
parents. Figure 13.1 demonstrates positive outcomes as a result of paediatric
and social-work intervention. As noted above, the multi-disciplinary work
reported by Hampton (1996) was organised and led by the social worker.
Again, methods based on social-learning theory were used successfully in
resolving nutritional/feeding and interactional problems.

Hathaway (1989) described the role that social workers play in a multi-
disciplinary team (consisting of physician, nutritionalist, and a social worker),
and the type of work they did with families whose children failed to thrive.
Cases were always discussed, tasks allocated according to skills and expertise, and progress reviewed on a regular basis. The social worker dealt with
matters such as economic difficulties, family functioning, relationships within
the family, attachment work with mother and FTT child, and general support
for parents during the time of intervention. In addition, arrangements were
made to provide necessary services if progress was slow at home, or if parents did not engage in treatment, either because they were not able to, or
because they did not want to. For example, if there was persistent lack of
progress at home, foster placements had to be provided. Because of the parents' emotional difficulties, support, encouragement, and supervision had to

be provided by the social worker in order to nurture the parents and teach them how to nurture their children.

While social workers are seldom involved at a *universal* level of intervention in relation to failure-to-thrive children, and only occasionally in *selective* intervention, they are always involved in *targeted* and *Civil Court* interventions. As *targeted* intervention is associated with child-protection procedures (such as case-conferencing and registration of children who are at risk of significant harm), social-work involvement is not only desirable but essential. In the United Kingdom, once a child is placed on the *Child Protection Register*, social workers have a duty, as stated in the Department of Health Guidance and Procedures (1991), to monitor the case and to provide necessary services and therapeutic help to resolve the problems which led to the child's registration in the first place. Additionally, children who are considered as 'at risk' and are registered as a result of a multi-disciplinary case-conference decision, have to be visited on a regular basis by a social worker. Their progress has to be formally reviewed, at least every six months, according to the social services' procedures. If the progress is considered as satisfactory (because of effective intervention), then the child is de-registered—in other words, the child's name is taken off the *Child Protection Register*.

A small percentage of children who fail to thrive require Court intervention should they be assessed as at serious risk of harm if they remain with their carers. Here again, social workers have a duty and responsibility to make application to the Court to obtain a Supervision Order, Care Order, or Freeing Order in respect of adoption. Apart from application to the Court, social workers have to prepare a Social Inquiry Report based on a comprehensive assessment and chronology of events leading to the Court appearance.

Familiarity with child care legislation, legal requirements, and a sound knowledge of regulations and procedures are essential to take the case through the Court system. Social workers are trained in child care law and they have experience in court work. They are the only professionals in the multi-disciplinary teams who have these skills, who can advise on the legal framework, and what is the process when targeted or Court intervention is required.

Another advantage of having a social worker included as a member of the intervention team dealing with failure-to-thrive cases is that it is possible to draw upon knowledge of services available and suitable to help the child and parents, inside and outside the home environment. Services outside the home include provision for placements with day-nurseries, family centres, daily minders, and short-term foster-care. Within the home, provision includes family aid to assist parents with regular child care, or home help, if required, which can be as important as therapeutic work itself.

It is argued that since social workers are associated with removing children from home (and all rather difficult aspects of child-protection work), they should not be involved in early interventions because such interventions may increase parental perceptions that they may be at fault, and anxieties that their children may be taken into care. These fears are real, as social workers do take children into care or rescue them from, at times, extremely dangerous homes—that is their job. Equally, they can alert others in the team as to what is happening to the child at home, and whether the devised management programme is put into practice. They may also advise on how the parents are coping with new child care and feeding-management strategies. Social workers, in order to work with FTT children, help them recognise FTT, to assess the extent of a problem, and to acquire skills in intervention methods.

## INTER-AGENCY WORK

Since failure to thrive is multi-factorial in nature and requires a multi-disciplinary approach, difficulties can arise with respect to the co-ordination and effective management of multiple agencies when working together on a case. Interagency management structures have been under-developed, exacerbated by a range of factors including interagency differences in definitions, conceptualisations, and approaches to the failure-to-thrive syndrome, together with differences in training and work practices. Often such differences can lead to defective service provision, with the risk that FTT children and their families may fall through gaps in care. A number of authors (e.g. Iwaniec, 1995; Taylor & Daniel, 1999; Wright, 2000) have stated the need for agencies to establish a system whereby co-operation and exchange of information occurs so that children in need, and children for whom child-protection issues are evident, are adequately managed.

Tensions that exist between professionals can obstruct speedy detection and intervention in failure-to-thrive cases, and cannot be over-estimated. However, in order to prevent children being overlooked by a series of multiple agencies, there is a need to develop clear formal procedures and protocols for interagency case management. It is argued that if children are to be provided with an opportunity to be brought up in their own families (in cases such as failure to thrive), sound inter-disciplinary co-operation and exchange of information must be in place.

Taylor and Daniel (1999), in a review of interagency practice concerning children with FTT, state their belief that FTT is a child-protection issue, with a potential to fall into the gap between the different professional groups. This, according to the authors, is due to overlapping professional definitions and classifications of failure to thrive, and the complex nature of FTT as a condition in which multiple causal roots and multiple approaches to intervention exist. The authors refer to a growing literature, based on failure-to-thrive intervention, for both the medical and social-work professions, and a corresponding lack of attention as to how these disciplines mesh together in the provision of services. A significant disparity exists between the ways in which the medical and social-work professions respond to failure to thrive: this could lead to a number of failure-to-thrive children not receiving the most appropriate intervention. This disparity is described as having a number of possible causes, including, at the most basic level, conceptualisations of FTT (for example, whether it is characterised as a symptom of abuse, neglect, stressful feeding interactions, or as a primarily nutritional outcome). Taylor and Daniel (1999) refer to the absence of an agreed co-ordinated inter-disciplinary protocol: problems include a lack of a clear framework for inter-disciplinary response; inconsistent definitions of FTT among different professions; and the composition of the multi-disciplinary team. They also argue that there is no agreement as to which specific team structure is most successful in failure-to-thrive intervention. Further, disparity exists in the source of referral: for instance, when the FTT is linked to child abuse and neglect, social-work systems are put into operation; however, where it is identified through child symptomatology, diagnosis and intervention are routed through the medical system. Disparity also exists in intervention settings, where both hospital and community interventions are in operation.

In order to bridge the gap and create more consistency between disciplines involved in failure-to-thrive diagnosis and intervention, early co-ordination should be established between different professional agencies, with attention to the division of skills and tasks. Care and response pathways should be clarified for children with FTT, particular attention being paid to routing of referrals and agreement of roles and responsibilities. Additionally, multi-agency training should be provided on identification and response to failure to thrive, and a dedicated team response should be based on initial evidence, in which some models have been shown to be more effective than others. Future research could explore the most appropriate structure of multi-disciplinary teams, and the most effective settings for treatment.

Undoubtedly, failure to thrive appears to be a very competitive area of work and research where medical professions often claim ownership, based on the premise that under-nutrition is a health issue, sometimes disregarding psychosocial factors (which are also in operation in every failure-to-thrive case). We still do not know what comes first: feeding difficulties and subsequent parenting problems; or parenting problems and subsequent feeding difficulties. In fact, it might be both.

Batchelor (1999), in a discussion of interagency failure-to-thrive collaboration, suggests that a prerequisite for successful multi-disciplinary work is a level of mutual respect and understanding across the professions which is likely to be fostered by the experience of joint training and moving beyond the stumbling-blocks of professional rivalries.

## SUMMARY

Several disciplines and approaches have been active in failure-to-thrive inter-vention, and have been outlined in this chapter together with examples from research. In addition to multi-disciplinary approaches to FTT intervention, programmes have included a focus on nutritional management, but as a part of a wider and more comprehensive picture of child care and parental nurtur-ing of the child. Health-visitor-led intervention has been explored in detail, emphasising advantages as well as existing gaps in such interventions. The role of social workers has been addressed, together with a look at interagency collaboration in failure-to-thrive intervention programmes.

# 14

# CONSIDERATIONS ARISING FROM FAILURE-TO-THRIVE INTERVENTION RESEARCH

*None thrives for long upon the happiest dream*
Coventry Kersey Dighton Patmore (1823–96)

## INTRODUCTION

A review of failure-to-thrive intervention research literature has revealed several issues worthy of consideration. In order to increase the chances of successful long-term outcomes resulting from FTT intervention, it is necessary to improve understanding of the multiple factors existing at every stage of the intervention process. With reference to examples from the research literature, a number of care-giver considerations (including parental beliefs, the parental history of nurturance, psychological factors, parent–child interactions, and facilitation of parental competence, as well as parental self-efficacy) will be discussed. In addition, it is important to take into account factors associated with parental co-operation (a prerequisite for long-term success), as well as the impact of differing characteristics and behaviour of individuals on the success (or otherwise) of failure-to-thrive intervention programmes. In addition, various methodological issues will be addressed. Finally, recommendations for future FTT intervention programmes will be put forward.

## PARENTAL BELIEFS AND ATTITUDES

At the assessment stage of intervention, parental attitudes towards a child's FTT, parents' food-beliefs, and their perceptions of eating should be fully explored in order to achieve a better understanding of the issues involved and to identify any misconceptions the care-giver may have that could act to negatively affect outcomes. Available facts, based on thorough investigation, should help to clarify parental (particularly maternal) beliefs, and it is important to establish what these are as essential parts of intervention. Moores (1996) alludes to traps into which some health-conscious parents may fall because they fail to understand that what is healthy for adults may not be appropriate (and may damage) young children. Commercial and ubiquitous advertisements insist on the importance of high-fibre, low-fat, low-calorie diets for good health, but do not mention that such diets are inadequate for children, who need a more calorie-dense diet to achieve adequate growth. Other findings, e.g. those of McCann *et al.* (1994), have shown that parental attitudes towards eating and food have an enormous influence on the eating habits of children, and that mothers of FTT children tend to restrict their own diets as well as the range and quantity of what they felt was appropriate for their children (Heffer & Kelley, 1994; Maggioni & Lifshitz, 1995; Moores, 1996). It is thus essential to address and correct misconceptions about diet: to facilitate successful interventions these misconceptions should be explored and explained in a sensitive yet convincing manner, and support and reassurance should be given to facilitate change.

Eating habits of parents whose children fail to thrive have been found to be disturbed in a number of studies (e.g. Stein *et al.*, 1995; Wolke, 1996; Russell *et al.*, 1998). There is evidence of a connection between eating disorders in parents and associated disturbances in parenting, mother–child interactions, development of eating difficulties, and children's experiences of food deprivation and enforced dieting.

Sturm and Drotar (1992) placed particular emphasis on the importance of addressing and developing a better understanding of the perspectives, beliefs, and attitudes of parents of FTT children: they devised a number of communication strategies to be considered by professionals working with these parents. These strategies included exploring parental health beliefs and prior experiences, and addressing expectations for outcomes and possible misconceptions that might affect the efficacy of any treatment prescribed. Iwaniec (1991; 1995) put forward cognitive restructuring as an effective way of dealing with faulty parental perceptions and attitudes regarding their own eating behaviour and that of their children.

## Parental History of Nurturance

Several studies have examined the influence of the history of nurturance, attachment, and experience of abuse on the abilities of FTT children. Using data based on maternal childhood histories, Haynes *et al.* (1984) found that parents' ability to adequately nurture their children was related to their own history of being nurtured. These authors also found that, while characteristics of children played a role in the mothers' ability to recognise, interpret, and respond to signals and cues, the primary influence was the mothers' own childhood experiences. A majority of mothers of FTT children reported negative memories of childhood, with 56% reporting inadequacies in nurturance, 22% reporting neglect, 40% reporting sexual abuse (22% confirmed), and 16% reporting physical abuse. Iwaniec (2000) reported that 40% of mothers whose children were failing to thrive had poor maternal nurturing as children in terms of limited warmth, lack of physical closeness, and feelings that they were not supported and were unloved, regardless of their personal circumstances.

Using the Adult Attachment Interview, Chatoor *et al.* (1997) investigated non-organic FTT parents' childhood experiences with their own parents in order to explore positive or negative influences of previous relationships on their own parenting abilities (including setting boundaries, and skills in conflict resolution). When asked to assess the efficacy of this exercise, 79% of the parents rated the experience as either somewhat or very helpful (47.4%, 31.6%), while 21% of the parents found the experience to be unhelpful.

Weston and Colloton (1993) found that a group of 59 mothers of children (under 5 years of age) with non-organic FTT reported a significantly higher level of history of abuse than in a comparison group of normally growing children, and recommended that consideration should be given to the parental history of abuse when designing an intervention. Available literature indicates that emotional abuse (in particular emotional neglect) is a frequent feature in the lives of failure-to-thrive children. Many parents seem to be low in warmth and high in resentment, impatience, and insensitivity. Such passive, emotional neglect, according to Iwaniec (1991, 1995, 2000), seems to stem from maternal experiences of undemonstrative emotional nurturing when they were children, and later unsupportive relationships as adults (particularly marital relationships). On the other hand, children classified as of psychosocial short stature (as a rule) are usually severely emotionally abused and rejected, and there is often a history of abuse in their mothers' lives, and such a history tends to be a common feature of their fathers' lives as well. Apart from physical abuse and neglect, parents of psychosocial short-stature children are not often emotionally available to them, some of whom are sexually abused. It is not surprising, therefore, that some of these parents are not able to nurture, as they seldom experienced a loving and warm relationship themselves. Yet some of them, in spite of their adverse childhood history, become very caring and loving parents. According to Iwaniec and Sneddon's (2001, 2002) 20-year follow-up study, such parents' changes of behaviour and parenting style were due to supportive marital relationships and to therapeutic help they received which heightened their self-efficacy and cognitive abilities. Some of them showed considerable resilience which helped to overcome the adversities from which they suffered in early life.

## PSYCHOLOGICAL ISSUES

A number of connections have been made in the failure-to-thrive intervention literature between FTT and increased parental psychological risk. Duniz *et al.* (1996) referred to a widespread tendency in paediatrics to imply a 'parentogenic' cause to non-organic FTT, and maintained that whilst it is important to recognise that the mental health of parents with non-organic FTT children is not necessarily questionable, and that they are not inaccurately and harmfully labelled with a psychological condition, failure to address the psychodynamic problems of parents can result in chronic problems in infants and the development and prolonging of secondary complications. The association of maternal psychopathology with FTT and with maternal attachment disturbances has been discussed in many studies (Woolston, 1985; Lachenmeyer & Davidovicz, 1987; Brinich *et al.*, 1989; Russell & Russell, 1989; Drotar *et al.*, 1990). According to psychoanlytical theory, traumatic memories might have an impact on parental functioning (Grossmann *et al.*, 1988; Crittenden, 1990). Parental stress has also been shown to have adverse effects on feeding behaviour. Polan *et al.* (1991) and Benoit *et al.* (1989) both found higher rates of psychopathology in mothers of failure-to-thrive babies than in mothers of normally thriving children.

Duniz *et al.* (1996) conducted a study based on a psychosomatic approach which aimed to investigate parental psychiatric disorders and their courses during the treatment of non-organic FTT infants in order to further explore findings that higher rates of psychopathology exist in mothers of failure-to-thrive babies. In this study (which aimed to stimulate the child to break a vicious circle of opposition against feeding under pressure), it was found that 70% of all care-givers showed pathology at baseline 93% (n = 46) of mothers and 38% (n = 7) of fathers. Feeding problems were found to be related to parental disorders. Throughout the course of the intervention, parental psychopathology was found to have been reduced to 37%, and after one year only 12% of the parents were still found to have psychiatric disorders. Whilst the majority of parents' psychiatric disorders were reactive in nature, their personality disorders were found to be more persistent, and therefore were regarded as a trait variable. This study presents a number of issues for failure-to-thrive intervention. First, an issue of causality is raised. Did the infants recover because the care-takers' anxiety and fears subsided through counselling? Or did the parents recover because the child's feeding behaviour was managed more effectively? The authors felt that one difficulty aggravates the other, and suggested that future research should address the connection between parental mental health and FTT. Such research, it is argued, should commence from the time when parents decide to have a baby.

Douglas's (1991) research findings indicated that failure to thrive in a child may affect the mental health of a care-giver. Bauman *et al.* (1997) and other investigators have reported that parents of children with poor health conditions have been found to be at increased psychological risk: the number of 'children and families' vulnerable to psychological problems 'secondary to' 'chronic illness' in 'children is large'. Skuse *et al.* (1994) also found a relationship between failure to thrive and depression whereby parents of children with later onset of FTT had significantly higher levels of depression than controls.

Hutcheson (1993), in an attempt to add to existing knowledge of the moderating effects of risk factors on intervention outcomes, examined maternal negative affectivity as a risk factor hypothesised to compromise benefits received from early home intervention, as well as cognitive development, motor development, and interactive behaviour. The outcome in this study was found to be determined by mothers' low or high levels of negative affectivity, with decline in cognitive development particularly noticeable in children of mothers with high levels of depression, hostility, and anxiety.

They concluded that intervention is most beneficial among mothers with relatively low levels of negative affectivity, and that parents with high levels of negative affectivity may benefit from specific attention directed towards ameliorating their condition in their parenting role. Later intervention, directed at improving parent–child attachment behaviour and mutual relationship, has proved to produce desirable results for failure-to-thrive children (Iwaniec & Sneddon, 2001).

## PARENT–CHILD INTERACTION

Whilst failure-to-thrive intervention research has moved away from a discredited focus on the role of maternal deprivation in the aetiology of failure to thrive (Duniz *et al.*, 1996; Batchelor, 1999), mother–infant interaction is still assessed and addressed in many interventions from a more encompassing multidimensional perspective. It is recognised that disturbed mother–child interaction is just one of many elements of the syndrome.

However, treatment should include a focus on the dysfunctional mother–infant interaction and assessment of family feeding interactions as a useful and critical element. Whether disrupted interaction is viewed as a symptom or a cause of the child's failure to thrive, attention to parent–child interaction patterns (including assessment of feeding) can be used to identify and break mutually destructive cycles, and strengthen relationships and communication strategies between these parents and their children, thus ensuring more rewarding and potentially more successful feeding experiences.

Heffer and Kelley (1994), in the presentation of an ideographic approach to failure-to-thrive intervention comprising psychosocial assessment and interventions, maintain that one of the many and complex factors that accentuate non-organic FTT is the presence of dysfunctional relationships. These authors list parent–child interaction as a necessary component in failure-to-thrive intervention, whereby both feeding interactions and non-feeding interactions should be assessed. According to many authors, structured assessment of parent–child meal-time interaction can be carried out using techniques (including videotaping), thus providing vital information that can be used to identify patterns in interaction. Observations of non-feeding interactions (including play vocalisations and home observations) can provide information regarding general behaviour, and contribute to an understanding of how child-specific, family, and situational variables interact in the triggering of non-organic FTT. This has also been postulated by Iwaniec (1991, 1995) and Iwaniec and Herbert (1982).

Haynes *et al.* (1984), in their study of 50 hospitalised non-organic FTT children and their families, examined the effect of short-term lay-health-visitor intervention (with additional community support), and included a component specifically focused on patterns of maternal care and how these patterns affected the mother–child relationship. In contrast to a control group of 25 thriving mother–infant dyads (who were found to have interactions characterised by the mothers' responses to their babies' actions and cues of feelings), the 50 failure-to-thrive mother–infant dyads were found to have less positive interaction styles. Based on videotaped feeding and play interactions (as well as maternal interviews), three interaction patterns were identified: benign neglect; incoordination; and overt hostility. Benign neglect was characterised by an absence of appropriate stimulation and guidance by the parent, together with a lack of understanding and adequate attention to the babies' nutritional needs. Inappropriate dependence on their babies for guidance and direction on care-giving activities was also evident, resulting in a vicious circle of reduced responsivity and unrewarding behaviour in the babies, with further associated reductions in maternal responsivity. Incoordination was the largest identified group, characterised by incoordination between the mothers' actions and babies' cues (with a tendency for parents, while showing some degree of awareness of cues, to respond inappropriately), including evidence of failure to respond to babies' cues of distress or pain. Incoordinated interaction was found to lead to a lack of persistence in babies' cues of hunger or dissatisfaction, and a tendency to give up, lose interest, and disengage from the feeding situation. The overtly hostile category of interaction was characterised by the failure of parents to recognise, and respond appropriately to, their babies' social signals and distress cues, combined with difficulties in carrying out the act of feeding. In addition, there was an underlying presence of hostility in interactions with their babies, including engagement in hostile actions (such as pinching, poking, and slapping them). These interaction profiles were again examined six months post-intake, and found to persist in all cases with few positive changes evidenced despite the intervening health-visitor intervention. The authors suggested that in cases where the mothers were more pathological, the children might not have been as negatively affected by parents' behaviours as might have been the case without the intervening diagnosis and intervention. They pointed out a need in FTT intervention to differentiate treatment goals and priorities based on assessment of the extent of disturbance present in the mother–child relationship.

In Duniz *et al.*'s (1996) study of changes in psychopathology of parents of non-organic FTT infants during treatment, the affective quality of the parent–infant relationship was assessed, with three degrees of severity identified at three assessment periods from baseline, and the following three months and one year. The three degrees were identified as those parents who were over-involved with their children, those who were under-involved with them, and those (all mothers) who were anxious/tense. There was a further group of 12 cases (9 mothers and 3 fathers), identified as mixed, with an additional angry/hostile father, and one abusive mother–infant relationship. Whilst the type of relationship disorder remained constant over time for each dyad, the authors found a correlation between the infant's recovery and simultaneous regression of tension in the dyadic relationship, with lesser severity of relationship disorder, indicating that the intervention had a positive effect on the parent–infant relationship.

Chatoor *et al.* (1997) describe infantile anorexia as a relationship disorder arising from conflictual care-giver–infant interactions. According to the transactional developmental model described by them:

> certain characteristics of the infant combine with certain vulnerabilities in the mother to bring out negative responses and conflict in their interactions; more specifically, the infant's temperament characteristics of emotional intensity, distractability, and stubbornness evoke conflicts over control and limit setting in a vulnerable mother who becomes anxious and insecure when faced with the infant's food refusal and oppositional behaviors during feeding.

They observed feeding interactions using the Feeding Scale. It was found that for the mother–infant dyads (17 of 20) who responded positively to the intervention, both dyadic reciprocity and interactional patterns improved to a level comparable with the non-feeding disorder control group.

Iwaniec and Sneddon (2002), in their 20-year prospective follow-up of the quality of parenting of individuals who had failed to thrive as children, examined inter-generational cycles of familial interaction. This study found interaction patterns whereby parents who had failed to thrive as children either did or did not emulate the care-giving environment in which they were brought up. This was found to be influenced by the particular type of family environment at the time of the intervention. In cases where the relationship between failure-to-thrive children and their parents had been characterised by interactional difficulties in specific contexts (such as feeding) and with such interactional difficulties addressed in the intervention with positive outcomes, the quality of parenting and family relationships was generally found to have improved in the next generation. However, in cases where the intervention had failed to result in long-term changes in interaction patterns, there was a greater incidence of failure to thrive in the next generation. In cases of unresolved neglectful care-giving, following the initial intervention, the next generation was found to be more likely to mirror its own parents' parenting styles, showing similar patterns of interaction. The authors pointed out the relevance of this finding for FTT practitioners (who should be aware of the difficulties in effecting long-term changes in neglectful families): therefore early decision-making is necessary.

## PARENTAL COMPETENCE

A number of failure-to-thrive researchers and practitioners have pointed to the mediating role of parental competence in achieving positive outcomes. Various findings indicate that the presence of FTT in a child can be a threat to a parent's feelings of competence—this needs to be addressed in failure-to-thrive intervention strategy development (Wolfe, 1990; Sturm & Drotar, 1992). With this in mind, recommendations have been made for good practice: for example, when working with parents it is important not to undermine their feelings of competence because increased parental competence has been linked to improved growth outcomes (Bithoney et al., 1995); and Batchelor (1999) refers to parental competence as a key component of FTT intervention, suggesting that building it up may be the key component to achieving the changes necessary to overcome a child's failure to thrive.

Many FTT intervention studies have attempted to increase feelings of parental competence through a number of different methods, including aiming to avoid inculcating a sense of guilt or blame in the parents, and involving them in the intervention to such an extent that they may achieve a sense of being at least partly responsible for improvements. Throughout intervention much emphasis tends to be placed on providing parents with support and encouragement. Some researchers have referred to the importance of establishing positive feelings in the mother and child, with improvements in parent–child interaction achieved as a result of the intervention leading to increased feelings of self-esteem. According to many intervention studies there is a need to emphasise that parents are not necessarily responsible for the problem, so emphasis should be placed on creating feelings that they have some degree of control over the situation, and can be effective in bringing about change. Maggioni and Lifshitz (1995) point to the importance of providing parents with reassurance, support, and education regarding nutrition: in order to promote parental competence, consideration for parents' feelings should be evident throughout the intervention, with care taken to avoid making the parents feel guilty or judged.

Chatoor et al. (1997) refer to the importance of increasing parents' confidence and helping them to overcome any feelings of guilt. In their intervention, work was undertaken with parents to develop their understanding of their infants' special temperamental characteristics, with a raising of parental awareness that such infants require special parenting skill. When parents were successful in facilitating the self-regulation of eating in their infants, confidence increased, and more positive parent–infant interactions ensued.

Failure-to-thrive interventions have evidenced trends towards the inclusion of parents as working members of the intervention team. From the start of the intervention, the parents should be encouraged to feel like effective members of the team, and involved in the decision-making process. Thus parental competence and self-confidence will be increased.

As alluded to earlier in this section, and reflecting a trend in the literature to place emphasis on the importance of the parent–professional relationship, Sturm and Drotar (1989) have devised communication strategies for working with parents. First, practitioners should be sensitive to the fact that a problem with weight gain in an infant or toddler poses a significant threat to parental feelings of competence. Time should be taken to enquire about the parents' views of their child's condition. Further, it should be understood that parents may voice a medical explanation for their child's poor growth in order to reduce anxiety. At the time of diagnosis professionals should be prepared for some degree of disagreement or conflict with parents of non-organic FTT infants, which may be due to their difficulty in accepting the diagnosis. If this occurs, it is important to work through those feelings with the parent. If there is disagreement, then staff should respect the parents' position and agree to disagree: where possible, a working compromise should be negotiated in order to promote parents' confidence in working in a team and being an important part of it. Finally, they suggest that when discussing the child's condition, the focus should be future-oriented, with emphasis on the working relationship between parents and professionals.

## PARENTAL SELF-EFFICACY

Self-efficacy theory is highly relevant to failure-to-thrive intervention research and management strategies. Whilst the role of parental competence has been applied to FTT intervention research, the role of parental self-efficacy remains a potentially fruitful unexplored avenue of research.

Lack of self-efficacy has been shown to impair parental competence. Parental self-efficacy is thus a powerful determinant of parental functioning, and is concerned with both parents' feelings of their ability to exercise control in their roles and to perform successfully and effectively in parenting scenarios (Teti & Gelfand, 1991). It may play an important part in helping parents' abilities to positively exert an influence on their child's behaviour and development (Coleman & Karraker, 1997).

Applied to failure to thrive, self-efficacy can be theorised to act at a number of levels. If a parent has experienced persistent difficulties in feeding interactions and behaviours, together with a perceived inability to cause an improvement in the child's weight acquisition, the child's failure to thrive may potentially impact on parents' abilities to exercise control, with associated feelings (such as helplessness or despair) simultaneously impacting on the parents' affective state. Self-efficacy in parents of FTT children thus can be affected by their perceptions of an inability to exercise control over feeding behaviour, and beliefs that they are unable to create conditions for an improvement in the child's weight. This can result in depressed feelings and reduced motivation (Iwaniec, 1995).

An exploration of further self-efficacy mechanisms has identified a number of ways in which this theory can be usefully applied to failure-to-thrive research and intervention strategies. Efficacy beliefs have been shown to have effects on goal-setting and cognitive appraisals of either success or failure scenarios. Applied to failure to thrive, this could indicate that high levels of self-efficacy may positively affect parents' motivation to maintain compliance with failure-to-thrive intervention, with increased coping behaviour, positive affect, and ability to perceive successful child outcomes (including more effective feeding behaviour, parent–child interactions, and achievement of weight goals). Conversely, low parental self-efficacy may have a negative effect on the above, thus reducing the chances of a successful outcome and parental compliance with an FTT intervention.

Research has indicated that self-efficacy can be positively influenced by a number of mechanisms. Bandura (1982) has identified four such mechanisms that may be usefully applied to failure-to-thrive theory. First, self-efficacy can be influenced positively or negatively due to experiences of success or failure. A parent of an FTT child who has put considerable effort into resolving feeding difficulties may have especially low levels of self-efficacy. An intervention that aims to provide parents with an experience of success rather than failure resulting from efforts that they themselves may have made may increase the parents' sense of efficacy. Second, self-efficacy has been shown to be positively influenced by modelling when the behaviours modelled are viewed as realistically achievable and within the parents' capabilities. Many failure-to-thrive interventions (as explored in Chapters 11, 12, and 13) make use of strategies based on modelling of parenting and feeding behaviours (where effective strategies are taught to the care-giver through example and guidance). The third strategy is verbal persuasion, which again is influenced by perceptions as to whether or not the appraisal is seen as realistic and achievable. As applied to failure-to-thrive intervention, this would relate to education of the parents or care-givers in a manner which is matched to the particular needs and characteristics of the parents. Feelings of competence could thereby be increased, and the strategy could include the establishment of achievable goals, targets, general advice, and guidance. The fourth and final mediating variable on self-efficacy is the influence of emotional arousal. High emotional arousal caused by, for example, parental distress associated with FTT may impair parental functioning and task performance, with higher levels of parental excitability. Examples of such strategies include providing the parents or care-givers with emotional support and facilitating contact with community-based sources of help. Further, a number of intervention methods include counselling and psychotherapy aimed at working through parents' worries and assisting parents to develop coping strategies in order to buffer the impact of the FTT on the parents' affective system.

With reference to mastery of occupational roles, and having direct applicability to failure-to-thrive intervention research, Iwaniec (1983) describes how competencies may be developed through mastery modelling, a process whereby knowledge and skills are enhanced through three elements that may be equally applicable to FTT intervention.

## PARENTAL CO-OPERATION

Parental compliance has been shown to be enhanced with inclusion of the parent in the intervention programme; matching treatment to parents' needs and preferences (empowering and equipping them to create change); avoiding negative labelling of the parent as pathogenic; avoiding conflict with the parents and reducing feelings of guilt or blame; providing support, education, role-modelling and encouragement; and avoiding conflicting advice if working in a multi-disciplinary team. Some parents benefit from, and are more likely to comply with, interventions that differ in timing and intensity. Willingness of the parents to invest time and effort in the intervention also affects co-operation, as do parents' attitudes and understanding towards the child. Finally, equipping parents with an understanding of their child's 'special characteristics', their role in the failure-to-thrive intervention, and the potential to achieve a positive outcome can be effective.

## INDIVIDUAL DIFFERENCES

The study of the effect of individual differences on the success of FTT intervention programmes has received increasing attention in the literature. While outcomes of non-organic failure-to-thrive interventions can be affected by factors such as nutrition, malnutrition, a thrust for autonomy, and the presence of an adverse social and psychological environment, a number of issues relating to individual differences have been found to impact on the ability of children to benefit from certain interventions.

Black et al. (1995) found significant age effects which they claim to be consistent with their ecological perspective of FTT, and conclude that interventions which may be effective for one age group may not be as effective for other age groups due to a number of age-related factors (including multiple changes in growth and development during the first several years of life). This occurs because feeding skills differ significantly according to children's ages and developmental levels. It has been pointed out that increased placidity in the first year of life compared to more differentiated development in toddlerhood (with more established behaviour and interaction patterns requiring a greater intensity of intervention strategies) requires different ways of managing the behaviour. If problems are not solved during the infancy of the child, they will grow with the child into the toddler stage, when they are more difficult to resolve.

Haynes *et al.* (1984), in their study assessing the effectiveness of lay-health-visitor intervention with failure-to-thrive children, found that the children who achieved satisfactory weight gain were those who were diagnosed early in life. While many of the FTT children were found to have persistent delays in development, these delays were less severe when diagnosis was made earlier.

Studies investigating predictive factors have been infrequent; however, early diagnosis, early intervention, a degree of psychological risk, and the duration of FTT have been shown to be predictive factors (Kristiansson & Fällström, 1987). Sturm and Drotar (1989), who conducted a predictive follow-up of growth outcome following intervention, found that the children (50%) who achieved the best levels of compensatory growth were more likely to be black, to have a lower birth order, a lower socio-economic status, and to have unmarried parents.

## METHODOLOGICAL ISSUES

A number of authors have pointed to methodological issues that need to be addressed regarding failure-to-thrive intervention research. At the most basic level, problems have been associated with the lack of a clear definition of FTT.

Sturm and Drotar (1989) refer to a number of limitations of studies addressing physical growth outcomes of non-organic failure-to-thrive children, including a tendency towards small sample sizes; lack of information concerning the course of physical growth or intervention effects; and failure to study a comprehensive set of predictor variables. According to these authors, lack of sequential assessment of progress prevents determining the point at which improvement in physical growth occurred and the degree to which recovery is maintained over time. In addition, these authors found that intervention effects have not been well described, and that non-organic FTT children's nutritional status has not been well documented in follow-up studies.

Bauman *et al.* (1997), in a review of psychosocial interventions for children with chronic health conditions, focused on a number of methodological issues. They found that few programmes evaluated were guided by theory. In addition, many reports included insufficient details about the interventions being evaluated, and a lack of attention to the clinical significance of findings.

Further, researchers were found to rarely analyse whether particular sub-groups benefited more than others. Based on such findings, these authors engaged in a discussion of ways in which the quality of intervention research could be improved. Echoing Sturm and Drotar (1989), these authors again referred to a tendency towards small sample sizes and associated limitations including impaired ability to show anything but the largest effects. They also recommended that power analysis should be conducted to ensure that studies have the statistical integrity to detect meaningful programme effects. Use of a control group to ensure that changes observed can be linked to the intervention, and the use of sufficiently sensitive measurement tools with adequate validity and reliability was also recommended. To help ensure successful outcomes, it has been suggested that programmes should be preceded by a process of evaluation, and to this end a further recommendation was that it should be made clear in advance which outcome variables must be improved in order for the intervention to qualify as a success.

Kendrick *et al.* (2000) conducted a systematic review and meta-analysis of studies assessing the impact of home visiting on parenting. In this review the authors referred to the inherent difficulty in measuring parenting due to the complex nature of the investigation. They found that a lack of availability of means and SDs of studies restricted their meta-analysis. They made a number of points, some of which closely corresponded to issues raised. First, many of the studies did not provide a theoretical framework that attempted to hypothesise how the interventions would improve parenting. As most interventions were multi-faceted or multi-disciplinary in nature, it was difficult to separate out the effect of each aspect of the intervention to establish which part was the essential ingredient for success. Rather, it was just possible to establish particular packages that were associated with improvements.

Heffer and Kelley (1994), in a discussion of FTT intervention techniques, recommended that to better identify biological and psychosocial risk variables which lead to poor developmental outcomes, statistical approaches should be extended to include multiple regression, structural modelling and path analysis (as opposed to a group-differences approach which is often used). In order to achieve a sample size large enough to provide more powerful statistics, they recommended that failure-to-thrive researchers collaborate. To track the developmental course of FTT infants and toddlers, and in so doing facilitate mapping of the developmental trajectories and outcomes, the authors suggested that researchers should also design longitudinal assessment procedures.

Raynor *et al.* (1999), in a discussion of methodological issues associated with failure to thrive, concluded that due to the complex nature of the FTT syndrome, methodological difficulties exist in carrying out randomised controlled trials, and pointed out the danger of assuming that absence of evidence necessarily indicates that an intervention is ineffective. As they have noted, 'absence of evidence is not evidence of absence'. They advocated that future

FTT intervention research should be carried out using larger multi-centre trials. In addition, the study of longer-term outcomes of failure to thrive, and a need for the development of better outcome measures were recommended. They further suggested the application of qualitative methodology to intervention research.

In summary, multi-centre collaboration may facilitate the use of larger sample sizes, with the added benefits of enabling detection of more subtle effects through the use of more rigorous statistical techniques. Clearer conceptualisation and mapping of the proposed trajectory of effects will be facilitated through the adoption of longitudinal designs. Increased development of theoretical underpinnings should also assist with this process. Finally, assessment and evaluation techniques should be sufficiently sensitive, valid, and reliable in order to detect a wider range of effects and outcomes.

## RECOMMENDATIONS FOR FAILURE-TO-THRIVE INTERVENTIONS

Research has demonstrated that early differential diagnosis and intervention lead to an increased likelihood of success (Haynes *et al.*, 1984; Hutcheson *et al.*, 1997). Due to individual differences affecting failure to thrive, the best results are achieved when intervention is tailored to meet the individual needs of the child and family. Programmes should also be theory-driven and comprehensive, and include proximal and distal variables (Black *et al.*, 1995; Iwaniec, 2000). On a related note, focus on empirically determined sub-types, including socio-economic status and psychosocial factors rather than aetiology, has been shown to result in improved outcomes. Parent variables (such as levels of maternal hostility, negative affectivity, parental competence, self-efficacy, their own experience of nurture as children, presence of psychological problems, degree of pathology, and, most significantly, willingness to comply with the intervention) have all been shown to impact on the success of non-organic FTT intervention (Haynes *et al.*, 1984; Duniz *et al.*, 1996; Hutcheson *et al.*, 1997).

Short-term intensive interventions have been shown to be effective in some cases (Moore, 1982). An active team approach of direct support and education has proved to have benefits over and above long-term counselling or therapy (McMillen, 1988; Hanks & Hobbs, 1993; Hampton, 1996).

It is suggested by many researchers that both assessment and intervention must include the multi-factorial aetiology of failure to thrive, addressing nutritional and psychosocial factors. Regarding composition of failure-to-thrive teams, a multi-disciplinary team may be best placed to provide the necessary breadth of response. FTT interventions need to be staged, flexible, based on aetiology, and should commence with the broadest, least intrusive methods, and then draw upon a step-by-step approach with input increased according to child and family needs and seriousness of presenting problems.

Because both nutritional and psychosocial dimensions must be addressed at assessment and intervention stages, and because assessment and intervention are beyond the expertise of any single group, a multi-disciplinary perspective is extremely valuable. For improved growth, interventions should be shaped to the needs of each child and its family on the basis of assessment. Intervention must take account of the multi-factorial nature of failure to thrive, and should include a full history of feeding, completion of a food diary, evaluation of oral-motor functioning, and (preferably) a video-recording of a meal-time (although this is not essential as good observation will provide the necessary data). Psychosocial factors should be attended to, together with nutritional factors, as focusing solely on nutrition has been shown to exacerbate problems.

Iwaniec (1995) drew attention to the value of negotiated agreements with parents and the establishment of a partnership in therapeutic endeavours in order to promote a sense of achievement and competence in parents. It has been demonstrated by many researchers that health visitors are particularly well placed to undertake failure-to-thrive work. They need to be trained, however, to deal with more serious cases which go beyond nutrition and feeding problems.

Iwaniec (2000), drawing from her 20-year follow-up study of children who failed to thrive, made a number of recommendations for changes at the decision-making, service-provision, and policy-making levels:

1. Early intervention is essential to prevent escalation of negative parent–child interaction and relationship and to prevent poor growth and development;
2. Family support in terms of service provision and direct therapeutic input is required at an early stage of failure to thrive;
3. Parental concerns and complaints regarding poor feeding and inadequate weight gain should be taken seriously, dealt with, and monitored until satisfactory weight gain for the child's chronological age is established and maintained for at least six months;
4. Repeated parental visits to physicians regarding worries about the child's poor physical health should be investigated, as in some cases the medical reason for failure to thrive is not recognised, risking a presumption that the cause was inadequate or neglectful parenting;
5. Regular monitoring of children's growth (weight, height, and head-circumference) should be mandatory for all children under 2 years of age. Many children were not referred for assessment and treatment until they were between 3 and 6 years of age, in spite of health-visiting records indicating growth failure: a growth and development chart is a good instrument to identify problems early on, and quickly respond to them;

6. Children who are identified as of severe psychosocial short stature should be removed from stressful, abusive environments. The prognosis of problem-solving at home is extremely poor;

7. Full psychosocial assessment is essential when FTT is persistent. There are many reasons why children fail to thrive. The assessment of problems and needs must be done comprehensively and promptly acted on. A care-plan addressing all aspects of identified difficulties should be devised on a multi-disciplinary basis, and tasks allocated to appropriate professions;

8. A multi-disciplinary approach in assessing and helping those children and their families is essential. Health visitors, GP, paediatricians, social workers, and dieticians are usually involved. Day-care services, such as family centres, day-nurseries, and community centres can help the child and parents;

9. Most serious cases of failure to thrive, especially those where rejection and emotional maltreatment are present, need to be conferenced promptly and an appropriate care-plan urgently put into action. These cases need to be monitored and followed up for a considerable time as the relapse rate is high;

10. Booster programmes need to be provided when progress is slow, or when deterioration is evident; and

11. Family support seems to benefit both child and family. Clear goals for intervention work best when an agreement of mutual obligations, tasks, and goals is written down and negotiated between the parties. Loosely defined support does not seem to work.

(Reproduced from Iwaniec, D. & Hill, M. (2000) *Child Welfare Policy and Practice* with permission from Jessica Kingsley Publishers. Copyright © 2000 Jessica Kingsley Publishers.)


## SUMMARY

While it is as yet unclear as to which particular mechanism holds the best ingredient for a successful failure-to-thrive intervention, types of interventions that have proved successful have been identified, as have factors affecting outcomes of parental considerations and individual differences. Also, while a multi-disciplinary team approach to intervention, involving inter-agency and parental collaboration, has been advocated, it remains unclear as to what is the best composition of such a team. We are still left without a clear specification of the most effective role structure within such teams. Nevertheless, health visitors have been increasingly identified as the most suitable to conduct FTT intervention, and parental compliance as the most important factor to have successful outcomes. It has been suggested in numerous writings that future failure-to-thrive research should be undertaken with larger sample sizes through multi-centre collaboration and the use of longitudinal prospective study design. This would provide greater statistical power and allow the use of more rigorous statistical techniques to facilitate more detailed examination of effects. Finally, future research should explore the application of self-efficacy theory to FTT research, an area that could have many beneficial applications to the design and implementation of intervention programmes.

# EPILOGUE

After many years of research and professional involvement in dealing with failure-to-thrive children and their families, the author became convinced that there should not be a division between organic and non-organic FTT. Both types can overlap, and therefore require equal attention. A child who fails to thrive because of illness can also be rejected, neglected, and poorly parented, so there is a danger of such children being overlooked in terms of their emotional welfare and safety.

Failure to thrive is much more complex than eating problems and faulty nutrition, so psychosocial factors have to be addressed as equally important in any investigation. It is strongly believed that dismissal of psychosocial factors can lead to misinterpretation of the presenting problems. Attempts to correct poor weight gain by attending purely to the intake of food (without considering the manner of feeding style and general parent–child interaction) can be counter-productive and of limited value. Because the aetiology of FTT tends to be multi-factorial, a multi-disciplinary approach is necessary in order to deal effectively and competently with a variety of problems. There is a need to develop better recognition of and respect for different professional disciplines which may play important parts in assessment and intervention where FTT children and their families are concerned. Failure-to-thrive research and practice appear to be very competitive, especially when the medical professions claim superiority and ownership in the understanding of and dealing with FTT children. Clearly, this is inappropriate.

There is a need to provide multi-disciplinary training for different professional groups so that they can learn what each profession can offer, and what expertise is needed to speedily and appropriately deal with emerging difficulties. Care needs to be taken when investigating and assessing cases not to over-react without evidence: making assumptions without carefully collected information is dangerous, and can lead to false diagnoses, which in turn can lead to damaging public criticism. Equally, careful consideration should be given during the assessment stage as to whether a child is failing to thrive because of illness, as there is tendency to believe that very few children fail to grow and develop because of illness, and tragic cases have been reported as a result of such dogmatic beliefs.

Further attention needs to be paid to long-term studies of the effects of FTT. It is difficult, and unwise, to make general assumptions based upon small research samples and short time-spans. The longitudinal study carried out by the author (and described in the text of the book) indicated that those children and families referred during or near the onset of the problems had a very good recovery rate and did not appear to carry forward any scars, whereas those who had suffered prolonged emotional neglect and abuse prior to referral had a very poor prognosis, carrying their difficulties with them into adulthood (and in some cases developing major emotional and behavioural problems). Furthermore, these individuals' children tended to fail to thrive as well. There is a need (as suggested by some researchers) to pull data together from several research projects to enhance statistical power for more sophisticated analysis.

More research is needed in the areas that remain murky, but dogmatic attitudes defending entrenched positions will not help: open-mindedness and a true spirit of unbiased scientific inquiry can only improve matters. We need to be more concerned about severe cases of failure to thrive, to study aetiological factors for prevention purposes, and to develop intervention and treatment strategies to avoid significant harm. Equally, emerging weight-faltering and poor developmental attainments need to be dealt with as soon as they are recognised by the front-line professionals charged with providing universal services for all children and their families. Only by stepping in at the onset of emerging problems and giving a helping hand to worried, and often stressed, parents can we prevent further deterioration in growth and the parent–child relationship.

# REFERENCES

Accardo, P.J. (1982) Growth and development: an interactional context for failure to thrive. In P.J. Accardo (Ed.) *Failure to Thrive in Infancy and Early Childhood, a Multidisciplinary Team Approach*, Baltimore, MD: University Park Press, 3–18.

Achenbach, T.M., Howell, C.T., Aoki, M.F., and Rauh, V.A. (1993) Nine year outcome of the Vermont Intervention program for low birth weight infants. *Pediatrics*, **91** (1), 45–55.

Adcock, M. (2001) *Significant Harm: Outcomes and Management*. Paper presented at Guardian Ad Litem Conference on Significant Harm, Belfast.

Ainsworth, M.D.S. (1982) Early caregiving and later patterns of attachment. In M.H. Klaus and M.O. Robertson (Eds) *Birth, Interaction and Attachment, Exploring the Foundations for Modern Perinatal Care*. Skillman, NJ: Johnson and Johnson Baby Products Pediatric Round Table Series.

Ainsworth, M.D.S. and Wittig, B.A. (1969) Attachment and exploratory behaviour of one year olds in a strange situation. In B.M. Foss (Ed.) *Determinants of Infant Behaviour*, London: Methuen, 113–136.

Ainsworth, M.D.S., Blehar, M.C., Waters, E. and Wall, S. (1978) *Patterns of Attachment*. Hillsdale, NJ: Lawrence Erlbaum.

Anderson, J. and McKane, J. (1996) Münchausen syndrome by proxy. *British Journal of Hospital Medicine*, **56** (1), 43–45.

Apley, J., Davies, J., Russell Davis, D., and Silk, B. (1971) Dwarfism without apparent cause. *Proceedings of the Royal Society of Medicine*, **64**, 135–138.

Ariès, P. (1973) *Centuries of Childhood*. Harmondsworth: Penguin Books.

Arnold, D. (Ed.) (2001) *The New Oxford Companion to Music*. Oxford: Oxford University Press, 1936–1938.

Asher, R. (1951) Münchausen's Syndrome. *Lancet*, **1**, 339–341.

Bakwin, H. (1949) Emotional deprivation in children. *Journal of Paediatrics*, **35**, 512–521.

Baldwin, C. (1996) Münchausen syndrome by proxy: problems of definition, diagnosis and treatment. *Health and Social Care in the Community*, **4** (3), 159–165.

Bandura, A. (1982) Recycling misconceptions of perceived self-efficacy. *Cognitive Therapy and Research*, **8** (3), 231–255.

Barbero, G. (1982) Failure to thrive. In M.H. Klaus, T. Leger, and M.A. Trause (Eds) *Maternal Attachment and Mothering Disorders*. Skillman, NJ: Johnson and Johnson Baby Products Pediatric Round Table Series: 3–5.

Barbero, G.J. and Shaheen, E. (1967) Environmental failure to thrive: a clinical view. *Journal of Paediatrics*, **71** (5), 639–644.

Batchelor, J.A. (1996) Has recognition of failure to thrive changed? *Child: Care, Health and Development*, **22** (4), 235–240.

Batchelor, J.A. (1999) *Failure to Thrive in Young Children: Research and Practice Evaluated*. London: The Children's Society.

Batchelor, J. and Kerslake, A. (1990) *Failure to Find Failure to Thrive: The Case for Improving Screening, Prevention and Treatment in Primary Care*. London: Whiting & Birch Ltd.

Bauman, L.J., Drotar, D., Leventhal, J.M., Perrin, E.C., and Pless, I.B. (1997) A review of psychosocial interventions for children with chronic health conditions. *Pediatrics,* **100** (2), 244–251.

Beck, A.T. and Weishaar, M. (1989) Cognitive Therapy. In H. Arkowitz, L.E. Beutler, A. Freeman, and K. Simon (Eds) *Handbook of Cognitive Therapy*. Dordrecht: Kluwer Academic.

Bee, H. (1985) *The Developing Child*. New York: Harper & Row.

Belsky, J. (1984). The determinants of parenting: a process model. *Child Development,* **55**, 83–96.

Belsky, I. and Cassidy, I. (1994) Attachment theory and evidence. In M. Rutter and D. Hay (Eds) *Development Through Life*. London: Blackwell Science, 373–402.

Benoit, D., Madigan, S., Lecce, S., Shea, B., and Goldberg, S. (2001) Atypical maternal behaviour toward feeding-disordered infants before and after intervention. *Infant Mental Health Journal,* **22** (6), 611–626.

Benoit, D., Zeanah, C., and Barton, M.L. (1989) Maternal attachment disturbances in failure to thrive. *Infant Mental Health Journal,* **10** (3), 185–193.

Bernstein, D.A., Clarke-Stewart, A.C., Roy, E.J., Srull, T.K., and Wickens, C. D. (1994) *Psychology*. Third Edition. Boston, MA: Houghton Mifflin Company.

Berwick, D.M. (1980) Non-organic failure to thrive. *Pediatrics in Review,* **1** (9), 265–270.

Birch, L.L. (1990) The control of food intake by young children: the role of learning. In E.D. Capadli and T.L. Powley (Eds) *Taste, experience and feeding*. Washington DC: APA: 116–138.

Bithoney, W.G. (1984) Organic concomitants of non-organic failure to thrive. Paper presented at the *Failure to Thrive Symposium*, Ontario Centre for the Prevention of Child Abuse. Toronto: Ontario Ministry of Community and Social Services: 32–69.

Bithoney, W.G. and Newberger, E.H. (1987) Child and family attributes of failure to thrive. *Journal of Developmental & Behavioural Pediatrics,* **8** (1), 32–36.

Bithoney, W.G., Van Sciver, M.M., Foster, S., *et al.* (1995) Parental stress and growth outcome in growth-deficient children. *Pediatrics,* **96** (4, part 1), 707–711.

Black, M.M. (1995) Failure to thrive: strategies for evaluation and intervention. *School Psychology Review,* **24** (2), 171–185.

Black, M.M., Dubowitz, H., Hutcheson, J., Berenson-Howard, J., and Starr, R.H. (1995) A randomized clinical trial of home intervention for children with failure to thrive. *Pediatrics,* **95** (6), 807–814.

Blizzard, R.M. and Bulatovic, A. (1993) Psychological short stature: a syndrome with many variables. *Baillière's Clinical Endocrinology and Metabolism,* **6** (3), 637–712.

Blom, E (Ed.) (1966) *Grove's Dictionary of Music and Musicians*. London: Macmillan & Co. Ltd.

Bools, C.N. (1996) Factitious illness by proxy, Münchausen syndrome by proxy. *British Journal of Psychiatry,* **169** (3), 268–275.

Bools, C.N., Neale, B., and Meadow, R. (1992) Co-morbidity associated with fabricated illness (Münchausen Syndrome by Proxy). *Archives of Disease in Childhood,* **67**, 77–79.

Bools, C.N., Neale, B., and Meadow, R. (1993) Follow up of victims of fabricated illness (Münchausen Syndrome by Proxy). *Archives of Disease in Childhood,* **69** (6), 625–630.

Bowlby, J. (1953) *Child Care and The Growth of Love*. Harmondsworth: Penguin Books Ltd.

Bowlby, J. (1973) *Attachment and Loss. Vol. 2: Separation, Anxiety and Anger*. New York: Basic Books.

Bowlby, J. (1982) *Attachment*. New York: Basic Books.

Bowlby, J. (1988a) *A Secure Base: Clinical Application of Attachment Theory.* London: Routledge.
Bowlby, J. (1988b) Developmental psychiatry comes of age. *The American Journal of Psychiatry*, **145** (1), 1–10.
Brazelton, T.B. (1981) Nutrition during early infancy. In R.M. Suskind (Ed.) *Textbook of Paediatric Nutrition.* New York: Raven Press.
Brazelton, T.B., Koslowski, B., and Main, M. (1974) The origins of reciprocity: the mother–infant interaction. In M. Lewis and L. Rosenblum (Eds) *The Effect of the Infant on its Caregiver.* New York: John Wiley & Sons.
Bremeau, J. (1932) The infant ward. *American Journal of Diseases in Children*, 578–584.
Bretherton, I. and Waters, E. (Eds) (1985) *Monographs of the Society for Research in Child Development.* Monograph 50, Serial No. 209, 3–35.
Brinich, E., Drotar, D., and Brinich, P. (1989) Security of attachment and outcome of preschoolers with histories of non-organic failure to thrive. *Journal of Clinical Child Psychology*, **18** (2), 142–152.
Bronfenbrenner, U. (1979) *The Ecology of Human Development.* Cambridge, MA: Harvard University Press.
Bronfenbrenner, U. (1993) *Parenting—An ecological perspective.* Hillsdale, NY, and London: Erlbaum Associates, vii–xii.
Bullard, D.M., Glaser, H.H., Heagarty, M.C., and Privchik, E.C. (1967) Failure to thrive in the neglected child. *American Journal of Orthopsychiatry*, **37** (4), 680–690.
Butler, N.R. and Golding, J. (1986) *From Birth to Five: A Study of the Health and Behaviour of Britain's Five-Year-Olds.* Oxford: Pergamon Press.
Cassidy, I. and Berlin, I.J. (1994) The insecure-ambivalent pattern of attachment: theory and research. *Child Development*, **65**, 971–991.
Chatoor, I., Schaefer, S., Dickson, L., and Egan, J. (1984) Non-organic failure to thrive: a developmental perspective. *Paediatric Annals*, **13** (11), 844, 847–848, 850.
Chatoor, I., Hirsch, R., and Persinger, M. (1997) Facilitating internal regulation of eating: a treatment model for infantile anorexia. *Infants and Young Children*, **9** (4), 12–22.
Chatoor, I., Ganiban, J., Hirsch, R., Borman-Spurrell, E., and Mrazek, D.A. (2000) Maternal characteristics and toddler temperament in infantile anorexia. *Journal of the American Academy of Child and Adolescent Psychiatry*, **39** (6), 743–751.
Chess, S. and Thomas, A. (1973) *Annual Progress in Child Psychiatry and Child Development.* New York: Brunner-Routledge.
Cicchetti, D. and Toth, S.L. (Eds) (1999) *Rochester Symposium on Developmental Psychopathology: Developmental Approaches to Prevention and Intervention.* Rochester, NY: University of Rochester Press, 195–219.
Clarke, A.M. and Clarke, D.B. (1992) How modifiable is the human life path? *International Review of Research in Mental Retardation*, **18**, 157–173.
Clarke, A.M. and Clarke, D.B. (1999) The prediction of early development. In David Messer and Fiona Jones (Eds) *Psychology for Social Carers.* London and Philadelphia, PA: Jessica Kingsley.
Cole, T.J. (1994) Do growth chart centiles need a face lift? *British Medical Journal*, **308** (6929), 641–642.
Coleman, P.K. and Karraker, H. (1997) Self-efficacy and parenting quality: findings and future applications. *Developmental Review*, **18** (1), 47–85.
Coleman, R. and Provence, S. (1957) Environmental retardation (hospitalism) in infants living with families. *Pediatrics*, **19**, 285–291.
Colombo, M., de la Para, A., and Lopez, I. (1992) Intellectual and physical outcome of children undernourished in early life is influenced by later environmental conditions. *Developmental Medicine and Child Neurology*, **34** (7), 611–622.

Coolbear, J. and Benoit, D. (1999) Failure to thrive: risk for clinical disturbance of attachment? *Infant Mental Health Journal*, **20** (1), 87–104.

Corbett, S.S., Drewett, R.F., and Wright, C.M. (1996) Does a fall down a centile chart matter? The growth and developmental sequelae of mild failure to thrive. *Acta Paediatrica*, **85**, 1278–1283.

Crickmay, M. (1955) *Speech and the Bobath Approach to Cerebral Palsy.* Springfield, IL: C.C. Thomas.

Crittenden, P.M. (1987) Non-organic failure to thrive: deprivation or distortion? *Infant Mental Health Journal*, **8** (1), 51–64.

Crittenden, P.M. (1990) Internal representational models of attachment relationships. *Infant Mental Health Journal*, **11** (3), 259–277.

Crittenden, P.M. (1992) Quality of attachment in the pre-school years. *Development and Psychopathology*, **4**, 28–33.

Dawson, P. (1992) Should the field of early child and family intervention address failure to thrive? *Zero to Three* (June): 20–24.

Department of Health (1991) *Patterns and Outcomes of Placement.* London: Department of Health.

De Wolff, M.S. and Van Ijzendoorn, M.H. (1997) Sensitivity and attachment: a meta analysis on parental antecedents of infant attachment. *Child Development*, **68** (4), 571–591.

Derivan, A.T. (1982) Disorders of bonding. In P.J. Accardo (Ed.) *Failure to Thrive in Infancy and Early Childhood, a Multi-disciplinary Team Approach.* Baltimore, MD: University Park Press, 91–103.

*Dictionary of National Biography* (*D.N.B.*) (1917) Oxford: Oxford University Press.

Diehl, M., Elnick, A.B., Bourbeau, L.S., and Labouvie-Vief, G. (1998) Adult attachment styles: their relations to family context and personality. *Journal of Personality and Social Psychology*, **74** (6), 1656–1669.

Douglas, J. (1991) Chronic and severe eating problems in young children. *Health Visitor*, **64** (10), 334–6.

Douglas, J.E. and Bryon, M. (1996) Interview data on severe behavioural eating difficulties in young children. *Archives of Disease in Childhood*, **75**, 304–308.

Dowdney, L., Skuse, D., Rutter, M., Quinton, D., and Mrazek, D. (1985) The nature and qualities of parenting provided by women raised in institutions. *Journal of Child Psychology and Psychiatry*, **26** (4), 599–625.

Dowdney, L., Skuse, D., Heptinstall, E., Puckering, C., and Zur-Szpiro, S. (1987) Growth retardation and developmental delay amongst inner city children. *Journal of Child Psychology and Psychiatry & Allied Disciplines*, **28** (4) , 529–541.

Dozier, M., Stovall, K., and Albus, K. (1999) Attachment and psychopathology in adulthood. In J. Cassidy and R. Shaver (Eds) *Handbook of Attachment Theory and Research.* New York: Guilford: 497–519.

Drotar, D. (1991) The family context of non-organic failure to thrive. *American Journal of Orthopsychiatry*, **6** (1), 23–34.

Drotar, D. and Crawford, P. (1985) Psychological adaptation of siblings of chronically ill children: research and practice implications. *Developmental and Behavioral Pediatrics*, **6** (6), 355–362.

Drotar, D. and Malone, C.A. (1982) Family-oriented intervention in failure to thrive. In M.H. Klaus and M.O. Robertson (Eds) *Birth Interaction and Attachment.* Skillman, NJ: Johnson & Johnson: 104–111.

Drotar, D. and Sturm, L. (1988) Prediction of intellectual development in young children with histories of non-organic failure to thrive. *Journal of Pediatric Psychology*, **13** (2), 218–296.

Drotar, D. and Sturm, L. (1992) Personality development, personality solving, and behavioral problems among preschool children with early histories of nonorganic failure to thrive: A controlled study. *Journal of Developmental and Behavioral Pediatrics*, **13** (4), 266–273.

Drotar, D., Malone, C.A., Negray, J., and Dennstedt, M. (1981) Psychosocial assessment and care for infants hospitalised for non-organic failure to thrive. *Journal of Clinical Child Psychology*, 63–66.

Drotar, D., Eckerle, D., Satola, J., Pallotta, J., and Wyatt, B. (1990) Maternal interactional behaviour with non-organic failure-to-thrive infants: a case comparison study. *Child Abuse and Neglect*, **14** (1), 41–51.

Duniz, M., Scheer, P.J., Trojovsky, A., Kaschnitz, W., Kvas, E., and Macari, S. (1996) Changes in psychopathology of parents of NOFT (non-organic failure to thrive) infants during treatment. *European Child and Adolescent Psychiatry*, **5** (2), 93–100.

Dykman, R.A., Ackerman, P.T., Loizou, P.C., and Casey, P.H. (2000) An event-related study of older children with an early history of failure to thrive. *Developmental Neuropsychology*, **18** (2), 187–212.

Edwards, A.G.K., Halse, P.C., and Parkin, J.M. (1990) Recognising failure to thrive in early childhood. *Archives of Disease in Childhood*, **65** (11), 1263–1265.

*Encyclopædia Britannica* (1959) London: Encyclopædia Britannica Ltd.

Evans-Morris, S. and Klein, M.D. (1987) *Pre-feeding Skills: A Comprehensive Resource for Feeding Development*. Tucson, AZ: Therapy Skill Builders.

Fahlberg, V. (1994) *A Child's Journey through Placement*. London: BAAF.

Feldman, K.W., Christopher, D.M., and Opheim, K.B. (1989) Münchausen syndrome/bulimia by proxy: ipecac as a toxin in child abuse. *Child Abuse and Neglect*, **13** (2), 257–261.

Field, T.M. (1984) Follow-up developmental status of infants hospitalised for non-organic failure to thrive. *Journal of Pediatric Psychology*, **9**, 241–256.

Field, T.M., Ignatoff, E., Stringer, S., Brennan, J., Greenberg, R., Widmayer, S., and Anderson, G.C. (1982) Non-nutritive sucking during tube feedings—effects on preterm neonates in an intensive care unit. *Pediatrics*, **70** (3), 381–384.

Fischhoff, J., Whitten, C.F., and Pettit, M.G. (1971) A psychiatric study of mothers of infants with growth failure, secondary to maternal deprivation. *Journal of Pediatrics*, **79** (2), 209–215.

Foy, T., Czyzewski, D., Phillips, S., Ligon, B., Baldwin, J. and Klish, W. (1997) Treatment of severe feeding refusal in infants and toddlers. *Infants and Young Children*, **9** (3), 26–35.

Frank, D. and Zeisel, S. (1988) Failure to thrive. *Paediatric Clinics of North America*, **35** (6): 1, 187–1, 206.

Galler, J.R. and Ramsey, F. (1987) A follow-up study of the influence of early malnutrition on development: Behaviour at home and at school. *Journal of the American Academy of Child Psychiatry*, **28**, 254–261.

Gibbons, J. (1995) Family Support in Child Protection. In M. Hill, R. Hawthorn Kirk, and D. Part, *Supporting Families*. Edinburgh: HMSO.

Gohlke, B.C., Khadilkar, V.V., Skuse, D., and Stanhope, R. (1998) Recognition of children with psychosocial short stature: a spectrum of presentation. *Journal of Pediatric Endocrinology and Metabolism*, **11**, 509–517.

Goldson, E. (1987) Failure to thrive; an old problem revisited. *Progress in Child Health*, **7**, 83–99.

Goldson, E. (1989) Neurological aspects of failure to thrive. *Developmental Medicine and Child Neurology*, **31** (6), 821–826.

Gordon, A.H. and Jameson, J.C. (1979) Infant–mother attachment in patients with nonorganic failure to thrive syndrome. *Journal of the American Academy of Child Psychiatry*, **18** (2), 251–259.

Gough, D. (2002) To or For Whom: A Social Policy Perspective on Child Abuse and Child Protection. In K. Brown, H. Hanks, P. Stratton, and C. Hamilton (Eds) *Early Prediction and Prevention of Child Abuse: A Handbook*. Chichester: John Wiley & Sons.

Grantham-McGregor, S.M. (1995) A review of studies of the effect of severe malnutrition on mental development. *Journal of Nutrition*, **125** (8 Suppl.), 2233S–2238S.

Grantham-McGregor, S.M., Walker, S.P., and Chang, S. (2000) Nutritional deficiencies and later behavioural development. *Proceedings of the Nutrition Society*, **59** (1), 47–54.

Gray, J. and Bentovim, A. (1996) Illness Induction Syndrome: Paper 1—A series of 41 children from 37 families identified at the Great Ormond Street Hospital for Children's NHS Trust. *Child Abuse and Neglect*, **20** (8), 655–673.

Green, W.H., Deutsch, S.I., and Campbell, M. (1987) Psychosocial dwarfism: psychological and aetiological considerations. In C.B. Nemesoff and P.T. Loosens (Eds) *Handbook of Psychoneuroendocrinology*. New York: Guilford Press.

Greenberg, M.T. (1999) Attachment and psychopathology in childhood. In J. Cassidy and P. Shaver (Eds) *Handbook of Attachment*. New York: Guilford Press, 469–491.

Greenspan, S.I. (1981) *The clinical interview with the child*. New York: McGraw-Hill.

Griffith, J.L. (1988) The family systems of Münchausen syndrome by proxy. *Family Process*, **27** (4), 423–437.

Grossmann, K., Fremmer-Bonbik, E., Rudolph, I., and Grossmann, K.E. (1988) Maternal attachment representations as related to child–mother attachment patterns and maternal sensitivity and acceptance of her infant. In R.A. Hinde (Ed.) *Relations within Families*. Oxford, Clarendon Press, 241–260.

Hampton, D. (1996) Resolving the feeding difficulties associated with non-organic failure to thrive. *Child: Care, Health & Development*, **22** (4), 261–271.

Hanks, H. and Hobbs, C. (1993) Failure to thrive: a model for treatment. In *Baillière's Clinical Paediatrics*, **1** (1), 101–119.

Harington, Sir John (1607) *The Englishman's Doctor. Or, The Schools of Salerne*. London: John Helme & John Busby. Reprinted in F.R. Packard and F.H. Garrison (Eds) (1920), *The School of Salernum: Regimen Sanitatis Salernitanum*. New York: P.B. Hoeber.

Harris, G. (1988) Determinants of the introduction of solid food. *Journal of Reproductive and Infant Psychology*, **6** (4), 241–249.

Harris, G. and Booth, I.W. (1992) The nature and management of eating problems in pre-school children. In P. Cooper and A. Stein (Eds) *The Nature and Management of Feeding Problems and Eating Disorders in Young People*. Monographs in Clinical Paediatrics (Lanzkowsky, P.: Ed.) New York: Harwood Academic, 61–84.

Hathaway, P. (1989) Failure to thrive: knowledge for social workers. *Health and Social Work*, **14** (2), 122–126.

Hawdon, J.M., Beauregard, N., Slattery, J., and Kennedy, G. (2000) Identification of neonates at risk of developing feeding problems in infancy. *Developmental Medicine and Child Neurology*, **42** (4), 235–239.

Haynes, C.F., Culter, C., Gray, J., and Kempe, R.S. (1984) Hospitalized cases of nonorganic failure to thrive: the scope of the problem and short-term lay health visitor intervention. *Child Abuse and Neglect*, **8** (2), 229–242.

Hazan, C. and Shaver, P.R. (1987) Romantic love conceptualised as an attachment process. *Journal of Personality and Social Psychology*, **52**, 511–524.

Heffer, R.W. and Kelley, M.L. (1994) Nonorganic Failure to Thrive: Developmental Outcomes and Psychosocial Assessment Issues. *Research in Developmental Disabilities*, **15** (4), 247–268.

Heptinstall, E., Puckering, C., Skuse, D., Start, K., Zur-Szpiro, S., and Dowdney, L. (1987) Nutrition and meal-time behaviour in families of growth retarded children. *Human Nutrition: Applied Nutrition*, **46** (6), 390–402.

Herbert, M. (1974) *Emotional Problems of Development in Children*. London: Academic Press.

Herbert, M. (1987) *Behavioural Treatment of Children with Problems: A Practice Manual*. London: Academic Press.

Herbert, M. (1993) *Working with Children and the Children Act*. Leicester: BPS Books.

Hinde, R.A. (Ed.) (1988) *Relations with Families*. Oxford: Clarendon Press.

Hobbs, C. and Hanks, H.G.I. (1996) A multi-disciplinary approach for the treatment of children with failure to thrive. *Child: Care, Health & Development*, **22** (4), 273–284.

Hollburn-Cobb, C. (1996) Adolescent–parents attachments and family problem-solving styles. *Family Process*, **35** (1), 57–82.

Holt, L.E. (1887) *The Diseases of Infancy and Childhood*. New York: Appleton–Century, 192–204.

Holt, L.E. and Fales, H.L. (1923) Observations on the health and growth of children in an institution. *American Journal of Diseases in Children*, **28** (1), 2–22.

Hufton, I. and Oates, R.K. (1977) Non-Organic failure to thrive: a long-term follow-up. *Pediatrics*, **59** (1), 73–77.

Humphry, R. (1995) The nature and diversity of problems leading to failure to thrive. *Occupational Therapy in Health Care*, **9**, 73–89.

Hutcheson, J.J., Black, M.M., and Starr, R.H. (1993) Developmental differences in inter-actional characteristics of mothers and their children with failure to thrive. *Journal of Pediatric Psychology*, **18** (4), 453–466.

Hutcheson, J.J., Black, M.M., Talley, M., Dubowitz, H., Berenson-Howard, J., Starr, R.H., and Thompson, B.S. (1997) Risk status and home intervention among children with failure-to-thrive: follow-up at age 4. *Journal of Pediatric Psychology*, **22** (5), 651–668.

Illingworth, D. (1983) *The Development of the Infant and Young Child* (8th edition). Edinburgh: Churchhill Livingstone.

Illingworth, R.S. and Lister, J. (1964) The critical or sensitive period, with special reference to certain feeding problems in infants and children. *Journal of Paediatrics*, **65**, 839–849.

Isabela, R.A., Belsky, J., and von Eye, A. (1989) Origins of infant–mother attachment: an examination of interactional synchrony during the infant's first year. *Developmental Psychology*, **25**, 12–21.

Iwaniec, D. (1983) *Social and psychological factors in the aetiology and management of children who fail-to-thrive*. PhD thesis. University of Leicester.

Iwaniec, D. (1991) Treatment of children who fail to grow in the light of the new Children Act. *Association for Child Psychology & Psychiatry Newsletter*, **13** (3), 21–27.

Iwaniec, D. (1995) *The Emotionally Abused and Neglected Child: Identification, Assessment and Intervention*. Chichester: John Wiley & Sons.

Iwaniec, D. (1997) Evaluating parent training for emotionally abusive and neglectful parents; comparing individual versus individual and group intervention. *Research on Social Work Practice*, **7** (3), 329–349.

Iwaniec, D. (1999) Lessons from 20-year follow-up study on children who failed to thrive. *Child Care in Practice*, **5** (2), 128–139.

Iwaniec, D. (2000) From childhood to adulthood: A 20-year follow-up study of children who failed-to-thrive. In D. Iwaniec and M. Hill (Eds) *Child Welfare Policy and Practice: Current Issues Emerging from Child Care Research*. London: Jessica Kingsley.

Iwaniec, D. (2002) Working with families who neglect their children. In G. Bell and C. Wilson (Eds) *Practice Guide for Working with Families*. London: Macmillan Press.

Iwaniec, D. and Herbert, M., (1982) The assessment and treatment of children who fail-to-thrive. *Social Work Today*, **13** (22), 8–12.

Iwaniec, D. and Sneddon, H. (2001) Attachment style in adults who failed-to-thrive as children: outcomes of a 20-year follow-up study of factors influencing maintenance or change in attachment style. *The British Journal of Social Work*, **31** (2), 179–195.

Iwaniec, D. and Sneddon, H. (2001a) *Failure to Thrive Children and their Families: Outcomes of a 20 Year Longitudinal Study*. Belfast: Centre for Child Care Research.

Iwaniec , D. and Sneddon, H. (2002) The quality of parenting of individuals who had failed to thrive as children. *The British Journal of Social Work*, **32** (3), 283–298.

Iwaniec, D., Herbert, M., and McNeish, A.S. (1985a) Social work with failure to thrive children and their families. Part 1: Psychosocial factors. *British Journal of Social Work*, **15** (4), 243–259.

Iwaniec, D., Herbert, M., and McNeish, A.S. (1985b) Social work with failure to thrive children and their families, Part II: Behavioural Social Work Intervention. *British Journal of Social Work*, **15** (4), 375–389.

Iwaniec, D., Herbert, M., and Sluckin, A. (2002) Helping emotionally abused and neglected children and abusive carers. In K. Browne, H. Hanks, P. Stratton, and C. Hamilton (Eds) *Early Prediction and Prevention of Child Abuse: A Handbook*. Chichester: John Wiley & Sons, Ltd., 249–265.

Iwaniec, D., Sneddon, H., and Allen, S. (in press) The outcomes of a longitudinal study of non-organic failure to thrive. *Child Abuse Review*.

Iwata, B.A., Riordan, M.M., Wohl, M.K., and Finney, J.W. (1982). Pediatric feeding disorders: a behavioural analysis and treatment. In P.J. Accardo (Ed.) *Failure to Thrive in Infancy and Early Childhood: A Multidisciplinary Team Approach*. Baltimore, MD: University Park Press, 297–329.

Jureidini, J. (1993) Obstetric factitious disorder and Münchausen Syndrome by Proxy. *Journal of Nervous and Mental Disease*, **181** (2), 135–137.

Kahng, S.W., Tarbox, J., and Wilke, A.E. (2001) Use of a multi-component treatment for food refusal. *Journal of Applied Behaviour Analaysis*, **34** (1), 93–96.

Kempe, H., Silverman, F.N., Steele, B.F., Droegmueller, W., and Silver, H.K. (1962) The battered child syndrome. *Journal of the American Medical Association*, **181**, 17–24.

Kendall, P.C. and Lockman, J. (1994) Cognitive-Behavioural Therapies. In M. Rutter, E. Taylor and L. Hersove (Eds) *Child and Adolescent Psychiatry—Modern Approaches*. Oxford: Blackwell.

Kendrick, D., Elkan, R., Dewey, M., Blair, M., Robinson, J., Williams, D., and Brummell, K. (2000) Does home visiting improve parenting and the quality of the home environment? A systematic review and meta analysis. *Archives of Disease in Childhood*, **82** (6), 443–451.

Kotelchuck, M., Gordon, A., Jamison, J., and Newberger, E.H. (1981) Behavioural observation of non-organic failure to thrive children: A pilot study of attachment. In E.H. Newberger and C.M. Kotelchuck (Eds) *The Symptom of Child Abuse*, Cambridge, MA: Harvard University Press.

Kristiansson, B. and Fällström, S.P. (1987) Growth at the age of 4 years subsequent to early failure to thrive. *Child Abuse and Neglect*, **11** (11), 35–40.

Lachenmeyer, J.R. and Davidovicz, H. (1987) Failure-to-thrive: a critical review. *Advancement of Clinical Child Psychology*, **10**, 335–358.

Leonard, M.F., Rhymes, J.P., and Solnit, A.J. (1966) Failure to thrive in infants. *American Journal of Diseases of Children*, **111** (6), 600–612.

Lernihan, U. (2003) *A Study of Kinship Foster Carers in Northern Ireland in relation to: (1) Selected characteristics in the Wider Context of Traditional Foster Carers; (2) The Attitude of Kinship Foster Carers to the Involvement of Social Services in their Lives*. PhD Thesis, The Queen's University of Belfast.

Lewis, J.A. (1982) Oral motor assessment and treatment of feeding difficulties. In P.J. Accardo (Ed.) *Failure to thrive in Infancy and Early Childhood, a Multi-disciplinary Approach.* Baltimore, MD: University Park Press, 265–298.

McCann, J.B., Stein, A., Fairburn, C.G., and Dunger, D.B. (1994) Eating habits and attitudes of mothers of children with non-organic failure to thrive. *Archives of Disease in Childhood*, **70** (3), 234–236.

MacCarthy, D. and Booth, E. (1970) Parental rejection and stunting of growth. *Journal of Psychosomatic Research*, **14** (3), 259–265.

McGuire, T.L. and Feldman, K.W. (1989) Psychologic morbidity of children subjected to Münchausen syndrome by proxy. *Pediatrics*, **83** (2), 289–292.

McJunkin, J.E., Bithoney, W.G., and McCormick, M.C. (1987) Errors in formula concentration in an out-patient population. *Journal of Pediatrics*, **111** (6), 824–850.

MacMillan, A.B. (1984) Failure to Thrive: An Historical Perspective. In *Failure to Thrive Symposium*, Ontario Centre for the Prevention of Child Abuse. Toronto: Ontario Ministry of Community and Social Services, 4–31.

McMillen, P. (1988) Infants thrive with failure-to-thrive program. *Health Progress*, **69** (1) (January–February), 70–71.

Mackner, L.M. and Starr, R.H. (1997) The cumulative effect of neglect and failure to thrive on cognitive functioning. *Child Abuse and Neglect*, **21** (7), 691–700.

Maggioni, A. and Lifshitz, F. (1995) Nutritional management of failure to thrive. *Pediatric Clinics of North America*, **42** (4), 791–810.

Mahler, M. S., Pine, F., and Bergman, A. (1975) *The psychological birth of the human infant.* New York: Basic Books.

Main, M. (1991) Metacognitive knowledge, metacognitive monitoring, and singular (coherent) vs. multiple (incoherent) models of attachment: some findings and some directions for future research. In C. Parkes, J. Stevenson-Hinde, and P. Marris (Eds) *Attachment Across the Life Cycle.* London: Routledge, 127–159.

Main, M. and Hesse, E. (1990) Parents unresolved traumatic experiences are related to infant disorganised attachment status: is frightened and/or frightening parental behaviour the linking mechanism? In M.T. Greenberg, D. Cicchetti and E.M. Cummings (Eds) *Attachment in the Preschool Years.* Chicago, IL: University of Chicago Press, 161–184.

Main, M. and Solomon, J. (1986) Discovery of an insecure, disorganised/disoriented attachment pattern: procedures, findings and implications for the classification of behaviour. In M. Yogman and T.B. Brazelton (Eds) *Effective Development in Infancy.* Norwood, NY: Ablex, 95–124.

Main, M., Kaplan, N., and Cassidy, J. (1985) Security in infancy, childhood and adulthood: a move to a level of representation. In I. Bretherton and E. Waters (Eds) *Growing Points of Attachment Theory and Research, Monographs of the Society for Research in Child Development*, **50** (1–2), No. 209.

Marino, R., Weinman, M.L., and Soudelier, K. (2001) Social Work Intervention and failure to thrive in infants and children. *Health and Social Work*, **26** (2), May, 90–97.

Mathisen, B., Skuse, D., Wolke, D., and Reilly, S. (1989) Oral-motor dysfunction and failure to thrive among inner-city infants. *Developmental Medicine and Child Neurology*, **31** (3) 239–302.

Meadow, R. (1977) Münchausen syndrome by proxy—the hinterland of child abuse. *Lancet*, **2** (8033), 343–345.

Meadow, R. (1984) Fictitious epilepsy. *Lancet*, **2** (8393), 25–28.

Meadow, R. (1990) Suffocation, recurrent apnea and sudden infant death. *Journal of Paediatrics*, **117** (3), 351–357.

Meadow, R. (1993) False allegations of abuse and Münchausen syndrome by proxy. *Archives of Disease in Childhood*, **68** (4), 444–447.

Mehl, A.L., Cable, L., and Johnson, S. (1990) Münchausen Syndrome by proxy: a family affair. *Child Abuse and Neglect*, **14** (4), 577–585.

Messer, D.J. (1999) Communication, bonding, attachment and separation. In D. Messer and F. Jones (Eds) *Psychology and Social Care*, London and Philadelphia, PA: Jessica Kingsley.

Minde, K. and Minde, R. (1986) *Infant Psychiatry: An Introductory Text*. London: Sage.

Money, J. and Werlass, J. (1976) Folie à deux in the parents of psychosocial dwarfs: two cases. *Bulletin: American Academy of Psychiatry and the Law*, **4** (4), 351–361.

Money, J., Annecillo, C., and Hutchinson, H.W. (1985) Forensic and family psychiatry in abuse dwarfism, Münchausen syndrome by proxy, atonement and addiction to abuse. *Journal of Sex and Marital Therapy*, **11** (1), 30–40.

Montagu, A. (1978) *Touching: the Human Significance of the Skin*. New York: Harper & Row, 77–79.

Moore, J.B. (1982) Project thrive: a supportive treatment approach to the parents of children with nonorganic failure to thrive. *Child Welfare*, **61** (6), 389–399.

Moores, J. (1996) Non-organic failure-to-thrive—dietic practice in a community setting. *Child: Care, Health and Development*, **22** (4), 251–259.

Muszkowicz, M. and Bjørnholm, K.I. (1998) Factitious illness by proxy presenting as anorexia and polydipsia by proxy. *Acta Paediatrica*, **87** (5), 601–602.

Novaco, R.W. (1975) *Anger Control: The Development and Evaluation of an Experimental Treatment*. Lexington, MA: D.C. Heath & Co., Lexington Books.

Oates, R.K. and Yu, J.S. (1971) Children with non-organic failure to thrive: a community problem. *Australian Medical Journal*, **2** (4), 199–203.

Oates, R.K., Peacock, A., and Forrest, D. (1985) Long-term effects of non-organic failure to thrive. *Pediatrics*, **75** (1), 36–40.

Olds, D.L., Henderson, C.R., and Kitzman, H. (1994) Does prenatal and infancy nurse home visitation have enduring effects on qualities of parental caregiving and child health at 25–50 months of life? *Pediatrics*, **93** (1), 89–98.

Palmer, M.M., Crawley, K., and Blanco, I.A. (1993) Neonatal oral-motor assessment scale: a reliability study. *Journal of Perinatology*, **13** (1), 28–35.

Patrick, M., Hobson, R.P., Cesde, D., Howard, R., and Vaughan, B. (1994) Personality disorder and the representation of early social experience. *Development and Psychopathology*, **6**, 375–388.

Patton, R.G. and Gardner, L.I. (1962) Influence of family environment on growth: the syndrome of maternal deprivation. *Paediatrics*, **30**, 957–962.

Polan, J.H., Kaplan, M.B., Shindledecker, R., Newmark, M., Stern, D.N., and Ward, M.J. (1991) Psychopathology in mothers of children with failure to thrive. *Journal of Infant Mental Health*, **12**, 55–64.

Pollitt, E. and Eichler, A.W. (1976) Behavioural disturbances among failure to thrive children. *American Journal of Diseases of Children*, **130** (1), 24–29.

Powell, G.F., Brasel, J.A., and Blizzard, R.M. (1967) Emotional deprivation and growth retardation simulating idiopathic hypopituitarism: I. Clinical evaluation of the syndrome. *New England Journal of Medicine*, **276** (23), 1271–1278.

Powell, G.F., Low, J.F., and Speers, M.A. (1987) Behaviour as a diagnostic aid in failure to thrive. *Journal of Developmental and Behavioural Paediatrics*, **8** (1), 18–24.

Prugh, D. and Harlow, R. (1962) *Marked Deprivation in Infants and Young Children in Deprivation of Maternal Care*. Public Health Paper No. 14. Geneva: World Health Organisation (WHO).

Pugliese, M.T., Weyman-Daum, M., Moses, N., and Lifschitz, F. (1987) Parental health beliefs as a cause of non-organic failure to thrive. *Pediatrics*, **80** (2), 175–182.

Ramsay, M. and Gisel, E. (1996) Neonatal sucking and maternal feeding practices. *Developmental Medicine and Child Neurology*, **38** (1), 34–47.

Ramsay, M., Gisel, E.G., and Boutry, M. (1993) Non-organic failure to thrive: growth failure secondary to feeding-skills disorder. *Development Medicine and Child Neurology*, **35** (4), 285–297.

Rausch, H.L. (1965) Interaction sequences. *Journal of Personality and Social Psychology*, **2** (4), 487–499.

Raynor, P. and Rudolf, M.C.J. (1996) What do we know about children who fail to thrive? *Child: Care, Health and Development*, **22** (4), 241–250.

Raynor, P. and Rudolf, M.C.J. (2002) Anthropometric indices of failure to thrive. *Archives of Disease in Childhood*, **82** (5), 364–365.

Raynor, P., Rudolf, M.C.J., Cooper, C., Marchant, P., and Cottrell, D. (1999) A randomized controlled trial of specialist health-visitor intervention for failure to thrive. *Archives of Disease in Childhood*, **80** (6), 500–506.

Reif, S., Beler, B., Villa, Y., and Spirer, L. (1995) Long-term follow-up and outcome of infants with non-organic failure to thrive. *Israel Journal of Medical Sciences*, **31** (8), 483–489.

Reifsnider, E. (1995) The use of human ecology and epidemiology in nonorganic failure to thrive. *Public Health Nursing*, **12** (4), 262–268.

Reifsnider, E., Allan, J., and Percy, M. (2000) Mothers' Explanatory Models of Lack of Child Growth. *Public Health Nursing*, **17** (6), 434–442.

Reilly, S.M., Skuse, D.H., Wolke, D., and Stevenson, J. (1999) Oral-motor dysfunction in children who fail to thrive: organic or non-organic. *Developmental Medicine and Child Neurology*, **41** (2), 115–122.

Ricciuti, H.H. (1991) Malnutrition and cognitive development: Research–policy linkages and current research directions. In L. Okagaki and R.J. Sternberg (Eds) *Directors of Development: Influences on the development of children's thinking*. New York: Lawrence Erlbaum, 59–80.

Richman, N., Stevenson, J., and Graham, P.J. (1982) *Pre-school to School: A Behavioural Study*. London: Academic Press.

Rosenberg, D.A. (1987) Web of deceit: a literature review of Münchausen syndrome by proxy. *Child Abuse and Neglect*, **11** (4), 547–563.

Russell, A. and Russell, G. (1989) Warmth in mother–child and father–child relationships in middle childhood. *British Journal of Developmental Psychology*, **7**, 219–235.

Russell, G.F., Treasure, J., and Eisler, I. (1998) Mothers with anorexic nervosa who underfeed their children: their recognition and management. *Psychological Medicine*, **28** (1), 93–108.

Rutter, M. (1995a) Psychosocial adversity: Risk, resilience and recovery. *South African Journal of Child and Adolescent Psychiatry*, **7** (2), 75–88.

Rutter, M. (1995b) Clinical implications of attachment concepts: Retrospect and prospect. *Journal of Child Psychology & Psychiatry*, **36** (4), 549–571.

Saarilehto, S., Keskinen, S., Lapinleimu, H., Helenius, H., and Simell, O. (2001) Connections between parental eating attitudes and children's meagre eating: questionnaire findings. *Acta Paediatrica*, **90** (3), 333–338.

Samuels, M. (2002) Fabricated and Induced Illness: Use of Video Surveillance and Lessons for Child Protection. *Cornwall and Isles of Scilly Area Child Protection Conference*, Truro, Cornwall, November 2002.

Samuels, M.P., McLaughlin, W., and Jacobson, R.R., *et al.* (1992) Fourteen cases of imposed upper airway obstruction. *Archives of Disease in Childhood*, **67** (2), 162–170.

Schuengel, C., Bakermans-Kranenburg, M.J., and Van Ijzendoorn, M.H. (1999) Frightening maternal behaviour linking unresolved loss and disorganised infant attachment. *Journal of Consulting and Clinical Psychology*, **67** (1), 54–63.

Selley, W. and Boxall, J. (1986) A new way to treat sucking and swallowing difficulties in babies. *Lancet*, **1** (8491), 1182–1184.

Silver, H.K. and Finkelstein, M. (1967) Deprivation-dwarfism. *Journal of Pediatrics*, **70** (3), 317–324.

Single, T. and Henry, R.L. (1991) An unusual case of Münchausen syndrome by proxy. *Australian/New Zealand Journal of Psychiatry*, **25** (3), 422–425.

Skau, K. and Mouridsen, S.E. (1995) Münchausen syndrome by proxy: a review. *Acta Paediatrica*, **84** (9), 977–982.

Skuse, D. (1988) Failure to thrive, failure to feed. *Community Paediatric Group Newsletter*, **6**, 525–537.

Skuse, D. (1992) The relationship between deprivation, physical growth and the impaired development of language. In P. Fletcher and D. Hall (Eds) *Specific Speech and Language Disorders in Children*. London: Whurr Publishers, 29–50.

Skuse, D. (1993) Identification and management of problem eaters. *Archives of Disease in Childhood*, **69**, 604–608.

Skuse, D., Wolke, D., and Reilly, S. (1992) Failure to thrive: clinical and developmental aspects. In H. Remschmidt and M.H. Schmidt (Eds) *Developmental Psychopathology*. Lewiston, NY: Hogrefe & Huber.

Skuse, D., Pickles, A., Wolke, D., and Reilly, S. (1994) Postnatal growth and mental development: evidence for a Sensitive Period. *Journal of Child Psychology & Psychiatry*, **35** (3), 521–546.

Skuse, D., Gilmour, J., Tian, C.S., and Hindmarsh, P. (1994a) Psychosocial assessment of children with short stature: a preliminary report. *Acta Paediatrica Supplement*, **406**, 11–16.

Skuse, D., Reilly, S., and Wolke, D. (1994b) Psychosocial adversity and growth during infancy. *European Journal of Clinical Nutrition*, **48** (Suppl. 1), S113–S130.

Skuse, D., Albanese, A., Stanhope, R., Gilmore, J., and Voss, L. (1996) A new stress-related syndrome of growth failure and hyperphagia in children associated with reversibility of growth-hormone insufficiency. *Lancet*, **348** (9024), 353–358.

Sneddon, H. and Iwaniec, D. (2002) *Characteristics of Failure-to-Thrive Cases*. Occasional Paper, No. 3. Belfast: Centre for Child Care Research.

Spinetta, J. and Rigler, D. (1972) The child-abusing parent: A psychological review. *Psychology Bulletin*, **77** (4), 296.

Spinner, M.R. and Siegel, L. (1987) Non-organic Failure to Thrive. *Journal of Preventive Psychiatry*, **3** (3), 279–297.

Spitz, R.A. (1945) Hospitalism: an inquiry into the genesis of psychiatric conditions in early childhood. *Psychoanalytic Study of the Child*, **1**, 53–74.

Stein, A.S., Stein, J., Walters, E.A., and Fairburn, C.G. (1995) Eating habits and attitudes among mothers of children with feeding disorders. *British Medical Journal*, **310** (6974), 228.

Stern, D. (1985) *The Interpersonal World of the Infant*. New York: Basic Books.

Steward, D.K. (2001) Biological vulnerability in infants with failure to thrive: the association with birthweight. *Child: Care, Health and Development*, **26** (6), 555–567.

Sturm, L. and Drotar, D. (1989) Prediction of weight for height following intervention in three-year-old children with early histories of nonorganic failure-to-thrive. *Child Abuse and Neglect*, **13** (1), 19–28.

Sturm, L. and Drotar, D. (1992) Communication strategies for working with parents of infants who fail to thrive. *Zero to Three* (June), 25–28.

Sutton, C. (1994) *Social Work, Community Work and Psychology*. Leicester: The British Psychological Society.

Talbot, N.B., Sobel, E.H., Burke, B.S., Lindeman, E., and Kaufman, S.B. (1947) Dwarfism in healthy children: its possible relation to emotional, nutritional and endocrine disturbances. *New England Journal of Medicine*, **263**, 783–793.

Taylor, J. and Daniel, B. (1999) Interagency Practice in Children with Non-Organic Failure to thrive: Is there a Gap between Health and Social Care? *Child Abuse Review*, **8** (5), 325–338.

Teti, D.M. and Gelfand, D.M. (1991) Behavioral competence among mothers of infants in the first year: the mediational role of maternal self-efficacy. *Child Development*, **62** (5), 918–929.

Thomas, A., Chess, S., and Birch, H.G. (1968) *Temperament and Behaviour Disorders in Children*. New York: New York University Press.

Tizard, B. and Hodges, J. (1978) The effect of early institutional rearing on the development of eight year old children. *Journal of Child Psychology, Psychiatry & Allied Disciplines*, **19**, 99–118.

Valenzuela, M. (1990) Attachment in chronically underweight young children. *Child Development*, **61** (6), 1994–1996.

Van Bakel, H. and Riksen-Walraven, M. (2002) Parenting and development of one-year-olds: links with parental, contextual and child characteristics. *Child Development*, **73** (1), 256–273.

Van Ijzendoorn, M. (1995) Adult attachment representations, parental responsiveness and infant attachment: A meta-analysis of the predictive validity of the Adult Attachment Interview. *Psychological Bulletin*, **117** (3), 387–403.

Voss, L. (1995) Can we measure growth? *Journal of Medical Screening*, **2** (3), 164–167.

Walker, S., Grantham-Mc Gregor, S., Powell, C., Himes, J., and Simeon, D. (1992) Morbidity and the growth of stunted and nonstunted children, and the effect of supplementation. *American Journal of Clinical Nutrition*, **56** (3), 504–510.

Ward, M.J., Kessler, D.B., and Altman, S.C. (1993) Infant–mother attachment in children with failure to thrive. *Infant Mental Health Journal*, **14**, 208–220.

Ward, M.J., Lee, S.S., and Lipper, E.G. (2000) Failure to thrive is associated with disorganised infant–mother attachment and unresolved maternal attachment. *Infant Mental Health Journal*, **21** (6), 428–442.

Warner, J.O. and Hathaway, M.J. (1984) The allergic form of Meadow's syndrome (Münchausen by proxy). *Archives of Disease in Childhood*, **59** (2), 151–156.

Waterlow, J. (1984) Current issues in nutritional assessment by anthropometry. In J. Brozek and B. Schürch (Eds), *Malnutrition and Behaviour: Critical Assessment of Key Issues*, Switzerland: Nestlé Foundation, 77–90.

Weston, J.A. and Colloton, M. (1993) A legacy of violence in non-organic failure to thrive. *Child Abuse and Neglect*, **17** (6), 709–714.

Whitten, C.F. (1976) Failure to thrive. Can treatment be effectively investigated? *American Journal of Diseases of Children*, **130** (1), 15.

Whitten, C.F., Pettit, M.G., and Fischoff, J. (1969) Evidence that growth failure from maternal deprivation is secondary to undereating. *Journal of the American Judicial Association*, **209** (11), 1675–1682.

Widdowson, E.M. (1951) Mental contentment and physical growth. *Lancet*, **260**, 1316–1318.

Wilensky, D.S., Ginsberg, G., Altman, M., Tulchinsky, T.H., Ben Yishay, F., and Auerbach, J. (1996) A community based study of failure to thrive in Israel. *Archives of Disease in Childhood*, **75** (2), 145–148.

Winick, M. (1976) *Malnutrition and Brain Development*. New York: Oxford University Press.

Wolfe, D.A. (1990) Preventing child abuse means enhancing family functioning. *Canadas Mental Health*, **38**, 27–29.

Wolfe, D.A. and Wekerle, C. (1993) Treatment strategies for child physical abuse and neglect—a critical progress report. *Clinical Psychology Review*, **13** (6), 473–500.

Wolff, G. and Money, J. (1973) Relationship between sleep and growth in patients with reversible somatotropin deficiency (psychosocial dwarfism). *Psychiatric Medicine*, 3, 18–27.

Wolke, D. (1996) Failure to thrive: the myth of maternal deprivation syndrome. *The Signal: Newsletter of the World Association for Infant Mental Health*, 4 (3/4), 1–6.

Wolke, D., Skuse, D., and Mathisen, B. (1990) Behavioural style in failure to thrive infants: A preliminary communication. *Journal of Pediatric Psychology*, 15 (2), 237–254.

Woolston, J. (1984) Failure to thrive syndrome: the current challenge of diagnostic classification. In *Failure to Thrive Symposium*, Ontario Centre for the Prevention of Child Abuse. Toronto: Ontario Ministry of Community and Social Services, 70–85.

Woolston, J.L. (1985) Diagnostic classification: The current challenge in failure to thrive. In D. Drotar (Ed.) *New Directions in Failure to Thrive—Implications for Research and Practice*. New York: Plenum Press, 225–33.

World Heath Organisation (WHO) (1991) Tenth Revision of the International Classification of Diseases, Chapter V(F): Mental and Behavioural Disorders, including Disorders of Psychological Development. *Clinical Description and Diagnostic Guidelines*. Geneva: WHO.

World Health Organisation (WHO) Expert Committee (1995) *Physical Status: The Use and Interpretation of Anthropometry*. Geneva: WHO.

World Health Organisation (WHO) (1999) *Report of the Consultation on Child Abuse Prevention*. Geneva, 29–31 March 1999.

Wright, C.M. (2000) Identification and management of failure to thrive: a community perspective. *Archives of Disease in Childhood*, 82, 5–9.

Wright, C.M. and Talbot, E. (1996) Screening for failure to thrive—what are we looking for? *Child: Care, Health and Development*, 22 (4), 223–234.

Wright, C.M., Callum, J., Birks, E., and Jarvis, S. (1998) Effect of community based management in failure to thrive: randomized controlled trial. *British Medical Journal*, 317 (7158), 571–574.

Wright, C.M., Matthews, J.N.S., Waterson, A., and Aynsley-Green, A. (1994) What is a normal rate of weight gain in infancy? *Acta Pediatrica*, 83 (4), 351–356.

Wright, J. (2000) A case study of failure to thrive and interagency work. *Child Abuse Review*, 9, 287–293.

Wynne, J. (1996) Failure to thrive—an introduction. *Child: Care, Health and Development*, 22 (4), 219–221.

Zamora, S.A. and Parsons, H.G. (2000) Growth Failure and Malnutrition. In A.B.R. Thompson and E.A. Shaffer (Eds) *First Principles of Gastroenterology: The Basis of Disease and an Approach to Management*. Internet version at http://gastroresource.com/GITextbook/En/Default.htm.

*Dictionary of National Biography* (D.N.B.) (Oxford: Oxford University Press, 1917). For details of Matthew Paris and Michael Scott. Paris (xv), 207–13. Scott (xvii), 997–1001.

For Harington, see *D.N.B.*, 1917 (viii), 1269–1272.

For Kaiser Frederick II see *Encyclopaedia Britannica* (London: Encyclopaedia Britannica Ltd., 1959), ix, 711–713.

For Foundling Hospitals see *Encyclopaedia Britannica* ix, 559–560.

For Coram see *D.N.B.*, 1917, iv, 1119–1120.

For Vivaldi see Blom, Eric (Ed.) (1966): *Grove's Dictionary of Music and Musicians* (London: Macmillan & Co. Ltd.) and Arnold, Denis (Ed.) (2001) *The New Oxford Companion to Music* (Oxford: Oxford University Press), 1936–1938.

# INDEX

Note: The abbreviation FTT stands for failure to thrive.

attachment behaviour (*cont.*)
  early interactions, 110
  FTT children, 105–112
    as adults, 114–119
    assessment, 154–155
    dismissing mothers, 113–114
    infantile anorexia, 57
    mother–child communication,
      110–111, 212–214, 232–233
    rejecting mothers, 113–114
  holding of children, 110–111, 233
  interventions, 117–118, 211–214,
    232–234
  Münchausen Syndrome by Proxy, 127
  parental sensitivity, 103–105, 154,
    212–213, 233–234
  psychosocial short stature, 53, 57, 63,
    113
  styles, 104–105
    adults', 106, 112–113, 114–119
    assessment, 154, 155

behaviour problems
  assessment, 156, 157, 158–159
  case study, 47
  combined FTT, 38–39
  developmental impairment, 44
  feeding *see* feeding/eating behaviour
    of children
  multidimensional interventions,
    234
  non-organic FTT, 37
  psychosocial short stature, 52, 53, 54,
    58, 59–63
behavioural development, 155–156,
  157–159
behavioural therapy, 202–206
biological rhythms, 54
bodily contact, 110–112, 233
boundary-setting, by parents, 174–175
bulimia, parental, 133, 220

case-conferences, 193–194, 195, 197, 251,
  270
case management, interagency, 252–253
child abuse, 9
  case study, 46–47
  Civil Court intervention, 195–198, 251
  early research into, 23, 24, 26, 27
  emotionally stunting *see* psychosocial
    short stature
  family relationships, 161

parents' experience of, 24, 177–178,
  256–257
safety considerations, 168–169, 220
targeted intervention, 193–194, 251
Victorian legislation on, 17
*see also* fabricated or induced illness
child neglect, 9
  Civil Court intervention, 195–198,
    251
  developmental effects, 43–44
    case studies, 46–48
    psychosocial short stature, 55–56
    social, 160
  early research into, 24–26, 27
  parents' experience of, 257
  safety considerations, 168–169, 220
  targeted intervention, 193–195, 251
child protection
  Civil Court intervention, 195–198, 251
  interagency work, 252–253
  social workers, 251–252, 253
  targeted intervention, 193–195, 251
Child Protection Plan, 194
Child Protection Register, 194, 195, 197,
  251
child–parent interactions *see*
  parent–child interactions
Children Act 1989, 191–192
Children's Society, Infant Support
  Project, 206, 241
Civil Court interventions, 190, 195–198,
  251
cognitive behavioural theory, 207
cognitive characteristics, parents',
  167
cognitive development, 43–44, 153
  assessment, 153
  case study, 47
  and maternal psychopathology, 259
  psychosocial short stature, 53, 57, 58,
    62, 69
  stimulation for, 171–174
cognitive distortions, 208
cognitive therapy, 206–210, 256
combined FTT, 36, 38–40
communication
  parent–child, 89–92, 98–99
    attachment, 110–111, 212–214,
      232–234
    eating behaviour, 76–77, 82–83, 95,
      212–214, 260
  parent–professional, 256, 263